Neuro-Oncology for Nurses

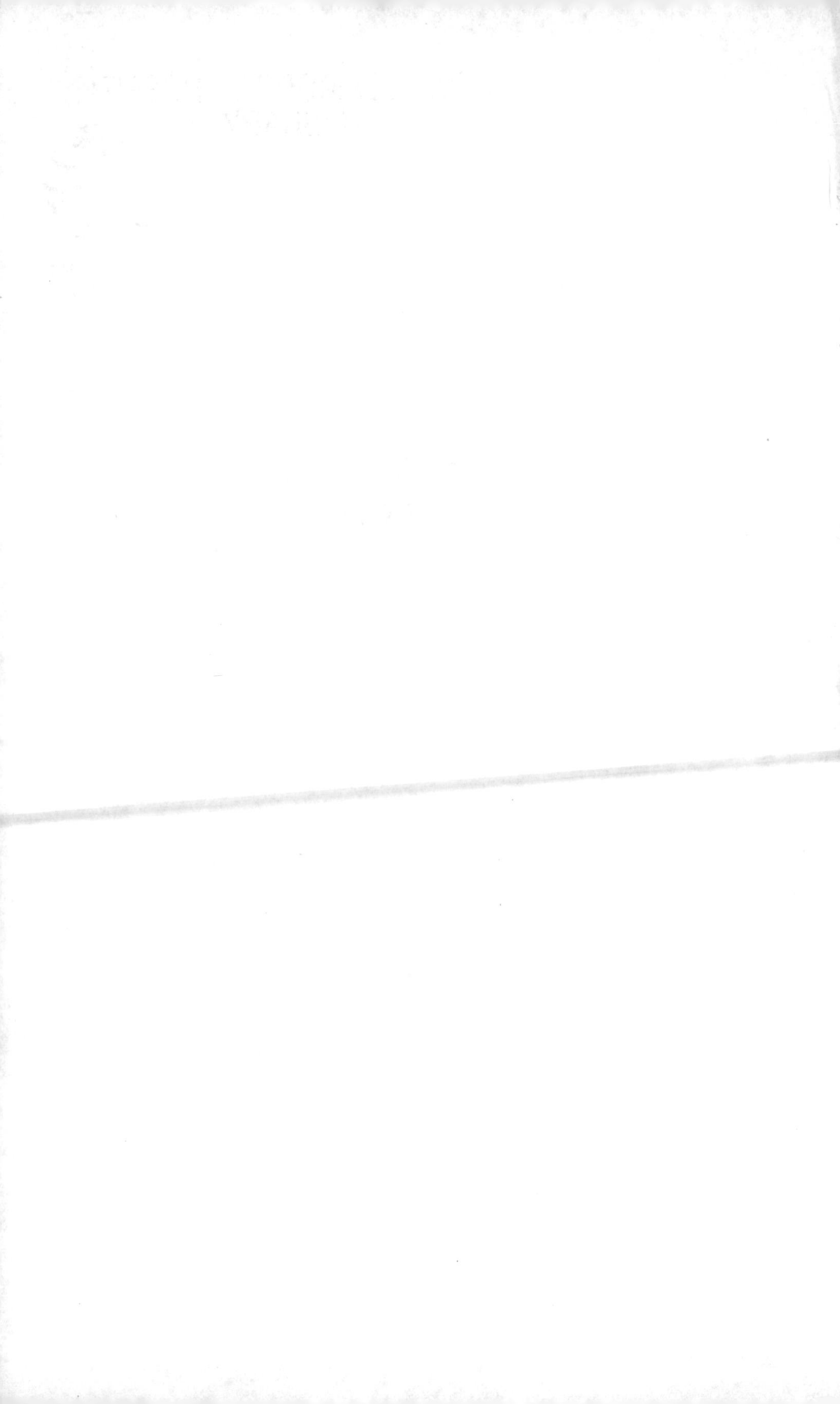

Neuro-Oncology for Nurses

Edited by
Douglas Guerrero

MSc (Clinical Neurosciences), BSc(Hons), RGN, NDN, Onc N Cert, COD Cert, Counselling Cert
Macmillan Clinical Nurse Specialist Neuro-Oncology, The Royal Marsden NHS Trust and Atkinson Morley's Hospital

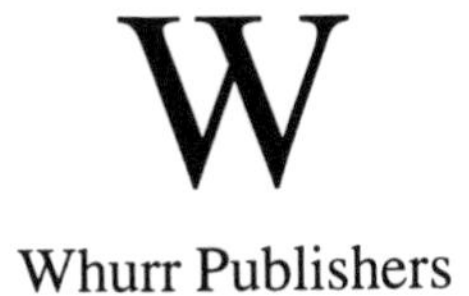

Whurr Publishers

First published 1998 by
Whurr Publishers Ltd
19b Compton Terrace, London N1 2UN, England

Reprinted 1999

British Library Cataloguing in Publication Data
A catalogue record for this book is available from the British Library.

ISBN: 1 86156 087 7

Printed and bound in the UK by Athenæum Press Ltd,
Gateshead, Tyne & Wear

Contents

Foreword vii
Preface ix
List of contributors xiii

Chapter 1. **1**

Anatomy and Physiology of the Nervous System
Katy Weldon

Chapter 2. **29**

Neurological Assessment
Sally Aucken and Belinda Crawford

Chapter 3. **66**

Pathological and Clinical Aspects of CNS Tumours
Geoffrey Sharpe

Chapter 4. **81**

Clinical Neuro-Imaging
Juliet Britton and Virginia Ng

Chapter 5. **124**

Neurosurgery
Clare Addison and Sarah Shah

Chapter 6. **151**

Radiotherapy
Douglas Guerrero

Chapter 7. **179**

Chemotherapy
Douglas Guerrero, Sue Sardell and Frances Hines

Chapter 8. **201**

Medication in the Symptom Management of CNS Tumours
Christopher Evans and Douglas Guerrero

Chapter 9. **221**

Multidisciplinary Teamwork
Sarah N Fisher

Chapter 10. **253**

Altered Body Image
Mave Salter

Chapter 11. **271**

Psychological Support
Sue Kibler

Chapter 12. **294**

Future Planning of Care
Mave Salter

Index **311**

Foreword

There are many books on the management of patients with central nervous system (CNS) tumours. They usually debate the technical issues of therapy and describe the latest technological feats. This book by Douglas Guerrero comes with a different philosophy. It recognises that the essential component of successful oncological management is care of the patient and the family, and this should be based on the knowledge and understanding of the disease and its treatment.

CNS tumours, epitomised by high-grade gliomas, the most common primary malignant brain tumours, are among the most complex and devastating of malignant diseases. Despite many years of research, treatment has advanced little beyond the limited tumour control achieved with surgery and conventional external beam radiotherapy. In the management of any malignant disease, therapy aimed at tumour control and patient care must be considered to be a part of a unified approach, and this is particularly true for patients with gliomas for which the treatment is largely palliative. Attention must focus on the multiple physical and cognitive disabilities, and their effect on patients and families in the face of a diagnosis with such a devastating prognosis.

This book is written largely by nurses and for nurses, and reflects the changing nursing skills in the late 1990s when the traditional boundaries between the medical and nursing professions are disappearing. Having had the privilege of working with some of the authors of this book, I am aware of the highly innovative changes in neuro-oncology nursing, combined with a dedication to patient care, which have transformed the pattern of nursing and medical care for the patient with a CNS tumour. Patient care delivered by nurses would, for example, be inadequate if prescribing remained within the province of the medical profession. It is a very positive aspect of the evolution of clinical practice that nurses have become skilled in the diagnosis and management of medical complications of disease and tumour-directed therapy, which includes giving medication traditionally prescribed by doctors. In many respects, experienced nurse specialists are better equipped to attend to symptom management and psychological support than are doctors, and this has long been recognised within the practice of palliative care in the UK.

Nursing has to take on new challenges and adapt to what the patient and health service require. However, changing a role steeped in history is not easy. The vision has to be shared by profession leaders and by doctors who may at times feel uncomfortable and threatened by new nursing practices. Transferring roles previously held by doctors to nurses may also be unsettling for patients and their views and wishes must be taken into account. The burden of a new role, however, falls on the practising nurse, and this will bring new demands and responsibilities, and a need for more education.

The current treatments of CNS tumours, in particular high-grade gliomas, are of limited efficacy, and it is important to be aware of the potential new directions. Research efforts to find more effective treatments must undoubtedly continue. For today's patients, we have to acknowledge the palliative nature of the available treatments and concentrate on improvement in quality of life. This is unlikely to be achieved with more radical and high-tech therapies but with improved care combined with a reduction in treatment intensity to minimise side-effects. There will undoubtedly be other new directions optimising treatment and care, which should be explored jointly by all the professionals involved in the care of patients with tumours of the CNS.

This book, which is at the forefront of the changing practice within a relatively small but demanding field of oncology, describes the present state of the art of management of CNS tumours from the nursing and medical perspective. It will serve as the foundation for nurses and other professionals involved in the care of patients with tumours of the CNS.

Michael Brada BSc, FRCP, FRCR
Senior Lecturer and Consultant in Clinical Oncology, The Royal Marsden NHS Trust; Chairman of the Medical Research Council Brain Tumour Working Party (UK); President, European Association of Neuro-Oncology

Preface

For many nurses, caring for patients with CNS malignancies poses major anxiety. This is because CNS tumours are, compared with other cancers, rare, and nurses (as well as many other health care professionals) often feel that are inappropriately prepared to deal with the complexities of care that can often be precipitated by such tumours.

The diagnosis of CNS tumours has major catastrophic consequences for patients and their families, which affect their entire life. For most patients, diagnosis is preceeded by neurological and physical deficits, and in most instances histology confirms a poor prognosis. The illness trajectory from diagnosis to palliative care is often steep. Problems are multiple, ranging from disease- to treatment-related issues, and often require skilled nursing intervention.

The major aim of nurses within a neuro-oncology setting is therefore to provide a service of education, management and support. This service should supply and maintain a programme of rehabilitation , community and palliative care utilising the skills and expertise of the other professionals within the multidisciplinary and primary health care team. As such, nurses involved in neuro-oncology care must have advanced skills in order to be able to support patients and families as well as to direct and educate other professionals involved in patient care.

This book provides a guide for those working with patients with CNS tumours. Although it has been written predominantly for nurses, other health care professionals may find individual chapters informative and interesting. Chapters can be used individually as self-contained units or in combination with other chapters.

This book has primarily been written to give nurses the skills and knowledge to be able to approach those patients with CNS tumours with a greater confidence and understanding in the hope that they can make an impact on total patient care.

The first four chapters outline the anatomy and physiology of the CNS, neurological assessment, pathological and clinical aspects of CNS tumours and clinical neuro-imaging. It is hoped that this will give nurses a better knowledge and understanding of the CNS, confidence in undertaking neurological examination and a knowledge of the different modes of tumour presentation types as well as grades of tumour. It will also explore the role of clinical neuro-imaging in the care of this group of patients.

Chapters 5–7 will guide the nurse through the different stages of treatment. They will discuss pre- and post-operative care and different surgical approaches, including the emotional and physical preparation of the patient and family prior to surgery. They will outline the role of radiotherapy and chemotherapy as adjuvant and palliative treatment for CNS tumours and discuss the unique role of the nurse in patient and family education and support throughout different stages of treatment. Chapter 8 aims to provide the nurse with a broader overview of the specific medication most commonly used in the treatment and management of CNS tumours. It will highlight potential drug side-effects and the nurses role of identification and prevention of the potential problems.

Chapters 9–12 will further explore issues of care. They will discuss the value of multidisciplinary teamwork and the major asset of early planning future care in order to prevent unnecessary crisis. They will explore issues surrounding altered body image in patients with CNS tumours, an area often ignored by many professionals. The role of the nurse as the patient's advocate and the psychological needs of patients, families and nurses will also be discussed.

This book aims to make the nurse aware of this group of patients' special needs and to indicate the unique contribution of nurses and other professionals in the delivery and planning of care.

Douglas Guerrero
1998

Acknowledgements

A book is never complete without thanking all the authors as well as those behind the scene who have made this publication possible. I therefore wish to express my heartfelt thanks to all the contributors as well as those colleagues both at the Royal Marsden NHS Trust and Atkinson Morley's Hospital for giving so generously of expertise and time. My particular thanks go to Dr Michael Brada, a friend and colleague who is a passionate believer in the therapeutic effects of expert nursing practice.

Douglas Guerrero
1998

This book is dedicated to all those patients who have taught us so much and to my parents Lourdes and Juan.

Contributors

Clare Addison BA(Hons), RGN, Dip. Prof. Nurse Studies
Education and Development Sister, Neurosurgery, Atkinson Morley's Hospital

Sally Aucken BSc(Hons), RGN
Senior Staff Nurse, Neuro-Intensive Care Unit, Atkinson Morley's Hospital

Juliet Britton MBBS, MRCP, FRCR
Consultant Neuroradiologist, Atkinson Morley's Hospital and Honorary Consultant Neuroradiologist, The Royal Marsden NHS Trust

Belinda Crawford BSc(Hons), RGN
Sister, Neuro-Intensive Care, Atkinson Morley's Hospital

Christopher Evans BSc, MRPharmS
Pharmacy Manager, The Royal Marsden NHS Trust

Sarah N Fisher MSc, Grad Dip Phys MCSP, SRP
Senior Physiotherapist, The Royal Marsden NHS Trust

Douglas Guerrero MSc (Clinical Neurosciences) BSc(Hons). RGN, NDN, Onc N Cert, COD Cert, Counselling Cert
Macmillan Clinical Nurse Specialist Neuro-Oncology, The Royal Marsden NHS Trust and Atkinson Morley's Hospital

Frances Hines RGN, Onc N Cert
Research Nurse Neuro-Oncology, The Royal Marsden NHS Trust

Sue Kibler MSc (PsychCouns), BA, RGN, Onc N Cert, COD Cert
Counsellor, Royal College of Nursing

Virginia Ng MBBS, MRCP, FRCR
Senior Registrar in Neuroradiology, Atkinson Morley's Hospital

Mave Salter MSc, BSc, RGN, NDN(Cert), CSCT, DipCounselling, CertEd
Clinical Nurse Specialist Community Liaison, The Royal Marsden NHS Trust

Sue Sardell RGN, Onc N Cert
Research Nurse, Neuro-Oncology, The Royal Marsden NHS Trust

Sarah Shah BSc(Hons), RGN
Teaching Sister, Neuro-Intensive Care, Atkinson Morley's Hospital

Geoffrey Sharpe BM. MRCP, FRCP
Consultant in Clinical Oncology, Wessex Cancer Centre, Southampton; formerly Senior Clinical Research Fellow and Honorary Senior Registrar, The Royal Marsden NHS Trust

Katy Weldon BSc(Hons), RGN PostGrad Dip Clinical Neurosciences
Clinical Nurse Specialist/Stroke Care, Epsom General Hospital, Surrey; formerly Neurology Sister, Atkinson Morley's Hospital

Chapter 1
Anatomy and physiology of the nervous system

Katy Weldon

Introduction

The nervous system endows us with the ability to appreciate, and to react to, the external environment and provides us with the means to control the internal state of our bodies. Hence the nervous system is said to have three principal functions:

- sensory;
- integrative;
- motor.

This chapter aims to provide nurses with an insight into how the nervous system is built and the nature of its functional organisation, which can then be related to patients with pathology of the nervous system.

Basic structure of the nervous system

There are two major divisions of the nervous system: the central nervous system (CNS) and the peripheral nervous system (PNS).

The central nervous system consists of two parts – the brain and the spinal cord – which are connected to structures in every part of the body by the peripheral nervous system.

The peripheral nervous system consists of the cranial and the spinal nerves. Nerves are either sensory or motor or both. Sensory (also known as afferent) nerve fibres convey sensory impulses from receptor structures, for example the skin, muscle, bones, joints, blood vessels, viscera and special sense organs, to different parts of the

CNS, where they are decoded and correlated. Motor (also known as efferent) nerve fibres transmit impulses that are initiated in the CNS in response to sensory impulses. Motor impulses produce an appropriate response such as muscular contraction or relaxation, glandular secretion or inhibition as well as other bodily activities.

Neurones and Neuroglia

The neurone is the basic unit of the nervous system. Neurones have four properties that distinguish them from other types of cell:

1. specialisation for the conduction of impulses;
2. great sensitivity to oxygen deprivation;
3. importance for many vital functions (such as cardiac and respiratory);
4. inability to divide and multiply (by mitosis).

Neurones are mainly grouped in the brain and spinal cord, but other collections of neuronal cell bodies, termed ganglia, are found in association with various peripheral nerves. Collections of neurone cell bodies are greyish in colour, and areas of the brain in which they predominate are sometimes referred to as the grey matter. Neurones are classified according to size, shape, polarity, function and the neurotransmitter utilised. It is estimated that the human brain contains in excess of over 100 billion neurones.

A typical neurone (see Figure 1.1) possesses a nucleated cell body and one or usually more branching processes. The neuronal processes are extensions of the cell body that conduct impulses to or from the cyton. Processes named dendrites conduct impulses to the cyton. Dendrites are variable in number per neurone, usually relatively short, branch freely and extend widely in the brain substance. Dendrites increase the surface area of the neurone and thus enhance the scope for it to be influenced by other neurones.

In a motor neurone, a single process conducts impulses away from the cell body; this is called the axon. Axons range in length from a few microns to a metre or more. The longest axons interconnect the brain and lower end of the spinal cord or extend from the cord to peripheral structures such as hands and feet. The site of contact between the axon of one neurone and the dendrites of another is the synapse and the site of contact between an axon and a muscle fibre is the motor end plate. However, the nerve impulse does not pass directly from neurone to neurone or neurone to muscle. Instead, it is transmitted by chemical mediators called neurotransmitters.

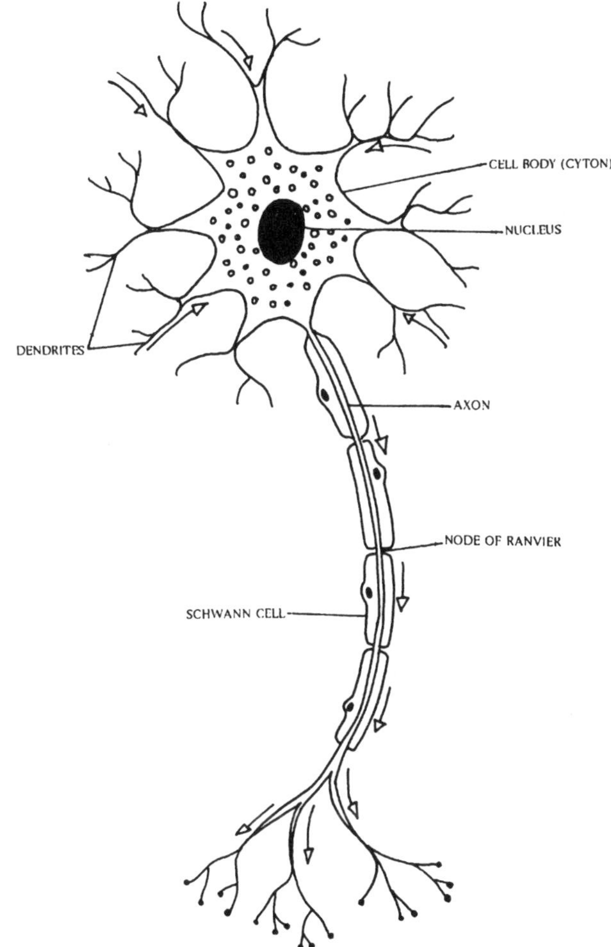

Figure 1.1 Typical efferent (motor) neurone. Arrows represent the direction of nerve impulse travel.

Neuroglia (neuro meaning nerve, and glia glue) make up approximately 40% of the CNS and are the supporting tissue of the brain and spinal cord. There are three main types of neuroglial cell:

- Astrocytes (astro meaning star, and cyte cell), which have many radiating processes. Their functions are to hold together the delicate neurones and to help to create the blood–brain barrier. Astrocytes are the largest and most numerous type.
- Oligodendrocytes (oligo meaning few, and dendro meaning tree), which are smaller cells with fewer branching processes. They tend to lie in rows between nerve fibres and are concerned with production and nourishment of myelin sheaths that surround axons in the CNS.

- Microglial cells (micro meaning small), which are smaller still and permeate the entire CNS. They are modified macrophages and act as scavengers by engulfing and destroying micro-organisms.

Neurones lose their mitotic capacity (ability to divide and multiply) at around the time of birth, whilst neuroglia maintain their mitotic capacity throughout life. This is why the great majority of neoplasms of the nervous system arise from glial cells (see Chapters 3 and 4).

Many axons are covered by multiple concentric layers of myelin. Myelin is a lipid-rich insulating material produced by Schwann cells in the peripheral nervous system and by oligodendrocytes in the CNS. Areas of the nervous system where myelinated axons predominate are known as white matter because of their colour.

The axons in peripheral nerves are protected and insulated by Schwann cells with or without the formation of a myelin sheath. Those axons which do not have a myelin sheath are called unmyelinated axons.

The myelin sheath is interrupted at the nodes of Ranvier at intervals of between 0.1 and 1.5 mm. The node of Ranvier is a gap between adjacent Schwann cells where the axon is covered only by a continuation of the basement membrane material that covers the Schwann cells.

Nerve signals are transmitted by action potentials, which are rapid changes in the membrane potential. At rest, there is a small excess of negative ions inside the axon membrane and an equal excess of positive ions outside, giving rise to a negative membrane potential. Each action potential begins with a sudden change to a positive membrane potential and then ends with a rapid change back again. In order to conduct a nerve signal, the action potential moves along the nerve until it comes to the end.

Ions cannot flow significantly through the thick myelin sheaths of myelinated nerves, but they can flow with ease through the nodes of Ranvier. Therefore action potentials can occur only at the nodes. Action potentials are conducted from node to node (saltatory conduction). The current flows through the surrounding extracellular fluids and through the axoplasm from node to node. Thus the impulse 'jumps' down the fibre, and the speed of transmission is faster than if there were no myelin sheath.

At the synapse, it causes the release of neurotransmitter from the end of the axon, and this passes through the ultramicroscopic synaptic gap to the adjacent dendrites where it triggers a new impulse that is transmitted in the next neurone.

Repolarisation, by which the resting potential is restored, is also fast in myelinated fibres.

The brain

Several different terminologies are used to describe the different parts of the brain. The most widely used terminology divides the brain into six parts (Figure 1.2):

1. the cerebrum (also known as the telencephalon);
2. the diencephalon (together with the cerebrum, also known as prosencephalon or forebrain);
3. the mesencephalon (also known as the midbrain);
4. the cerebellum;
5. the pons;
6. the medulla oblongata (which, together with the cerebellum and pons, constitutes the rhombencephalon or hindbrain).

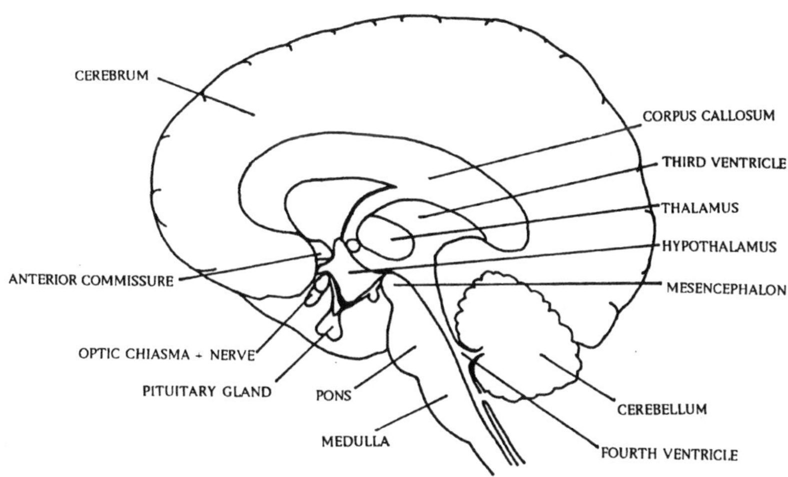

Figure 1.2 Medial view of the right half of the brain.

The cerebrum

The cerebrum is the centre for the highest functions (those associated with intellect) and is therefore most developed in humans.

It is composed of two cerebral hemispheres that are connected to each other through several bundles of nerve fibres. The two most important connections are made by:

1. the corpus callosum, which extends almost half the length of the cerebral hemisphere;
2. the anterior commissure, which interconnects, amongst other structures, the anterior and medial portions of the two temporal lobes.

Corresponding points in almost all areas of the two hemispheres interconnect with each other in both directions via the fibres in these two bundles, which allows continuous communication between the two hemispheres.

If the corpus callosum and anterior commissure are destroyed, each of the two hemispheres functions as a separate brain, even thinking separate thoughts and causing separate reactions in the two sides of the body.

Cerebral convolutions

A distinctive feature of the cerebrum is the folds in its surface. During embryonic development, when there is a rapid increase in brain size, the grey matter of the cortex enlarges out of proportion to the underlying white matter. As a result, the cortical region rolls and folds upon itself. These are called cerebral convolutions and each convolution is called a gyrus. The grooves between the gyri are called either fissures or sulci, the larger and deeper ones generally being called fissures.

Although certain gyri and sulci are present in almost every human brain, no two brains or even the hemispheres of the same brain have exactly the same pattern of gyri and sulci.

To some extent, these fissures and sulci demarcate separate functional parts of the cerebrum (Figure 1.3).

Grey and white matter

Grey matter consists of collections of great numbers of neuronal cell bodies that, all together, give it a greyish hue. A thin layer of grey matter covers the entire surface of the cerebrum. This is the cerebral cortex. One of the principal advantages of having the many fissures and sulci is that they triple the total surface area.

The white matter comprises great bundles of myelinated nerve fibres leading to or from the nerve cells in the grey matter.

Lobes of the cerebrum

Each cerebral hemisphere is subdivided into lobes by deep sulci or fissures. The four major lobes are:

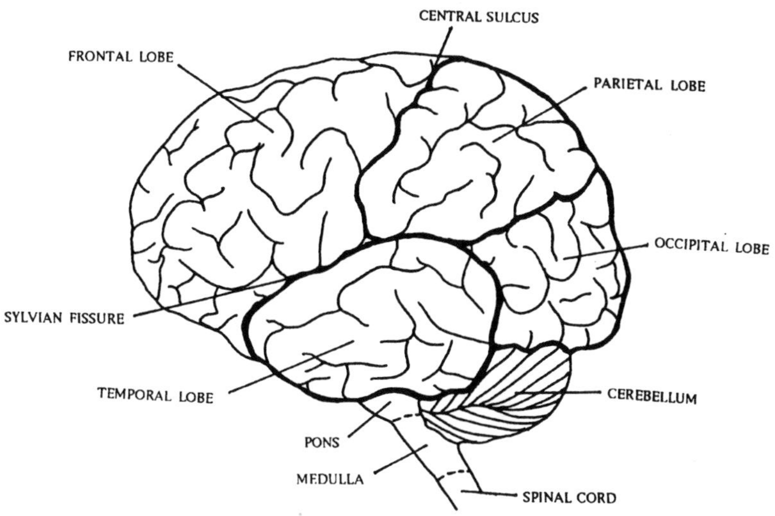

Figure 1.3 The lobes of the cerebrum.

1. the frontal lobe;
2. the parietal lobe;
3. the occipital lobe;
4. the temporal lobe.

Functional areas of the cerebral cortex

Functions of specific areas of the cortex have been discovered by neurosurgeons, neurologists and neuropathologists using techniques such as electrical stimulation of the cortex in awake patients and examination of patients after portions of the cortex have been removed.

Functional areas of the cerebral cortex are described as primary, secondary and association (Figure 1.4).

The primary areas have direct connections with specific muscles or specific sensory receptors for causing discrete muscle movement or experiencing a sensation (visual, auditory or somatic) from a receptor area.

The secondary areas interpret the functions of the primary areas so that patterns of motor activity can be carried out and sensory information can be interpreted.

Association areas receive and analyse impulses from multiple regions of the cortex and subcortical structures. There are three important association areas: the parieto-occipitotemporal, the prefrontal and the limbic.

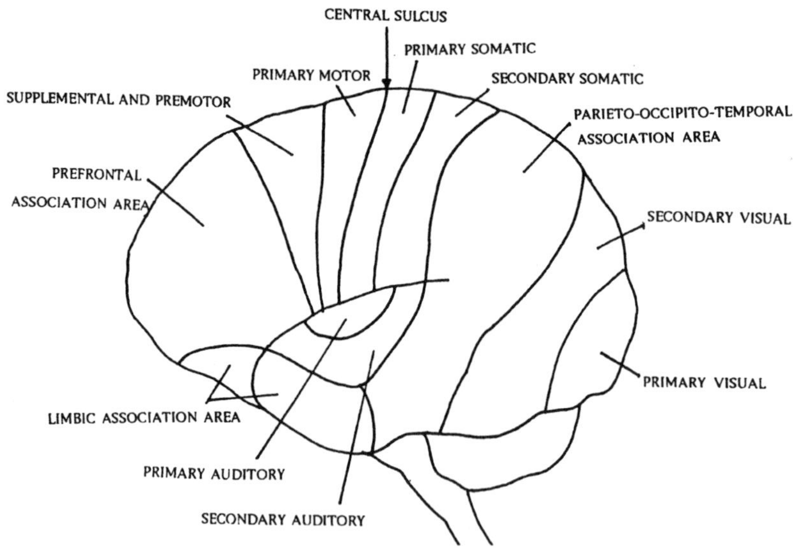

Figure 1.4 Locations of the primary, secondary and association areas.

The parieto-occipitotemporal association area provides interpretative meaning for the signals from surrounding sensory areas. One part analyses the spatial co-ordinates of all parts of the body as well as its surroundings. This is essential for planning movement and for awareness of the environment in association with that movement. Another part, called Wernicke's area, is concerned with language comprehension and, because almost all intellectual functions are language based, is considered to be the most important region of the brain for higher intellectual function. A third part deals with interpretation of visually perceived words, without which written words have no meaning. A fourth part has the function of naming objects.

The prefrontal association area functions in association with the motor cortex to plan complex patterns and sequences of movement. This area is also essential to carrying out prolonged thought processes. A special area called Broca's area is concerned with word formation and works in association with Wernicke's area.

The limbic association area is concerned with emotions such as anger, fear and sexual feeling as well as other behaviours and motivation. The limbic system itself is discussed below.

The dominant hemisphere

Generally, one cerebral hemisphere is more highly developed than the other for the functions of speech and motor control. This is referred to as the dominant hemisphere. In approximately 95% of people, it is the left hemisphere that is the dominant one. Dominance is primarily for language but also the motor areas for the hands, which results in the majority of people being right handed. However, if the left hemisphere of the brain is damaged or removed in early childhood, the right hemisphere can develop full dominant characteristics.

Basal ganglia

The basal ganglia are paired masses of grey matter situated deep within the cerebral hemispheres. In lower forms of animals, such as birds, who do not have a cerebral motor cortex, movement is initiated by the basal ganglia together with other subcortical areas. Such movement is highly co-ordinated and often very quick, but it is instinctive and crude. Humans have, in addition to this old system, a new, more advanced one known as the cerebral motor cortex. This advanced motor system enables us to perform exceptionally skilled and purposeful movements. This 'higher' system is called the pyramidal system, whereas the older, cruder system is the extrapyramidal.

The extrapyramidal system is concerned with associated movements, postural adjustments and autonomic integration. Lesions at any level of the extrapyramidal system may make voluntary movements difficult or even impossible, and involuntary movements can take over.

The limbic system

Certain components of the cerebral hemispheres and diencephalon constitute the limbic system. The limbic system is a wishbone-shaped group of structures that is concerned with the emotional aspects of behaviour and motivational drive. It also has a function in memory. The cortical components of the limbic system include the cingulate, parahippocampal and subcallosal gyri as well as the hippocampal formation. The hypothalamus also forms a major part of the limbic system.

Diencephalon

The diencephalon is a small area between the cerebral hemispheres that is divided into the thalamus – the main relay centre for the nervous system – and below it the hypothalamus.

The third ventricle bisects the thalamus into two halves. Each half of the thalamus functions separately within the cerebral hemisphere on the same side. The thalamus rather than the sensory cortex may be the crucial structure for the perception of some types of sensation, and the sensory (somatic) cortex may function to give finer detail to the sensation.

The cerebral cortex has extensive connections with structures situated deep within the brain. The thalamus is particularly important as it has been demonstrated that the loss of cerebral function is much greater when the thalamus is damaged along with the cerebral cortex than if the cerebral cortex is damaged alone. This is because thalamic excitation of the cortex is necessary for almost all cortical activity.

The hypothalamus is a vital area concerned with temperature control, emotional states, some neuroendocrine control, appetite and control over the autonomic nervous system. Information from the external environment comes to the hypothalamus via afferent pathways originating in the peripheral sense organs.

Also included in the diencephalon are the subthalamic nucleus and the pineal body.

Mesencephalon

The midbrain is located between the diencephalon and the pons. Together with the pons and the medulla oblongata, it forms a wedge-shaped structure extending down from the base of the brain to the foramen magnum of the skull. The mesencephalon contains the nuclei for the IIIrd (oculomotor) and IVth (trochlear) cranial nerves.

The reticular formation of the midbrain controls many of the stereotyped body movements, such as postural movements of the limbs. A major nucleus of the reticular formation is the red nucleus, which functions with the basal ganglia and cerebellum to co-ordinate muscle movements of the body. The reticular formation is also a major centre for control of the brain's overall activity.

Cerebellum

The cerebellum is found under the occipital lobe in the posterior fossa of the skull. The cerebellum is a control centre for the co-ordination of voluntary muscle activity, equilibrium and muscle tone. The names of the subdivisions and fissures of the cerebellum are very numerous. The archicerebellum is the most primitive and has the function of keeping the individual orientated in space. The paleocerebellum controls the antigravity muscles of the body. The neocerebellum acts as a brake on volitional movements, especially those requiring checking or halting activity and fine movements of the hands.

The cerebellum does not initiate movement. A person with cerebellar injury therefore does not become paralysed but his or her movements become slow, clumsy, tremulous and unco-ordinated. In order to work effectively, the cerebellum needs information concerning:

- the position and state of the muscles and joints and the amount of muscle tone present (this information being supplied by spinocerebellar pathways, which are nerve tracts that transmit messages from the periphery up the spinal cord to the cerebellum);
- the equilibrium state of the body (this information being supplied by the vestibulocerebellar tract, which is the pathway of nerves taking sensory information from special centres in the ears to the cerebellum);
- what messages are being sent to the muscles from the cerebral motor cortex (this information is supplied by corticopontocerebellar tracts).

The cerebellum integrates this information and, by means of feedback pathways, regulates and controls motor activity, equilibrium and muscle tone automatically and at an unconscious level.

Lesions of the cerebellum or its sensory or motor tracts can produce several characteristic signs (not always at the same time but usually on the same side of the body as the injury):

- abnormal gait and asynergia (jerky, unco-ordinated movement);
- falling, especially to the injured side;
- dysmetria (the inability to judge distance and to stop movement at a chosen point);
- intention tremor (tremor occurring during a voluntary movement);
- dysdiadochokinesia (the inability to perform rapidly alternating movements);
- dysphonic speech (slurred and explosive in nature);
- nystagmus (involuntary, rhythmical movements of the eyes).

Pons

Located between the midbrain and the medulla oblongata, and separated from the overlying cerebellum by the fourth ventricle, is the pons. Various ascending and descending tracts pass through the pons, which also contains nuclei of the Vth (trigeminal), VIth (abducens) and VIIth (facial) cranial nerves.

Nuclei of the reticular formation of the pons, together with the medullary rhythmicity area in the medulla oblongata, help to control respiration.

Medulla oblongata

The medulla oblongata is the last division of the brain, which becomes continuous with the spinal cord at the foramen magnum. The medulla contains all the ascending and descending tracts that communicate between the spinal cord and various parts of the brain.

On the ventral (anterior) side of the medulla are two roughly triangular structures called pyramids, composed of the largest motor tracts. At the base of the medulla, most of the fibres of the left pyramid cross to the right side, and most of the fibres of the right side cross to the left, before descending the spinal cord. This crossing is called decussation of the pyramids. As a result, fibres originating in the right cerebral cortex activate muscles on the left side of the body and vice versa.

The medulla also contains nuclei of the VIIIth (at the junction of the pons and medulla) to the XIIth cranial nerves, that is, the acoustovestibular (auditory), glossopharyngeal, vagus, accessory and hypoglossal nerves.

Within the medulla are three vital reflex centres of the reticular system. The cardiac centre regulates heartbeat and force of myocardial contraction, the medullary rhythmicity area adjusts the basic rhythm of breathing, and the vasomotor (vasoconstrictor) centre regulates the diameter of blood vessels.

Brain circulation

A constant flow of blood to the brain must be maintained at all times to meet the needs of neurones for oxygen and nutrients. Although the brain comprises approximately only 2% of total body weight, it utilises about 20% of the oxygen used by the entire body. Some of the oxygen supplied is used for the oxidation (metabolism) of glucose. In the brain, glucose is the chief source of energy.

The circle of Willis at the base of the brain is the principal arterial supply (Figure 1.5). It is formed by the junction of the internal carotid, basilar, anterior cerebral, anterior communicating, posterior cerebral and posterior communicating arteries.

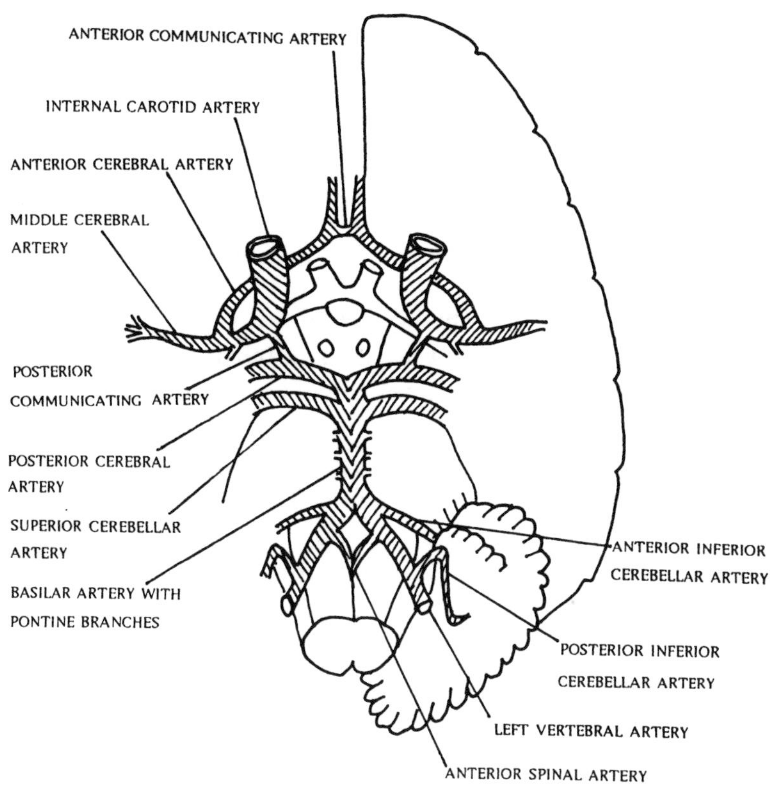

Figure 1.5 Circle of Willis and principal arteries of the brain stem.

In normal circumstances, each internal carotid artery supplies the ipsilateral (same side) cerebral hemisphere, whereas the basilar artery carries blood to structures within the posterior fossa and occipital areas.

Blood vessels pass along the surface of the brain and, as they penetrate inwards, they are surrounded by a loose-fitting layer of pia mater.

There are differential rates of passage of certain substances from the blood into most parts of the brain because of the blood–brain barrier. The capillaries of the brain differ structurally from other capillaries in that they are constructed of more densely packed cells and are surrounded by large numbers of neuroglial cells and a continuous basement membrane. The blood–brain barrier protects the brain from harmful substances and allows the rapid entry of glucose and oxygen.

The venous drainage from the brain is chiefly into the dural sinuses, vascular channels lying within the tough structure of the dura.

Spinal cord

The spinal cord is a long cylindrical structure beginning at the foramen magnum and descending in the vertebral canal to about the level of the first lumbar vertebra. The cord serves as the main pathway for the ascending and descending fibre tracts that connect the peripheral and spinal nerves with the brain. However, the spinal cord is not merely a conduit for sensory signals to the brain or for motor signals from the brain back to the periphery. There are special neuronal circuits within the cord, without which motor control systems in the brain could not bring about purposeful muscle movement such as the to-and-fro movement of the legs required for walking.

A cross-section of the cord reveals grey matter in the form of an H surrounded on all sides by white matter. The grey matter is the integrative area for the cord reflexes and other motor functions. Sensory signals enter the cord almost entirely through the posterior (dorsal) roots. After entering the cord, each sensory signal travels to two separate destinations, one branch terminating in the grey matter of the cord, which elicits reflexes, the other branch travelling to higher centres of the nervous system (Figure 1.6).

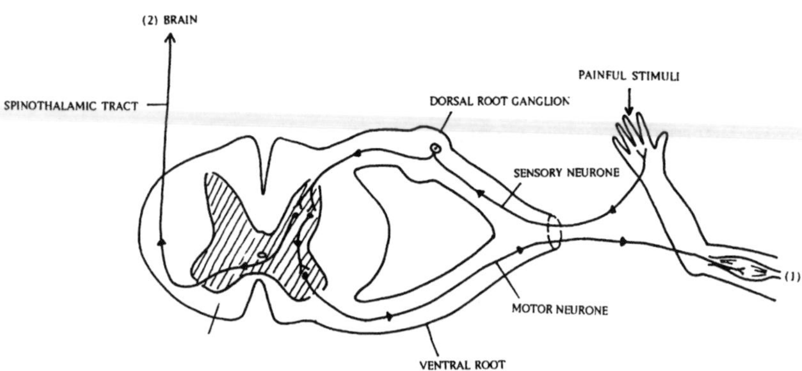

Figure 1.6 Diagram illustrating how sensory signals travel to two different destinations. (1) eliciting reflex, (2) to the brain.

The peripheral nerves are attached to the spinal cord by 31 pairs of spinal nerves.

Meninges

Both the brain and the spinal cord are enclosed and protected by three membranes known as meninges:

- the dura mater;
- the arachnoid mater;
- the pia mater.

All of these are continuous through the foramen magnum. The dura mater, which is the external layer, is tough and fibrous, the arachnoid or intermediate layer is avascular, loose and tenuous, and the pia is a thin connective tissue membrane close to the brain that carries blood vessels supplying the nervous tissue.

Cerebrospinal fluid

The brain and spinal cord are extremely delicate structures that require a special protective system. This protection is achieved by the encasement of both the brain and spinal cord in a rigid, bony vault comprising the cranial cavity in the skull and the vertebral canal in the vertebral column. Within this vault, the brain and spinal cord 'float' in a bath of fluid called the cerebrospinal fluid (CSF). Within the brain substance is a communicating system of four ventricles filled with CSF.

CSF is formed primarily by filtration and secretion from networks of capillaries, called choroid plexuses, located in the ventricles. The CSF formed in the choroid plexuses of the lateral ventricles circulates through the interventricular foramina to the third ventricle, where more CSF is added. It then flows through the cerebral aqueduct into the fourth ventricle where still further CSF is added. The CSF then circulates through the apertures of the fourth ventricle into the subarachnoid space around the back of the brain. It passes downwards in the subarachnoid space around the spinal cord and up over the surface of the brain. From there, it is gradually absorbed into veins. The absorption takes place through arachnoid villi, which are finger-like projections of the arachnoid mater that push into the dural venous sinuses. In an adult, approximately 500 ml of CSF are produced and reabsorbed each day.

Sensation

Sensation can be divided into four types: superficial, deep, visceral and special. Superficial sensation is concerned with touch, pain, temperature and two-point discrimination (the ability to perceive, separately, two points being touched simultaneously and in close proximity). Deep sensation includes muscle and joint position sense, deep muscle pain and vibration sense. Visceral sensations are relayed by the autonomic nervous system and include hunger, nausea and visceral pain. The special senses (sight, sound, taste and smell) are conveyed by the cranial nerves.

Pain and temperature pathway

Receptors for pain and temperature are found in the dermis and the epidermis of the skin. Sensory nerves pass from the skin to the spinal cord. The cell bodies are situated in the dorsal root ganglia. The neurones end in the dorsal horn of the grey matter. Here the first neurone synapses with a second neurone, which then crosses to the opposite side of the cord, entering the lateral white column, and ascends to the thalamus. This ascending bundle of crossed pain and temperature fibres is known as the lateral spinothalamic tract (Figure 1.7). In the thalamus, the axons synapse with tertiary neurones that ascend in the internal capsule to reach the postcentral gyrus. The cortical grey matter of the postcentral gyrus is the primary somatic sensory area of the brain and is concerned with interpreting pain and temperature sensations as well as other cutaneous sensations such as pressure and touch.

The primary pain and temperature axons have branches that synapse in the dorsal horn with short neurones that pass down to the

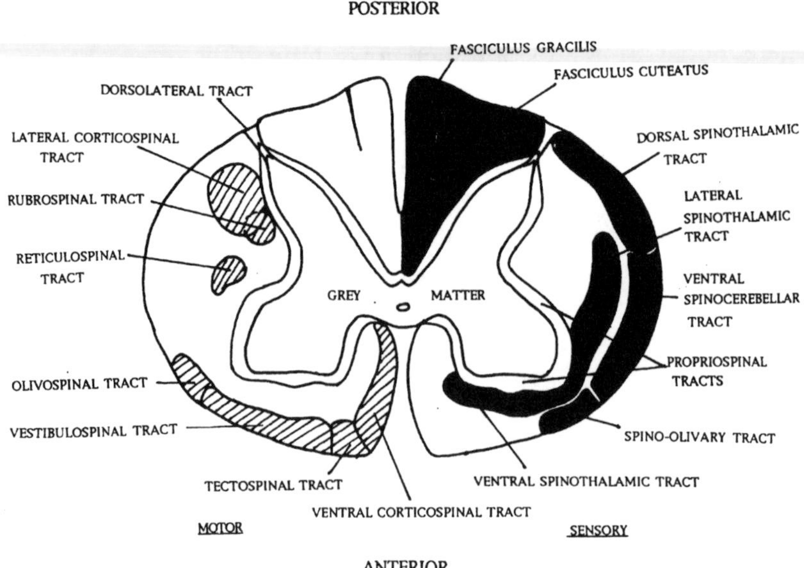

Figure 1.7 Cross-sectional view of the spinal cord.

ventral horn. Here they synapse with motor neurones, which proceed to voluntary muscles, initiating movement. This involuntary motor response to a sensory stimulus is called a reflex. A reflex is a defence mechanism of the nervous system that permits a quick, automatic response to a painful and potentially damaging situation.

The neurones of each dorsal root come from a fairly discrete area of skin known as a dermatome (Figure 1.8). There is, however, at each boundary of the dermatome, an area that is supplied by the adjacent segmental nerves. This overlap acts as a kind of biological insurance so that if one nerve root is damaged, sensation from the area served is not lost altogether.

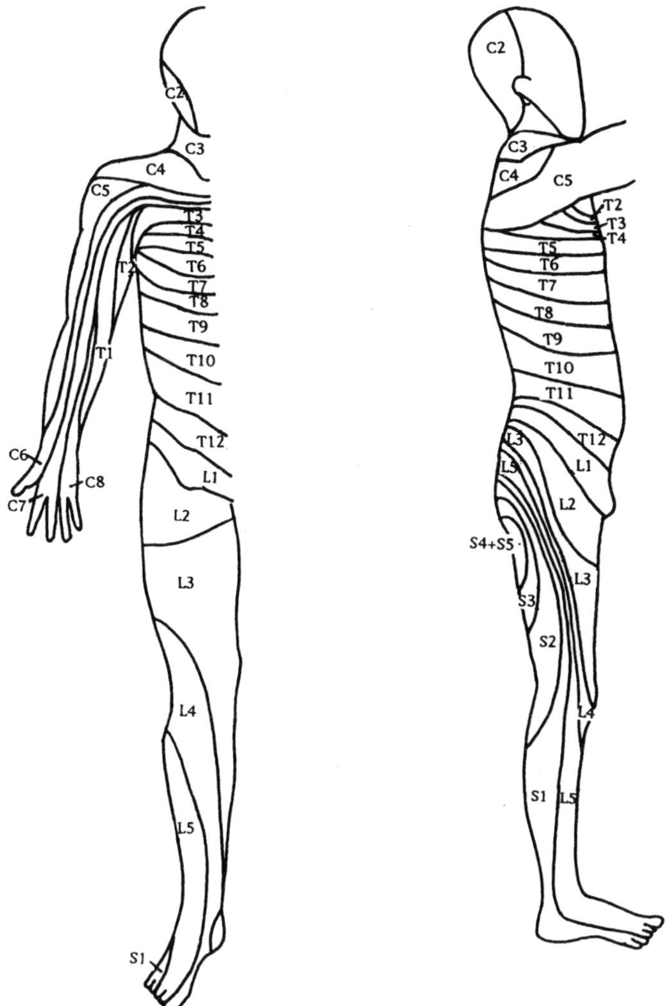

Figure 1.8 The dermatomes.

Pathway for pressure and simple touch from the extremities and trunk

The receptors for pressure and simple touch are found in the dermis of the skin. When pressure is applied, impulses travel in the peripheral nerves toward the spinal cord. The cell bodies are gathered in the dorsal root ganglion, and from here the axons enter the cord through the dorsal root. Upon entering, the axons pass into the ipsilateral dorsal white column and bifurcate. One branch enters the dorsal horn grey matter and synapses with a second neurone. The other branch ascends in the ipsilateral dorsal column for as many as ten spinal segments and then enters the dorsal horn grey matter to synapse with a second neurone. In both cases, the secondary neurones cross over and enter the ventral white column, where they form the ventral spinothalamic tract (see Figure 1.7).

Pathway for proprioception, fine touch and vibratory sense

The same pathway is used for the three different sensations of proprioception, fine touch and vibratory sense. The sense of proprioception enables a person to know at all times where the parts of the body are in space and in relation to each other. It enables a person, with the eyes closed, to touch the tip of the nose with the end of a finger. Proprioception receptors are located in muscles, tendons and joints. Fine touch is the sense that enables a person, with the eyes closed, to identify various objects and to discriminate between two points when touched simultaneously.

The sensory fibres pass towards the spinal cord in the peripheral nerves, and the cell bodies are aggregated in the dorsal root ganglion. The axons then enter the spinal cord and pass into the ipsilateral dorsal white columns, where they ascend to the medulla. The second neurones cross over to the other side of the medulla, where they form a bundle that ascends to the thalamus. Here the neurones synapse with third neurones that ascend through the internal capsule to reach the postcentral gyrus.

Facial sensation

The trigeminal nerve, the Vth cranial nerve, is the major somatic sensory nerve for the face. There are several reflexes involving the trigeminal nerve, of which the most important is the corneal or 'blink' reflex. If the cornea of one eye is touched, both eyes will blink immediately. Reflexes are not only a defence mechanism, but are also useful diagnostically, enabling the integrity of nerve pathways to be tested.

If the trigeminal nerve is transected, facial sensation will be lost on the same (ipsilateral) side as the injury. However, if there is a low pontine/medullary lesion, pain and temperature sensation is lost on the opposite (contralateral) side, although pressure and touch discrimination remain (dissociated sensory loss) as there are two trigeminal nuclei within the brain stem and the sensations of pressure and touch are projected bilaterally to the brain from each. This is known as lateral medullary syndrome.

The brain itself does not sense pain. Headaches are usually the result of pressure or pain in non-nervous structures on or within the brain or skull, such as the arteries or the meninges. Tumours can also cause headaches as a result of increased intracranial pressure.

The vestibular system

Maintenance of equilibrium is the function of the vestibular division of the VIIIth cranial nerve, the acoustovestibular (auditory) nerve. This is the system that attempts to save us if we trip and begin to fall. Its actions are reflexive. The cerebral motor cortex is not involved in its actions.

The inner ear houses the receptor organ. It consists of two fluid-filled sacks and three fluid-filled semicircular canals. The fluid is endolymph, suspended in which are specialised receptor cells sensitive to fluid currents. When there is a change of head position, the endolymph is set in motion. It then stimulates the receptors, which transmit this information to the brain, which in turn sets off the appropriate reflex responses.

Neuronal pathways from the inner ear have five major connections:

1. Vestibulocerebellar connections are vital as the cerebellum is the co-ordination centre for motor activity and equilibrium.
2. Vestibulospinal tracts descend in the spinal cord and discharge reflexively to maintain body equilibrium.
3. The vestibular system also regulates eyeball movements via the vestibulo-ocular tracts, which allows an individual to maintain a steady gaze despite head movement. Branches from the proximal end of the vestibulospinal tract enter the pons and midbrain where they synapse with the VIth (abducens), IVth (trochlear) and IIIrd (oculomotor) cranial nerve nuclei, which are all concerned with eyeball muscle movement.

4. Vestibulocortical connections allow us to sense a loss of equilibrium.
5. The cerebellum is involved in an additional pathway to maintain equilibrium via the reticulospinal tract, called the accessory pathway.

Symptoms of vestibular injury include abnormal to-and-fro movements of the eyes (nystagmus) and the inability to walk straight (ataxia).

Pathway for voluntary muscle activity

The corticospinal tract is the main tract for the majority of voluntary muscle activity. It originates in the motor cortex situated in the precentral gyrus of the frontal lobe. This tract is also known as the pyramidal tract.

Axons exit the motor cortex and pass down through the internal capsule, which is the main passageway for ascending and descending fibre tracts. From here, the axons pass through the midbrain into the medulla oblongata of the brain stem. At this point about 80–90% of the axons cross over (decussate) to the opposite side of the medulla and descend in the lateral aspect of the spinal cord (the lateral corticospinal tract). Those axons which do not decussate continue down the same side to enter the ventral white columns of the spinal cord (the ventral corticospinal tract).

At each level of the cord, some of the axons separate from the lateral corticospinal tract and enter the grey matter of the ventral horn, where they terminate by synapsing with second-order neurones. At each corresponding level of the cord, axons of the ventral corticospinal tract separate off from the main tract and cross over to the other side of the cord. Here, they enter and terminate upon second-order neurones in the ventral horn.

From the precentral gyrus to the ventral horns, these tracts are made up of uninterrupted single neurones known as the upper motor neurones. The upper motor neurones synapse with second-order neurones and send their axons out of the spinal cord via the ventral roots. These neurones then branch out in the peripheral nerves and supply voluntary muscles. They are known as lower motor neurones and the differentiation between them is important as upper motor neurone lesions result in different clinical signs from lower ones.

The nerve cell bodies of the upper motor neurones are arranged in a specific pattern in the motor cortex. The body is represented upside down, the areas for the head and neck being inferior, and those for the leg and foot superior. The areas of cortical representation for the face and hands, with their finely graded movements, are relatively large.

Lower motor neurones supplying the voluntary muscles of the head are not situated in the spinal nerves but are associated with cranial nerves originating in the brain stem. The basic framework is the same as for the corticospinal tracts. It is a two-neurone pathway consisting of an upper motor neurone originating in the cerebral cortex and a lower motor neurone that stimulates voluntary muscles. Upper motor neurones synapse with lower motor neurones in the brain stem and these are collectively called the corticobulbar tract. The cell bodies of the lower motor neurones are concentrated into specific areas of the brain stem called nuclei, and their axons form many of the cranial nerves.

The autonomic nervous system

The autonomic nervous system (ANS) stimulates and controls structures not under conscious influence. This system helps to control arterial blood pressure, gastrointestinal motility and secretion, urinary bladder emptying, sweating, body temperature and many other activities. It is divided into two parts – the sympathetic nervous system and the parasympathetic nervous system – which supply the same organs but act in ways antagonistic to each other (Table 1.1). The nervous system, acting through the autonomic nervous fibres, can exert rapid and effective control of most internal functions of the body.

The autonomic nervous system is activated mainly by centres located in the spinal cord, brain stem and hypothalamus. In addition, areas of the cerebral cortex, especially of the limbic system, can transmit impulses to the lower centres and in this way influence autonomic control.

The sympathetic nervous system

This dominates in a stress situation, be it physical or psychological. The body automatically responds to stress by preparing for 'fight or flight'. These responses will require the muscles to work harder, needing more oxygen and utilising more energy. The individual breathes faster and the bronchioles dilate for a quicker and greater passage of air; the heart beats stronger and faster to increase cardiac output; the arteries to the heart and voluntary muscles dilate in order

Table 1.1 Examples of autonomic effects on various organs of the body

Organ	**Effect on sympathetic stimulation**	**Effect on parasympathetic stimulation**
Eye: Pupil	Dilation	Constriction
Glands:		
Nasal, lacrimal, parotid, submandibular, gastric, pancreatic	Vasoconstriction + slight secretion	Stimulation of copious (except pancreas) secretion
Sweat glands	Copious sweating	None
Heart: muscle	Increased rate, increased force of contraction	Slowed rate, decreased force of contraction
Lungs: bronchi	Dilation	Constriction
Blood:		
Coagulation	Increased	None
Glucose	Increased	None

to increase their supply; the arteries to the skin and peripheral areas of the body constrict, thereby diverting more blood to the active muscles; the liver secretes glycogen; bowel peristalsis slows; the pupils dilate to get a better view of the surroundings; the hair stands on end and the individual sweats.

The chemical transmitter between the sympathetic axons and the structures they innervate is noradrenaline. If an individual is given an injection of adrenaline, the reaction is the same as if the sympathetic nervous system had been discharged.

The parasympathetic nervous system

In contrast to the sympathetic nervous system, the parasympathetic nervous system is most active when a person is relaxed and resting: the heart slows down, peristalsis and other digestive functions are active. The chemical transmitter between the parasympathetic axons and the structures that they innervate is acetylcholine.

The relative balance of noradrenaline and acetylcholine determines which part of the autonomic nervous system is dominant at any time.

The hypothalamus is the control and integrative centre for the autonomic nervous system, and its actions are automatic.

Cranial nerves

There are 12 pairs of cranial nerves (which are discussed in detail in Chapter 2). Cranial nerves are represented by Roman numerals and their functions can be summarised as follows:

- I The olfactory nerve conveys the sense of smell.
- II The optic nerve deals with vision.
- III The oculomotor nerve controls pupillary constriction, lens accommodation, elevation of the eyelid, and four of the six muscles for eyeball movement, which allow medial gaze, upward gaze, downward gaze and upward-lateral gaze.
- IV The trochlear nerve innervates the superior oblique muscle of the eyeball controlling downward-medial gaze.
- V The trigeminal nerve conveys sensations from the face, cornea, mouth, nose sinuses, tongue, teeth, meninges, eardrum and supplies motor fibres to the muscles of mastication.
- VI The abducens nerve innervates the lateral rectus muscle of the eyeball, controlling lateral gaze.
- VII The facial nerve has three major components: sensory fibres for taste, parasympathetic fibres to the sublingual, submandibular and lacrimal glands, and voluntary motor fibres to the muscles of facial expression.
- VIII The acoustovestibular (or auditory) nerve is concerned with hearing and equilibrium.
- IX The glossopharyngeal nerve has three major components: sensory taste neurones, parasympathetic fibres to the parotid gland, and sensory neurones from the ear, the tongue, the pharynx and the carotid sinus.
- X The vagus nerve has three major components: parasympathetic fibres to the autonomic structures of the chest and abdomen, voluntary motor fibres to the muscles of the larynx and pharynx, and sensory fibres from the larynx, the viscera, the carotid body, the carotid sinus, the dura of the posterior cranial fossa and the lower pharynx.
- XI The accessory nerve innervates the trapezius and sternomastoid muscles, whose contraction cause shrugging of the shoulders and turning of the head.
- XII The hypoglossal nerve supplies the muscles of the tongue.

The visual pathways and optic reflexes (sight)

Light rays from an object in the visual field strike the retina, having first being inverted by the lens. The inversion means that images in the temporal field of vision are projected onto the nasal retinal field and vice versa.

The retina is made up of various types of neurone, including the light-sensitive rods and cones. Axons from the nerve cells in the eye pass posteriorly to the optic nerve (Figure 1.9a). At the optic

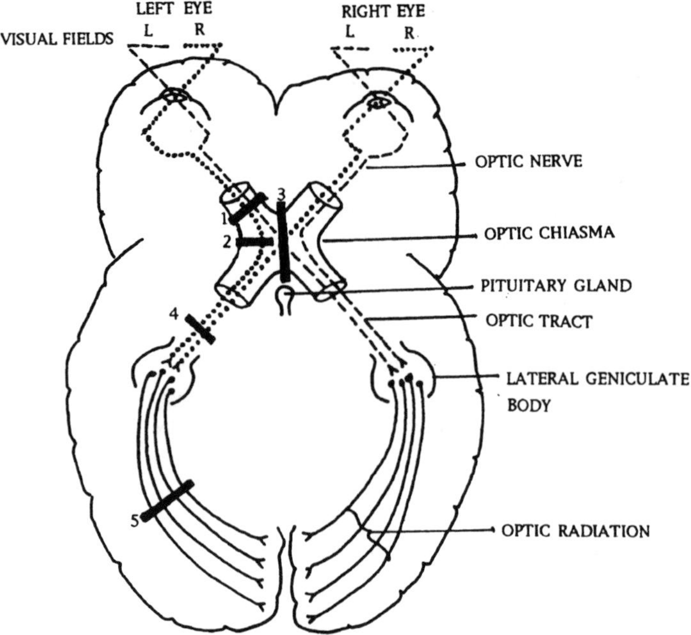

Figure 1.9a Optic pathways.

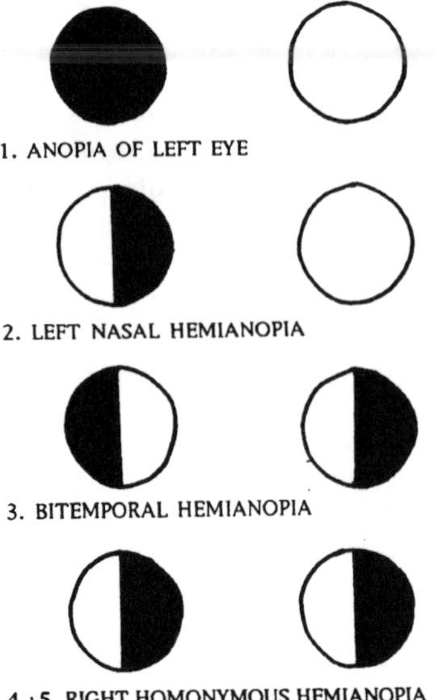

Figure 1.9b Resultant visual field loss from destruction of visual pathways as shown in Figure 1.9a.

chiasma, axons from the nasal retinal field cross over to join the axons of the temporal retinal field, which do not cross. Axons continue to the lateral geniculate body of the diencephalon. Here they synapse with neurones that sweep out to form the optic radiations, which end in the visual cortex of the occipital lobe.

Lesions at different points in the visual pathways affect vision (see Figure 1.9b). It should be noted that loss of vision is always described with reference to the visual fields rather than the retinal fields.

The pupillary light reflex is also known as the consensual reflex. It refers to pupillary constriction of both eyes when light is shone into only one. This is due to the interconnection of the nervous pathways for each eye. If this reflex cannot be elicited, a serious condition in the CNS, particularly the brainstem, is indicated.

The olfactory system (smell)

Smell is the least understood sense for several reasons. First, it has no obvious physical end-organ, as occurs in the touch or auditory systems, and second, the olfactory membrane located high in the nose makes it difficult to assess.

Receptor cells for smell are located in the epithelial tissue of the nasal cavity. From here, the first-order neurones travel up to the olfactory bulb (which rests on the cribriform plate of the ethmoid bone), where they synapse with second-order neurones whose axons form the olfactory tract. The olfactory tract runs along the olfactory groove of the cribriform plate to the cerebrum. Posterior to the olfactory nuclei, the olfactory tract divides into well-defined medial and lateral striae. The medial striae pass to the opposite side of the cerebrum by way of the anterior commissure. Most of the fibres of the olfactory bulb enter the lateral olfactory striae, which terminate in the medial and cortical nuclei of the amygdaloid complex (of the limbic system) and the lateral olfactory gyrus, also known as the prepiriform area. Similar to other sensory systems, the olfactory system has an area of associated neocortex. This neocortex is located posteriorly on the orbital surface of the frontal lobe and extends onto the anterior insular, which is adjacent to the gustatory cortex.

Damage to the receptor cells or olfactory tract (cranial nerve I) will result in a loss of the sense of smell (anosmia). Lesions of the temporal lobe can produce olfactory hallucinations, which sometimes take the form of an aura preceding a seizure.

The reticular system

There are many different states of brain activity, including sleep, wakefulness, excitement and different levels of mood. All these states result from different activating or inhibiting forces that are usually generated within the brain itself.

Areas of diffuse neurones (some grouped into nuclei) throughout the brain stem make up the reticular formation. Many of the ascending and descending fibre tracts between the brain and the spinal cord pass through the reticular formation, and as they do so, they provide collateral nerve endings to all reticular areas. In turn, the reticular formation provides multiple efferent (motor) fibres that pass both upward and downward in the axis of the nervous system.

The descending reticular formation is a system that has two main functions. The first is that of relaying impulses from the hypothalamus to various target organs of the autonomic nervous system. The second function is that of relaying involuntary motor impulses from the extrapyramidal systems to voluntary muscles. Stimuli are received from the hypothalamus, various basal ganglia, and the vestibular system by the reticular nuclei. Axons leaving the reticular nuclei form the reticulospinal tracts.

The ascending reticular formation is better known as the reticular activating system. It is concerned with degrees of conscious alertness and sleep. All of the major sensory pathways send collateral axons that terminate in the nuclei of the reticular activating system. The nuclei then send the sensory stimuli up the multisynaptic chain to the thalamus. From the thalamus, impulses are relayed up to the cerebral cortex, where they influence states of consciousness. Emphasis should be put on the word 'influence' as other factors also have a role.

Intellectual functions of the brain

In the past, it was believed that the prefrontal cortex was the area for higher intellect in humans because of its size in comparison with that of primates. However, damage to Wernicke's area (the language comprehension area) in the temporal lobe and the angular gyrus region in the dominant hemisphere causes a great deal more harm to the intellect than does damage to the prefrontal area. This is because much of our sensory experience is converted to its language equivalent before being stored in the memory areas of the brain. For example, when we read, we do not store the visual images of the words themselves but convert the words into language in order to discern meaning, storing the information in this form. If Wernicke's area in the dominant hemisphere is destroyed, the person normally loses all intellectual functions associated with language or verbal symbolism, including reading, solving mathematical problems and thinking through logical problems. Damage to the non-dominant hemisphere in this region affects ability to interpret all kinds of stimuli, for example music, non-verbal visual experiences such as patterns, body language and intonation of voice.

Prior to the development of modern medicine for the treatment of psychotic depression, patients with this condition were treated with prefrontal lobotomy. From the mental changes noted in these individuals, the function of the prefrontal cortex was determined. Post-prefrontal lobotomy patients were found to be unable to progress toward goals or to carry through with sequential thoughts, abilities that are associated with higher intelligence. They also expressed decreased aggressiveness and inappropriate social responses, lack of elaboration of thought and prognostication.

Memory is also associated with intellect. Physiologically, memories are caused by changes in the capability of synaptic transmission from one neurone to the next as a result of previous neuronal activity. The changes cause new pathways, called memory traces, to develop. Once they are established, they can be activated by the thinking mind to reproduce the memories. Memories are classified into their relative life spans: immediate, short term and long term. Immediate memory lasts as long as the individual continues to think about the subject and is then lost. Its mechanism is not fully understood. Short-term memories last from minutes to weeks but are lost unless memory traces become permanent, i.e. long-term. Long-term memory is thought to result from actual structural changes at the synapses.

The hippocampus has been found to have a role in the storage of memories. Patients who have had their hippocampus removed for the treatment of epilepsy subsequently experience difficulty storing new memories of verbal or symbolic type.

Intelligence, as with other functions of the nervous system, is not well understood. The neural mechanism for thought is not known, and there is still a great deal to learn about this highly complex system.

Conclusion

In this chapter, the nervous system has been reduced to its component parts in order that its structure may be understood. However, it is important to view the nervous system as a continuum. Neurones form the basic units of the system at the microscopic level and are supported by glial cells. Neurones are gathered together to form larger structures, with specific functions, which communicate with each other at many different levels. An individual's abilities and characteristics are a direct result of these interactions. In essence, our nervous system makes us what we are.

Further reading

ChusidJG (1985) Correlative Neuroanatomy and Functional Neurology, 19th edn. California: Lange Medical Publications.

DeGrootJ (1991) Correlative Neuroanatomy, 21st edn. California: Lange Medical Publications.

Guyton AC (1991) Basic Neuroscience. Anatomy and Physiology, 2nd edn. Philadelphia: WB Saunders.

Haines DE (1997) Fundamental Neuroscience. Edinburgh: Churchill Livingstone.

Liebman M (1986) Neuroanatomy Made Easy and Understandable, 3rd edn. Maryland: Aspen Publishers.

Mitchell GAG, Mayor D (1983) The Essentials of Neuroanatomy, 4th edn. Edinburgh: Churchill Livingstone.

Tortora GJ, Anagnostakos NP (1987) Principles of Anatomy and Physiology, 5th edn. New York: Harper & Row.

Chapter 2 Neurological assessment

Sally Aucken and Belinda Crawford

Introduction

A full neurological examination, as described in this chapter, is time-consuming. However, a well-conducted neurological assessment provides vast quantities of useful information that can be used towards the comprehensive planning of patient care. For routine, repeated observations, the neurological examination can be tailored to give a sufficient overview of a patient's condition to detect any changes (Hickey, 1992). This chapter aims to demystify the neurological examination, often seen as the domain of doctors, and will provide nurses with the information and confidence to undertake neurological examination appropriate to individual patients' needs.

Routine repeated observations for intracranial pathology should include:

- level of consciousness;
- general motor function to detect localising signs;
- pupillary reactions to light;
- vital signs;
- areas of specific dysfunction (such as cranial nerve dysfunction, for example visual field assessment in pituitary adenomas and craniopharyngiomas).

Routine repeated observations for spinal pathology should include:

- full motor assessment;
- sensory assessment;
- vital signs;
- recording of bladder and bowel dysfunction.

Changes in neurological status can be rapid and dramatic or subtle, developing over minutes, hours, days, weeks or even months depending on the insult. The frequency of these repeated neurological observations will therefore depend on the patient's condition and the underlying pathology.

Neurological assessment

A full neurological assessment provides details of a patient's neurological function and is carried out for a number of reasons. It is used by doctors to locate the site of any CNS dysfunction and to determine possible diagnoses. The main reasons for nurses carrying out assessments are to determine the effect of the nervous system dysfunction on activities of daily living and independent function, to establish a baseline for that patient with which to compare subsequent assessments, to determine changes in the condition over time and to detect life-threatening situations and those requiring intervention (Jennett and Teasdale, 1974; Hickey, 1992).

Although the full assessment is usually the responsibility of the doctors, nurses need to understand what it entails so that they can glean useful information to guide their own assessment of the patient's neurological status on a day-to-day basis. The nurse is usually the most consistent member of the multidisciplinary team, interacting with the patient, and is therefore in a unique position to regularly assess for subtle but important changes in condition (Hickey, 1992; Ackerman, 1993).

The neurological examination

Surveillance is the purposeful acquisition, interpretation and synthesis of patient data for clinical decision-making. The whole process of the systematic collection of valid and reliable data about neurological function, and the interpretation and evaluation of the findings against baseline recordings, constitutes neurological assessment (Ackerman, 1993; Stenger, 1993).

Watching for signs of recognised, potential and anticipated changes in neurological condition is an important nursing intervention when caring for patients with CNS malignancies. A delay in nurses identifying changes in neurological status can make a difference in the subsequent management of the patient in terms of recovery of function and prevention of further neurological damage.

A complete neurological examination includes:

- level of consciousness and higher cerebral function (including speech and memory);
- cranial nerve function;
- cerebellar function;
- motor function;
- sensory function;
- reflexes.

It is carried out in a systematic manner from the highest to the lowest level of function, that is from cerebral function to reflexes. A comprehensive neurological examination may take up to 1 hour to complete (Beveridge, 1995).

History

The first step in conducting the examination is to obtain a full patient history in order to chronicle the course of the neurological symptoms. If patients are unable to give specific details themselves, a relative or friend should be present to give information (Pressman et al, 1995).

Questions regarding symptoms should include the presence of the following:

- headaches, noting when in the day they are worst, the site of the headache and any relieving factors;
- blackouts, fits, epileptic seizures, convulsions;
- blurred vision;
- speech problems;
- swallowing difficulties;
- loss of memory;
- nausea and vomiting;
- clumsiness;
- falls;
- bladder or bowel problems;
- sexual dysfunction;
- limb weaknesses and/or sensory changes.

The significance of these observations will be demonstrated when discussing specific elements of the examination.

The history assessment must also include details of other illnesses and present medication as well as social and family history, noting any familial neurological history.

Equipment

The basic equipment to conduct the neurological examination includes:

- an ophthalmoscope;
- an otoscope;
- a tongue depressor blade;
- a cotton bud;
- a tuning fork (128 Hz);
- a Neuro-tip (disposable, one blunt and one sharp end);
- a pen-torch;
- a reflex hammer;
- cotton-wool;
- a Snellen chart.

Cerebral function

Observations of mental state (cerebral function) begin as soon as the nurse meets the patient. Facial expressions, behaviour and mood are noted, along with their appropriateness to the situation, taking into account the patient's education and social situation. By asking questions that require more elaborate answers than a monosyllabic response, it is possible to assess the patient's fluency, pace, coherence and congruency of speech and highlight any problems with concentration (Lower, 1992; Beveridge, 1995).

Consciousness

Consciousness is defined as a general awareness of oneself and the surrounding environment. It is a dynamic state and is therefore subject to change. Consciousness is traditionally described as having two components: arousal and cognition. Arousal is a state of wakefulness and is a function of the reticular activating system in the brain stem (see Chapter 1). Cognition is largely a function of the cerebral cortex, although if arousal is significantly altered or absent, cognition cannot take place (Lindsay et al, 1991; Hickey, 1992).

Assessing consciousness is difficult because it cannot be measured directly. It is estimated by the subjective observation of arousability and behaviour in response to stimuli (Ellis and Cavanagh, 1992).

Alterations in level of consciousness can vary from slight to severe changes, indicating the degree of brain dysfunction. The various stages of consciousness can be described on a crude continuum from full consciousness at one end to deep coma at the other. Coma is defined as a state of unrousable unresponsiveness.

Coma itself is not a disease process; instead, it reflects some underlying process resulting from a primary CNS insult or a metabolic or systemic disorder (including hypoxia following cardiac arrest, hypoglycaemia, diseases of major organs and the effects of pharmacological agents). Although all CNS lesions may cause an alteration in the level of consciousness, only those with diffuse hemispheric conditions, such as diffuse oedema or bleeding from a tumour, will actually result in coma. Lesions localised to one area of the brain may produce neurological symptoms, such as hemiplegia, without any deterioration in level of consciousness (Hickey, 1992).

The Glasgow Coma Scale

The Glasgow Coma Scale (GCS) was developed in 1974 at the University of Glasgow by Jennett and Teasdale. It was designed as a system to grade the severity of impaired consciousness in patients with traumatic head injuries or intracranial surgery. It aimed to provide an objective assessment and uniform labelling for the stages of the continuum, to minimise observer variability when comparing series of patients during the evaluation of different managements of pathologies and to provide a guide to estimating prognoses (Jennett and Teasdale, 1974).

As a standardised clinical assessment of consciousness, it has been adapted world wide in the care of patients with all forms of CNS dysfunction. Its application as a prognostic indicator is still a focus of research. The main advantages of the GCS are that:

- it provides a standardised, consistent assessment of conscious level;
- assessment results should be the same irrespective of the observer's status;
- it can be used serially to provide repeated assessments vital to the care of patients with any intracranial surgery or damage, allowing an accurate evaluation of any change in a patient's condition;
- using a graphic scale allows quick and easy evaluation of trends in

a patient's clinical condition;

- once the observer is familiar with the scale, it is quick to use;
- it can performed with patients ambulant or bed bound;
- it can be used by both medical and nursing staff, thus facilitating efficient and consistent communication and terminology.

The GCS describes the levels of consciousness by assessing arousal, awareness and activity in terms of eye-opening, verbal response and motor response of the upper limbs in response to verbal and tactile stimuli. Each activity is allocated a score depending on the response to the different stimuli (Table 2.1), giving a patient a total score of between 3 and 15. Numerical scores avoid subjective assessments such as stupor, light coma and deep coma. A score of 15 depicts a patient who is awake, alert, fully orientated and fully responsive, 7-8 is taken as denoting coma, and 3 is the lowest score possible, signifying unresponsiveness to any stimulus. The results are recorded graphically, enabling a rapid comparison of serial recordings against the baseline assessment (Jennett and Teasdale, 1974; Jennett et al, 1979).

Eye opening

When performing GCS assessment, begin by evaluating arousal (eye opening), as without arousal, cognition cannot occur. Once the degree of eye opening is assessed, orientation can be evaluated. The fact that the patient opens his or her eyes in response to a stimulus indicates that the brain stem is functioning (Lower, 1992).

Assessing verbal response

Orientation is a specific cognitive function assessed as part of the GCS. In order for patients to be completely orientated, they must be able to give accurate personal details, such as their full name, date of birth and home address, know where they are and be able to give the day of the week, month and year. It is important to remember that a patient who has been in hospital for a long time may not be able to pinpoint the actual day, but the month should be correctly identified (Beveridge, 1995; Stewart, 1996). Similarly, patients admitted as an emergency may not know exactly which hospital ward they are in.

Some patients may need a lot of stimulation to maintain their concentration to answer questions, even though they can answer them correctly. It is therefore important to note the amount of stimulation that the patient required as part of the baseline assessment. Subtle changes in the amount of stimulation required may indicate

Table 2.1 Scoring the activities of the Glasgow Coma Scale

Eye opening		*scored 1–4*
spontaneously	4	eyes open without need of stimulus
to speech	3	eyes open to verbal stimulation (normal, raised or repeated)
to pain	2	eyes open to central pain only
none	1	no eye opening to verbal or painful stimuli
Verbal response		*scored 1–5*
orientated	5	able to accurately describe details of time, person and place
sentences	4	can speak in sentences but does not answer orientation questions correctly
words	3	speaking incomprehensible, inappropriate words only
sounds	2	incomprehensible sounds following both verbal and painful stimuli
none	1	no verbal response following verbal and painful stimuli
Motor response		*scored 1–6*
obeys commands	6	follows and acts out commands, e.g. lift up right arm
localises	5	purposeful movement to remove noxious stimulus
normal flexion	4	flexes arm at elbow without wrist rotation in response to central painful stimulus
abnormal flexion	3	flexes arm at elbow with accompanying rotation of the wrist into spastic posturing in response to central pain
extension	2	extends arm at elbow with some inward rotation in response to central pain
none	1	no response to central painful stimulus

an increase in intracranial pressure despite a lack of actual change in their score of conscious level (Lower, 1992). Such changes are important and should be reported immediately.

It may be necessary to vary questions when frequent, serial assessments of conscious level are carried out, in order to avoid the patient memorising the responses, thus masking any deterioration. Further information about the patient's orientation may be gathered by general conversation (Shpritz, 1994; Sullivan, 1990).

Evaluation of response to an applied stimulus relies on the application of an adequate stimulus to elicit the best response. Inadequate stimulation, either verbal or tactile, may result in an inaccurate baseline assessment being recorded, so future neurological deterioration may not be noted on subsequent assessments. Verbal stimulation should be escalated from speaking in a normal voice to speaking loudly and shouting. If no response is elicited from the patient with verbal stimulation, tactile stimulation is performed. This begins with gentle touching, leading to applying pain. If no response is noted immediately, the stimulus should be continued for at least 30 seconds to ensure that it has been adequately applied (Lower, 1992). It is important to note when applying a painful stimulus that the brain responds to central stimulation, described below, and the spine responds first to peripheral stimulation, such as nail bed pressure.

Central stimulation can be applied in three ways (Lindsay et al, 1991; Lower, 1992):

1. Trapezium squeeze. Using the thumb and two fingers, hold 2 inches of the trapezius muscle where the neck meets the shoulder and twist the muscle.
2. Supraorbital pressure. Running a finger along the supraorbital margin, a notch is felt. Applying pressure to the notch causes an ipsilateral (on that side) sinus headache. This method must not be used if the facial bones are unstable, facial fractures are suspected or the assessor has sharp fingernails.
3. Sternal rub. Using the knuckles of a clenched fist to grind on the centre of the sternum. When applied adequately, marks are left on the skin as sternal tissue is tender and bruises easily, so this method should not be used for repeated assessments.

Nail bed pressure is a peripheral stimulus and should only be used to assess limbs that have not moved in response to a central stimulus.

Whichever method is used to provide stimulation, it is necessary to escalate it, making it painful, if it is to be adequate to elicit a response. To avoid anxiety in any relatives present during the assessment, it must be explained why this is important.

Assessing motor response

To obtain an accurate picture of brain function, motor response is tested by using the upper limbs. Responses in the lower limbs may reflect spinal function. If a spinal lesion is suspected, spinal function is evaluated using the assessment of motor function described below.

The best motor response is the ability to follow simple commands, for example asking the patient to lift her right arm or hold up her thumb. If gripping the examiner's hand is assessed, it must be in terms of the patient's ability to release the grip. Some patients with cerebral dysfunction may show an involuntary grasp reflex where stimulation of the palm of their hand causes them to grip. This is most frequently seen with diffuse brain disease, often involving the frontal lobes (Bates, 1987; Hickey, 1992).

Patients unable to obey commands should be tested in response to a central tactile stimulus. In order to be recorded as localising, the patient must make attempts to remove the noxious stimulus. Localising is a purposeful movement, for example trying to remove a nasogastric tube, or raising a hand to chin level when a central painful stimulus is applied.

If the patient does not localise to adequate central painful stimulation, the best arm response in terms of flexion (normal or abnormal) or extension is recorded (see Table 2.1 and Figure 2.1). A degree of arousal and orientation is necessary for the patient to be able to participate and co-operate in other areas of examination of cerebral function, particularly speech and memory.

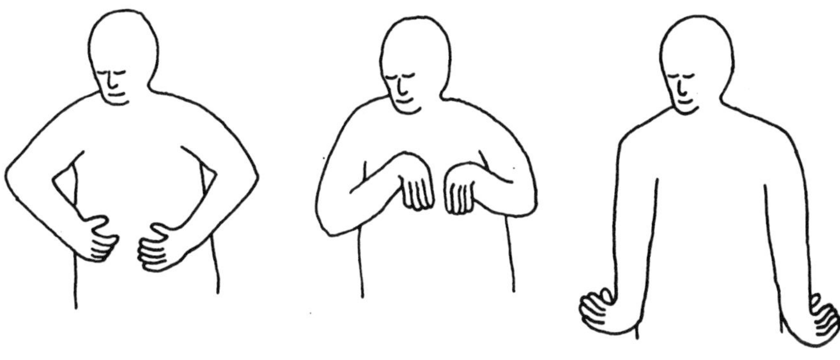

Figure 2.1 Motor response: (a) Normal flexion (b) Abnormal flexion (c) Extension.

Speech

Speech is a specific, complex cognitive function. Normal speech is clear, well paced and appropriate for the person's educational level. In-depth evaluation of speech requires intricate processes best suited to speech and language therapists (see Chapter 9), but for the purpose of the neurological examination, certain aspects of language can be assessed. Most of the evaluation can be picked up in conversation, while taking the patient's history or during the assessment of conscious level (Hickey, 1992; Sullivan, 1990).

Anatomically, the left cerebral hemisphere is dominant for language in right-handed people. Even in 80% of left handed people the left hemisphere is still dominant. There are two main language areas in the brain known as Broca's and Wernicke's areas. Broca's area in the frontal lobe is responsible for speech production and articulation. Pressure on or lesions of Broca's area cause an inability to produce speech. This is known as expressive dysphasia. Patients' understanding remains intact but they have difficulty finding the appropriate words. Expressive dysphasia can be tested by holding up an object (such as a pen or watch) and asking the patient questions related to that object.

Comprehension of spoken words is a function of Wernicke's area in the temporoparietal lobe. A lesion or damage to Wernicke's area causes an inability to understand spoken words. This is known as receptive dysphasia. When assessing for receptive dysphasia, non-verbal cues must be kept to a minimum and the patient's hearing must be known to be intact (Hickey, 1992; Sullivan, 1990).

Both expressive and receptive dysphasia can occur together or separately. Dysphasia is an extremely frustrating condition for both the patient and his or her family and carers. Aphasia denotes an inability to speak and is a combination of receptive and expressive dysphasia.

Other aspects of patients' speech that should be noted are fluency, enunciation, comprehension and their ability to correct their own speech errors. In the presence of major speech deficits, the patient should be referred to a speech and language therapist for expert evaluation. It is often more difficult to complete cerebral function tests in the presence of major speech disorders (Lower, 1992; Sullivan, 1990).

Attention and concentration

The patient's attention and concentration should be noted throughout the neurological examination. Aspects to observe are how coherent the patients are when answering questions, how easily they are distracted and what type of stimulation they require (voice, shaking, painful stimulus) and how often, in order to complete the examination (Mitchell et al, 1984).

Simple tests to evaluate attention and concentration include repeating digit lists: the patient is asked to repeat a random digit list, for example 1, 9, 7, 8, 3, 6, both backwards and forwards. Normally, between five and eight numbers can be repeated forwards and four to six backwards. Poor results may indicate organic brain disease in the absence of known mental retardation. Asking a patient to count backwards from 100 in decrements of threes or sevens can also be used, which can usually be completed in around 60 seconds. This test also evaluates short-term memory (Hickey, 1992).

Nurses can also assess for other changes in attention and concentration during day-to-day care by observing the patient undertaking aspects of daily living such as dressing and eating.

Memory

Memory consists of short- and long-term recall. The medial temporal lobes of the brain are the sites of memory storage and retrieval, the left temporal lobe for verbal information and the right for shapes, faces and spatial information (Mitchell et al, 1984).

Long-term memory can be adequately tested during conversation by asking patients their past medical history and questions such as 'Where were you born?' It is important to include other family members during the neurological examination if possible in order to verify the answers. Long-term memory is rarely lost with organic disease (Lindsay et al, 1991; Lower, 1992).

Short-term memory is also easily tested through conversation by asking questions that require the use of immediate memory, for example asking patients about recent events prior to admission, what they had to eat yesterday or who has visited them in hospital. Tests to examine speech also require the use of short-term memory. In addition, tests for verbal memory include the examiner giving patients a list of three unconnected items or a short sentence, and asking them to repeat and remember them. This will indicate whether the patient has heard and retained the information. At a later stage in the examination, usually after 15-30 minutes, the patient is asked to repeat the sentence or list again. Visual memory can be assessed by asking the patient to recollect items on a tray after 15 minutes. Loss of short-term memory can be an indication of organic brain disease (Hickey, 1992).

Memory is closely linked with other aspects of cerebral functions. With impaired concentration, memory is likely to be reduced, as attention and concentration are closely linked with memory. Cortical motor integration involves the understanding and interpretation of instructions, and the ability to remember them long enough to undertake them. Cortical motor integration is tested by giving a patient a three-step instruction to carry out, for example picking up a cup with the left hand, passing it to the right hand and then drinking out of the cup. An inability to perform such a task is known as apraxia (Barker and Moore, 1992; Beveridge, 1995).

Judgement and reasoning

The patient's educational and cultural background needs to be taken into consideration when evaluating judgement and reasoning. Judgement can be assessed by asking questions such as 'What would you do if you were locked out of your house?' or 'What would you do if this room was on fire?' Reasoning can be evaluated by asking the patient to explain a proverb such as 'Don't count your chickens before they have hatched' (Mitchell et al, 1984; Barker and Moore, 1992).

Emotions, mood and behaviour

Emotions, mood and behaviour are governed by the interactions between the frontal lobes and the limbic system. The frontal lobes are concerned with the inhibition of primitive emotions. Evaluation of affect can be observed throughout interactions with patients and by asking questions about how they are feeling. Further information can be obtained by monitoring the congruency of answers and facial expressions. Patients with frontal lobe lesions can present with altered, often labile personality and temperament, changes that are often noted by family and friends rather than the patients themselves. Lesions in the right frontal lobe tend to cause patients to be unconcerned about their situation, lesions in the left frontal lobe tending to promote very strong, sometimes inappropriate, expressions of emotion (Hickey, 1992; Beveridge, 1995).

Spatial perception

Spatial perception is a function of the right cerebral hemisphere and is the ability to recognise oneself and interact with the environment. General observation of the patient is usually all that is required to identify spatial perception deficits. Lesions of the right parietal lobe may cause neglect of the contralateral side of the body. Patients may ignore that side when washing and dressing, or fail to stop the affected limb knocking into objects (Beveridge, 1995).

Other tools for assessing memory, behaviour and cognition include Mini Mental State Examination and the Galveston Orientation and Amnesia Test (Hilton, 1991).

Cranial nerve assessment

Nurses often consider cranial nerve assessment to be complex and outside their scope of practice. However, an understanding of the location and function of the cranial nerves will indicate where lesions are in the brain. Such knowledge will allow nurses to anticipate and deal with deficits arising from tumours and/or raised intracranial pressure that could be exacerbated by surgery or radiotherapy. If nurses rely solely on the GCS for their information regarding the patient's neurological status, they will often miss subtle changes that suggest deterioration in the patient's condition, for example deteriorating visual acuity in patients with pituitary tumours.

There are 12 pairs of cranial nerves that relay information from the special centres and somatosensory receptors to the brain (see Chapter 1). Therefore assessment is always bilateral. The cranial nerves are part of the peripheral nervous system, each nerve arising from clusters of neurones called nuclei within the brain stem (Figure 2.2). Roman numerals are used to indicate the sequential order in which they emerge from the brain: cranial nerves I-II in the frontal region, III-IV in the midbrain, V-VIII in the pons and IX-XII in the medulla (Guyton, 1992).

Some cranial nerves are solely sensory in function, others elicit motor responses and some convey both sensory and motor information. Cranial nerves III, VII, IX and X are also associated with autonomic functions (Butler, 1993).

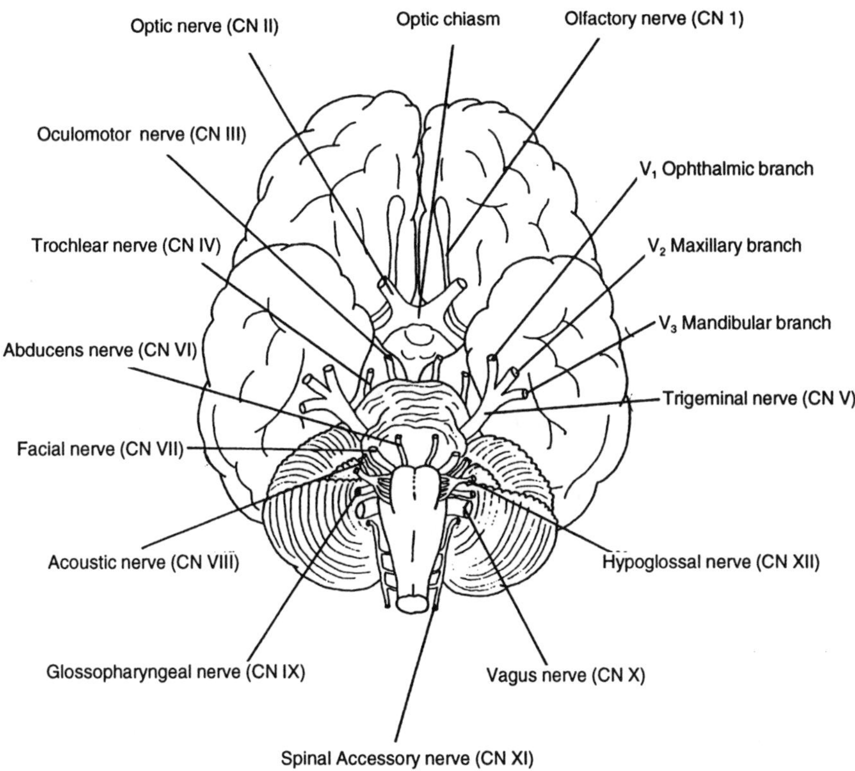

Figure 2.2 Basal view of the brain: schematic representation of gross anatomy.

An easy way to remember the 12 cranial nerves is the mnenomic:

On	**O**lfactory
old	**O**ptic
Olympus	**O**culomotor
towering	**T**rochlear
top	**T**rigeminal
a	**A**bducens
Finn	**F**acial
and	**A**uditory
German	**G**lossopharyngeal
viewed	**V**agus
some	**S**pinal accessory
hawks	**H**ypoglossal

Table 2.2 summarises the normal function of each of the cranial nerves. A guide to assessing each cranial nerve's function follows.

Assessment of Cranial Nerve Function

I Olfactory nerve

First ask the patient to blow his or her nose gently to ensure that the nasal passages are clear. Then ask the patient to close his or her eyes and occlude one nostril. Familiar smells such as coffee, oil of cloves or peppermint are used to test the recognition of smell. Repeat the test with the other nostril.

Avoid using pungent smells such as ammonia as this triggers pain fibres along the trigeminal nerve.

Points to note

- Anosmia is the absence of the sense of smell. It can arise from obstruction, for example by polyps or infection but is also seen in olfactory groove meningiomas and other frontal tumours or after a head injury.
- Parosmia is an alteration in the sense of smell, pleasant smells becoming offensive and vice versa, and is also noted with such tumours.

II Optic nerve

The optic nerve is described in many nursing texts as being responsible for vision, but it should be noted that 'normal' visual function depends on a full and conjugate range of eye movements (cranial nerves III, IV and VI) in addition to normally functioning optic and oculomotor nerves and an intact visual centre in the occipital cortex (see Chapter 1).

Table 2.2 Normal function of the cranial nerves

Cranial nerve	Function
I Olfactory	
Sensory	• Smell
II Optic	
Sensory	• Vision • Visual acuity • Field of vision • Pupillary response (afferent impulse)
III Oculomotor	
Motor	• Vertical and medial eye movement • Eyelid elevation • Convergence
Autonomic	• Focusing and pupil constriction (efferent impulse)
IV Trochlear	
Motor	• Downward and inward movement of the eyeball
V Trigeminal	
Motor	• Mastication and movement of the soft palate
Sensory	• Cutaneous sensation from the cornea, teeth, mouth, meninges and anterior two thirds of tongue (touch, heat, cold, pain)
VI Abducens	
Motor	• Lateral eye movement
VII Facial	
Sensory	• Taste on front two thirds of tongue • Sensation from back of external ear
Motor	• Facial expression • Elevates hyoid • Tenses stapes
Autonomic	• Lacrimation and salivation
VIII Auditory	
(or Acoustic-vestibular) *Sensory*	• Hearing (cochlear portion) • Detects orientation / position in 'space' and balance (vestibular portion)
IX Glossopharyngeal	
Sensory	• Sensation and taste from posterior tongue
Motor	• Swallowing (raises larynx and pharynx)
Autonomic	• Salivation
X Vagus	
Sensory	• Taste and general sensation from upper alimentary tract • Swallowing and gagging • Phonation (vocal quality) • Control of heart rate (inhibits)
Autonomic	• Secretory to stomach and other abdominal organs
XI Accessory	
Motor	• Rotates head • Elevates shoulder
XII Hypoglossal	
Motor	• Movement of the tongue • Speech (articulation)

The optic disc (end of the optic nerve) can be examined using an ophthalmoscope to observe for papilloedema. Papilloedema is a sign of raised intracranial pressure and is indicated by blurring of the disc margins, bulging of the optic cup and possible haemorrhages around the disc margin.

Point to note

- Not all patients with raised intracranial pressure will demonstrate papilloedema (Fuller, 1993).

Three components of vision can be then be assessed: visual acuity, visual fields and colour sense, although the latter is not routinely tested.

Visual acuity is assessed using a Snellen chart at a distance of 6 m. Patients who normally wear glasses or contact lenses should do so during the examination. Each eye is tested separately, and the patient should be able to correctly identify the letters on the sixth line down at a distance of 6 m.

Near vision is assessed by asking the patient to read from a newspaper or prepared reading chart with a range of print fonts, but this is a more subjective test to analyse and needs to be applied consistently in order to provide accurate information.

If the patient has a severe visual deficit, it may only be possible to assess his ability to count fingers or identify light or dark.

Colour perception is assessed using Ishihara plates, which require the patient to distinguish numbers from a background of coloured dots.

Visual fields can be formally examined by using Bjerrman screens or a Goldmann perimeter (descriptions of these can be found in an allied medical text, for example Lindsay et al, 1991) or can be evaluated by the nurse or doctor at the bedside using a confrontation technique.

Visual field assessment by confrontation

Patients are asked to sit or stand directly opposite the examiner at a distance of 1 m and to cover their left eye and to look at the examiner's left eye while the examiner covers his or her right eye. The examiner then introduces an object, such as a red-topped pin, into the peripheral field of vision. The object is moved slowly from the periphery into the centre of the visual field and patients are asked to say 'Now' when they can see it. The test is repeated from several angles for each eye (Figure 2.3). The physiological blind spot may be detected in the temporal portion of the visual field.

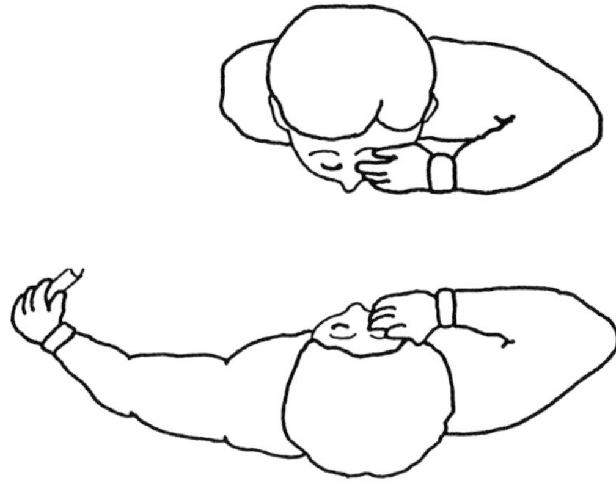

Figure 2.3 Testing visual fields by confrontation

Points to note

- The pattern of field loss depends on the site of the lesion. For example, bitemporal hemianopia indicates a tumour, such as a pituitary adenoma, near the optic chiasm.
- Visual field loss may or may not have been evident to the patient as non-dominant lesions often result in inattention.
- In the unco-operative patient, the examiner may detect a field deficit when moving the finger towards the patient's eye in a menancing way fails to elicit a blink.
- Orbital tumours often present with diplopia, pain (either in or behind the eye), visual disturbance and proptosis (bulging of the orbit).

III Oculomotor, IV trochlear and VI abducens

The eyes are examined for size, shape and symmetry. The eyelid should normally cover approximately one-third of the iris, more than this being considered to be a ptosis. Normal pupils are round and equal in diameter.

Oculomotor testing

The direct pupillary response to light is examined by shining a bright pen-torch into one eye and observing constriction; if the other pupil also constricts at this time, the consensual reaction is also present. The speed of reaction is usually indicated on the neuro-assessment chart as + = brisk, sl = sluggish and fl = flicker. The normal diameter of a pupil is 2-6 mm, the average being 3.5 mm (Evans, 1988).

To test for accommodation (the ability to focus on an object at various distances), the patient is asked to focus on some distant point and then to look at the examiner's finger placed 12 inches in front of the patient. The change in focus should constrict the pupil. These tests evaluate oculomotor function.

Points to note

- Because of its anatomical position, the IIIrd cranial nerve is damaged during uncal (tentorial) herniation; hence pupil dilation is an important sign of raised intracranial pressure, but pupil dilation is not always due to raised intracranial pressure.
- Drugs may affect the pupil reaction; for example atropine dilates the pupil whereas pilocarpine and opiate analgesia constrict it. However, the pupil reaction is not affected by neuromuscular blockers such as vecuronium.
- Cataracts and certain lens implants may prevent constriction to light.
- A complete IIIrd nerve palsy will occur on the same side as the lesion/mass. The pupil will be fixed and dilated, the eye is deviated laterally and downward, and the patient is unable to open his or her eyelids (ptosis). If the lesion is not complete, the symptoms may be less evident.
- In Horner's syndrome, the affected pupil is smaller than the other pupil and does not dilate in response to decreased light. Ptosis is present on the affected side but is not as evident as in a IIIrd nerve palsy. Sweating may be absent on the affected side of the face (anhydrosis). Horner's syndrome may be a symptom of various tumours.
- Because of its anatomical relationship with the oculomotor nerve, a posterior communicating artery aneurysm, even without rupture, may be the cause of a IIIrd nerve palsy.

As eye movement is regulated by the oculomotor, trochlear and abducens nerves, these are tested together. The patient is asked to look up, then down, then to each side and then diagonally (Figure 2.4).

Conjugate movement is the ability of the eyes to move together. At the same time, the nurse should observe for nystagmus (rapid involuntary movement of the eyes).

Points to note

- A lesion affecting the IVth cranial nerve causes double vision (diplopia) when the patient looks down and away from the side of the lesion. This is not always evident to the patient but is often evident when descending stairs or reading.
- Lesions of the VIth cranial nerve can result from brain stem disorders or from more peripheral lesions as the VIth cranial

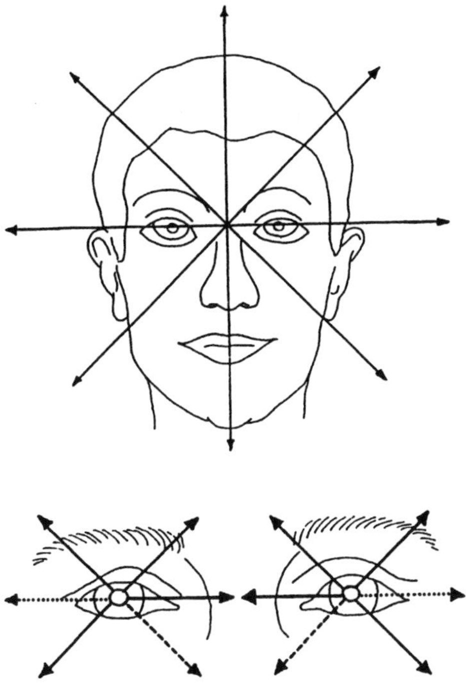

Figure 2.4 Assessing eye movement. Key: CN VI ······· CN III —— CN IV - - -

nerve has a long intracranial path.

- Tumours of the midbrain, petrous temporal, cavernous sinus and superior orbital fissure may exhibit VIth nerve signs.

V Trigeminal nerve

There are three divisions of the trigeminal nerve: the ophthalmic (V_1), maxillary (V_2) and mandibular (V_3). These branches have sensory and motor components.

Sensation is tested with patients' eyes closed. A wisp of cotton-wool is used to touch the forehead, cheeks and chin, and patients are asked to indicate when they feel the touch.

In unconscious patients, the cornea itself is lightly touched with cotton-wool; the normal response should be bilateral blinking and lacrimation.

Point to note

- Absence of the corneal reflex may result in corneal damage if eye care is not performed vigilantly.

Testing of sensation may also include perception of gentle pinpricks across the face or of the sensation of temperature.

Motor examination includes observation of any temporal muscle wasting. The patient is then asked to close the mouth tightly while the examiner attempts to open it by pulling the chin. Any deficits in function will make the jaw deviate to the weak side.

Points to note

- The trigeminal ganglion lies in the cerebropontine angle and may be compressed by tumours in this area.
- Trigeminal neuralgia (tic douloureux) or recurrent attacks of burning pain on one side of the face can be seen with tumour, infarction or multiple sclerosis but is most commonly due to compression of the nerve by a blood vessel.
- Tumours of the petrous temporal bone can cause Vth and VIth cranial nerve lesions (Gradenigro's syndrome).

VII Facial nerve

VIIth cranial nerve lesions cause facial weakness with a variable weakness of eye closure. The face is observed for symmetry at rest, and the patient is then asked to smile, showing the teeth, to wrinkle the forehead and to try to close the eyes while the examiner tries to open them.

Points to note

- Impaired eye closure again merits vigilant eye care, eye patch, taping or tarsorrhaphy being an option.
- Facial weakness may have a marked psychological effect as watering of the eye is common in severe upper facial weakness. Lower facial weakness is often accompanied by 'drooling'. Such problems, combined with a reduced ability to provide facial expressions that actually reflect the person's mood, cause much anxiety to patients.
- Taste is not routinely assessed but can be tested by placing sugar on the sides of the tongue and asking the patient to identify the taste. Alteration in taste rarely occurs on its own. Mealtimes are a particular problem, especially if taste and salivation are also impaired.
- Bell's palsy is an acute inflammation of the facial nerve that causes paralysis either unilaterally or, rarely, bilaterally. The precise aetiology is unknown, but it may be associated with viral infections. It is treated by high-dose steroids, 80% of patients tending to recover in 4-8 weeks (Lindsay et al, 1991).

VIII Auditory (or acoustic vestibular) nerve

The VIIIth cranial nerve is composed of two divisions: the vestibular and the cochlear. The vestibular branch helps to orientate the body in terms of its sense of balance and position in space. Sensory information is relayed from many parts of the body, including the labyrinths in the ears, to the cerebellum. The cochlear branch allows nervous conduction of sound to the auditory centre, that is, it is responsible for hearing.

Vestibular division

To check the function of the vestibular portion of the VIIIth cranial nerve, co-operative patients are asked whether they have experienced any dizziness, vertigo or loss of balance. In the unconscious patient, the oculovestibular reflex can be assessed by caloric testing. Both ear canals are inspected to ensure that the tympanic membranes are intact and are not occluded by wax, and the head is elevated to 30° to bring the semicircular canals into appropriate alignment. Then 30 ml of iced water is injected into each external auditory canal (at least 5 minutes apart). In a patient with intact function, the response would initially be slow nystagmus and eye movement towards the stimulated side quickly followed by rapid nystagmus and movement to the opposite side. If there is no movement noted, this brain stem reflex is absent.

Oculocephalic reflex (doll's eyes)

In deeply comatose patients, the oculocephalic reflex is used to assess the connection between the vestibular apparatus and the relay pathways to the cranial nerves controlling eye movement. In alert patients, this reflex is inhibited. Before performing the test, it must be determined that the patient has no cervical injury. Whilst keeping both of the patient's eyes open, the examiner turns the head briskly to one side and then the other. In an alert patient, the eyes point in the direction in which the head is turned; in the comatose patient with intact reflexes, the eyes will appear to look in the direction opposite to that in which the head has been turned. In the patient with absent brain stem reflexes, the eyes appear to remain stationary in the centre.

Cochlear division

Examination of the cochlear portion in the conscious patient is achieved by the assessment of hearing. This can be tested in a rudimentary way by whispering into each ear and asking the patient to repeat what has been heard.

Nerve conduction deafness causes a loss of high tone, whilst middle ear disease results in a loss of low tones. Detailed information about pitch and tone perception requires formal audiometry testing. Useful information can, however, be gained at the bedside by assessing perception of a vibrating tuning fork using Weber's and Rinne's tests. Hearing loss as a result of tumours such as acoustic neuromas occurs gradually over time, and these tests only need to be carried out on admission.

Weber's test assesses bone conduction of sound. The tuning fork is placed on the forehead in the midline and should be heard equally on each side. If the sound is louder in the affected ear, there is conductive (middle ear) deafness; if the sound is louder in the normal ear, there is nerve deafness as there is no transmission of sound impulses to the auditory cortex.

Rinne's test compares air and bone conduction. The base of a vibrating tuning fork is held against the mastoid bone. When the patient is no longer able to hear the sound, the fork is moved near the external meatus and the sound should once again be heard as air conduction via the ossicles should be better than bone conduction. In conductive deafness, bone conduction is better than air conduction and the sound will not reappear when the tuning fork is placed by the external meatus. In nerve deafness, the conduction of sound is impaired equally at the mastoid or the external meatus.

IX Glossopharyngeal and X vagus nerves

The glossopharyngeal and vagus nerves are usually tested together as their functions overlap. Muscle innervation of the palate is from the vagus, whilst sensation is supplied by the glossopharyngeal.

The vagus nerve can be assessed by listening to the patient's speech. A hoarse or nasal voice might indicate vocal cord paralysis. Glossopharyngeal function is assessed by asking patients to open their mouth, the tongue being depressed using a spatula, and then asked to say 'Ahh'. The uvula should elevate but not deviate to either side. Dilorio and Price (1990) do not advocate testing the gag reflex if there is an impaired swallowing or cough reflex as it provides little useful information on its own and there is a risk of aspiration.

The cough reflex is under voluntary and involuntary control, and both should be tested. Voluntary cough is assessed by asking the patient to cough twice; involuntary coughing may be elicited by gently rubbing the laryngeal protuberance.

To assess the swallowing reflex, patients are asked to swallow their saliva while the examiner assesses laryngeal elevation by placing thumb and index finger on the laryngeal protuberance. An intact swallow and cough are the most important aspects in determining whether a patient should receive oral food or fluids. If there is any doubt or evidence of dysfunction, the advice of the speech and language therapist should be sought to formally review the patient; assessment might include radiological studies such as videofluoroscopy.

Asking the patient to repeat sentences before and after swallowing 5 ml water may indicate silent aspiration if a difference in speech fluency occurs (DiIorio and Price, 1990).

The gag reflex is then assessed (with the patient sitting upright) by touching the back of the throat with a cotton-tipped applicator. This should contract the pharyngeal muscles, causing the patient to gag.

Points to note

- Isolated IXth cranial nerve tumours are virtually unknown. Glomus jugulare tumours tend to affect IXth, Xth and XIth cranial nerve function.
- Bulbar palsy refers to bilateral weakness of the muscles supplied by the IXth, Xth and XIIth cranial nerves, but some difficulty in swallowing (dysphagia) may occur when any of the motor components of cranial nerves V, VII, IX, XI and XII are affected.

An intact gag reflex only protects the patient from aspirating large boluses of food material into the respiratory system. In patients in coma (a GCS of less than 8), there is often flaccid paralysis of the pharynx, and such patients are best nursed in modified recovery positions rather than on their backs.

XI Spinal accessory nerve

To test the nerve supplying the trapezius muscle, the nurse places his or her hands on the patients' shoulders and asks them to try to raise their shoulders while observing for any localised weakness. To assess the nerve supply to the sternomastoid muscle, patients are asked to turn their heads while the nurse attempts to resist the movement by placing his or her hand against the patient's cheek; this should be repeated with the other cheek and any asymmetry of strength noted.

XII Hypoglossal nerve

The patient's tongue is examined for fasciculation (flickering motion). On sticking out the tongue, any deviation will be towards the affected side. Atrophy may also be present on the affected side of the tongue. Patients are then asked to move their tongues from one side of mouth to the other as quickly as possible; if spasticity is present, movement is either impossible or sluggish. The patient's speech may also be affected (dysarthria).

Brain stem function and brain stem death

Disorders of cranial nerves can result from a variety of neurological disorders such as head injury, subarachnoid haemorrhage, cerebrovascular incidents, tumours or infection. Cranial nerve assessment is an important part of evaluating brain stem function and forms the basis for determining brain stem death, providing the following preconditions have been met:

1. There is no doubt that the patient's condition is a result of irremediable structural brain damage.
2. At least 6 hours has passed from the onset of coma, or if the coma is due to cardiac arrest, 24 hours has elapsed from the onset of cardiac arrest.
3. The patient is maintained on a ventilator (and muscle relaxants and other relevant drugs have been excluded as a cause of respiratory inadequacy or failure).
4. All reversible causes of brain stem depression have been excluded:
   - No depressant drugs (especially those used to paralyse and sedate) are still present in the patient's system.
   - There is no hypothermia (i.e. the core temperature must be over 35°C).
   - There is no metabolic or endocrine disturbance (i.e. urea, electrolyte and glucose levels are in the normal range).

     (NB from March 1998, potentially reversible circulatory, metabolic and endocrine disturbances must have been excluded as the cause of the continuation of unconciousness. It is recognised that circulatory, metabolic and endocrine disturbances are a likely accompaniment of brain stem death (e.g. hypernatraemia, diabetes insipidus) but these are the effect rather than the cause of that condition and do not preclude the diagnosis of brain stem death.) Point 2.2.3 'Code of Practice for the Diagnosis of Brain Stem Death'.
5. There is no evidence of any brain stem function:
   - fixed dilated pupils with no response to light;
   - no corneal reflex to stimulation;
   - no oculocephalic reflex;

- no vestibulo-ocular reflex on caloric testing;
- no gag or cough reflex on bronchial stimulation by suction catheter;
- no motor response in response to *central* painful stimulus (pressure on the periorbital ridge), although other stimuli may provoke spinal reflexes that can persist in brain stem dead patients ;
- no respiratory effort when the patient is disconnected from the ventilator (apnoea test) (oxygen being given during disconnection via a suction catheter and endotracheal tube). The $PaCO_2$ should be within normal limits at the beginning of the test, that is, above 6 kPa or 45 mmHg, and should be allowed to rise to a level sufficient to stimulate respiration (that is, to a level of 6.66 kPa or 50 mmHg).
- The tests should be conducted by two experienced doctors, and the guidelines suggest that testing is repeated. Brain stem testing is mandatory prior to organ donation, and doctors involved in the transplant teams are precluded from being involved in determining brain stem death. There is no recommendation as to when testing should be repeated, but a minimum of 30 minutes between bouts of testing has been suggested.

It should be noted that the time of death is legally the time of completion of the second set of negative tests rather than the time at which ventilation is discontinued.

Organ donation

It should be remembered that patients with primary brain tumours may still donate their organs and that this may be a comfort to relatives. If there is any doubt or question about a patient's suitability to donate organs, the local transplant co-ordinators are always approachable via an aircall for any queries that staff or relatives may have. For a full description of brain stem testing and donation guidelines the reader is directed to the March 1998 'Code of Practice for the Diagnosis of Brain Stem Death including guidelines for the identification of potential organ and tissue donors' published by the Department of Health.

Cerebellar function

Examination of cerebellar function evaluates balance and co-ordination, which are both vital aspects of the smooth execution of voluntary movement. Unco-ordination of voluntary muscle actions, especially in walking and reaching, is known as ataxia and is a prominent feature of cerebellar disease.

The upper limbs are assessed for ataxia by asking patients to repeatedly reach out with their forefinger and alternately touch the examiner's forefinger, then their own nose, as quickly as possible. Rapid alternating movements are also observed, for example rapid pronation and supination of each hand, or tapping the thigh with the hand of the same side, as quickly as possible. Fine finger co-ordination is assessed by the patient rapidly tapping each finger of one hand in turn with the thumb of the same hand.

The balance and co-ordination of the lower limbs are assessed by observing the patient's walking, noting any unsteadiness, shuffling, dragging of either leg or swerving on turning corners. Further evaluation involves the Romberg test. Patients are asked to stand with their feet together, their arms by their sides and their eyes open. After 30 seconds, they are asked to close their eyes for another 30 seconds. The examiner should stay in close proximity to patients in case they lose their balance. Loss of balance only occurring when the eyes are closed indicates a positive Romberg test and denotes cerebellar dysfunction or disease. If unsteadiness is noted when patients have their eyes open, they should not be asked to close them (Lindsay et al, 1991). If the patient is unable to stand, an alternative to the Romberg test is to ask him or her to run the heel of one leg down the shin of the other, observing the ability to keep the heel on the shin.

Importance of motor and sensory assessment

Nurses working in the field of oncology must be alert to deterioration in motor or sensory function as many tumours, in particular those of breast and prostate, spread to the thoracic and lumbar vertebrae respectively. Prompt surgical intervention for cord compression can mean the difference between complete paralysis with associated bladder and bowel dysfunction and the maintenance of an independent lifestyle.

If a cranial malignancy is under investigation, the aim of the motor function examination is to assess for any localising signs of a lesion or its effects on surrounding cerebral tissue. Where a spinal pathology is involved, such as with cord compression from a spinal metastasis, the motor function assessment can be more detailed to locate the level of the lesion and the extent of the effects on function below that level.

Motor function

Motor function evaluation is assessment of voluntary muscle. Initial gross examination involves looking at muscle size, symmetry of the sides and position of the limbs at rest. A difference between the two sides may indicate a central nervous system deficit. Size differences resulting from atrophy and abnormal positioning of the limbs may indicate the presence of a hemiplegia. Any involuntary movements, tremors or fasciculation are noted, and strength and tone are then assessed (Hickey, 1992).

Tone is evaluated in both the conscious and unconscious patient by performing a passive range of movement exercises on all the limbs and noting any resistance to the movements. Abnormal tone can be described as spastic or rigid, or as showing hypertonicity, which usually occurs with upper motor neurone lesions, and as flaccid or showing hypotonicity for lower motor neurone lesions (Stevens and Becker, 1988; Lindsay et al, 1991).

Assessment of strength is carried out in the upper limbs and then the neck, trunk and lower limbs, at all times noting the symmetry of both sides. A test for upper limb weakness is that of pronator drift. This is assessed by asking patients to hold their arms straight out in front of them with the palms facing upwards. They are then asked to close their eyes while keeping their arms out in front. If an arm starts to drift downwards and/or the palm turns downwards, this indicates a hemiplegia on that side. The eyes must be closed for the test to avoid the use of visual cues to compensate for any weakness. This test can be performed sitting as well as lying in bed (Hickey, 1992; Lower, 1992).

In a full assessment of motor function in the conscious patient, movements are graded using the Medical Research Council (MRC)

Table 2.3 Scoring of motor power

Grade	Description
0	No evidence of muscle contraction (complete paralysis)
1	Flicker/trace of contraction only but no joint movement
2	Active joint movement with gravity eliminated (for patients lying on their backs in bed, for example, any movement of their arm across their body in a horizontal plane is occurring with gravity eliminated)
3	Joint movement against gravity only (in the above example, movement of the arm vertically is against gravity)
4	Joint movement against gravity and against some resistance
5	Normal power against gravity and full resistance

Adapted MRC grading scale (Marr and Reid, 1988).

Table 2.4 Tests performed at each spinal level

Spinal level	Test performed
C2–4	Shoulder shrug
C5	Shoulder abduction
C6	Elbow flexion
C7	Elbow extension
C5–7	Wrist extension
C8–T1	Finger abduction
L1–3	Hip flexion
L2–4	Knee extension
L4–5	Ankle dorsiflexion
S1–2	Ankle plantar flexion

Note: There are eight paired cervical nerve roots but only seven cervical vertebrae.

grading scale (Kendall, 1916) or an adapted version (Marr and Reid, 1988). Scores for each muscle group tested are recorded out of 5 (Table 2.3).

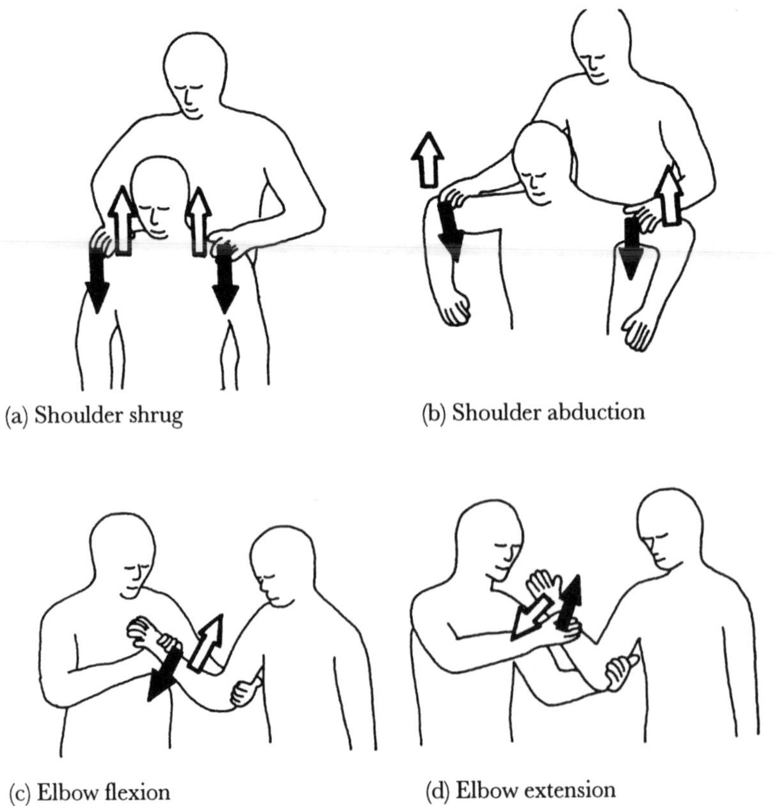

Figure 2.5 Performing assessments of motor function.

➡ Resistance by examiner ⇨ Movement by patient

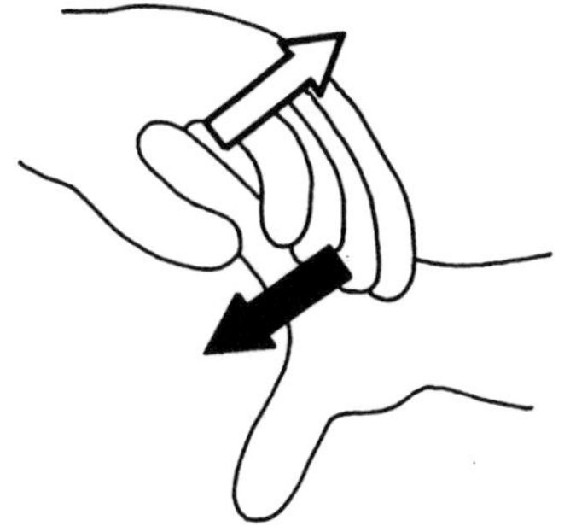

(e) Wrist extension

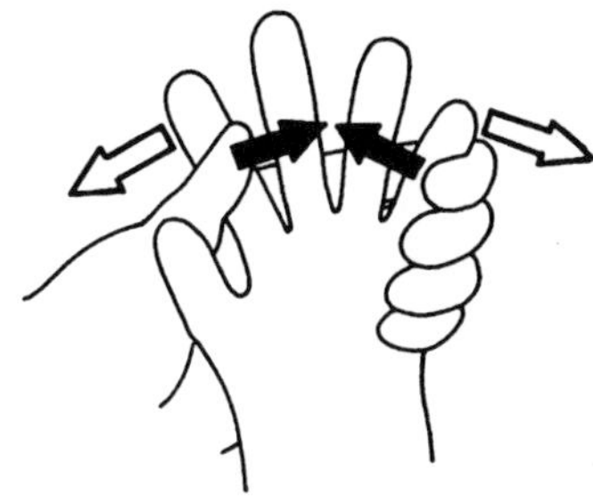

(f) Finger abduction

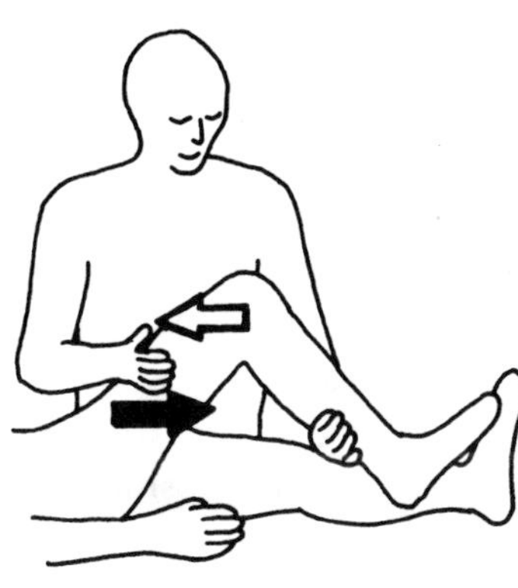

(g) Hip flexion

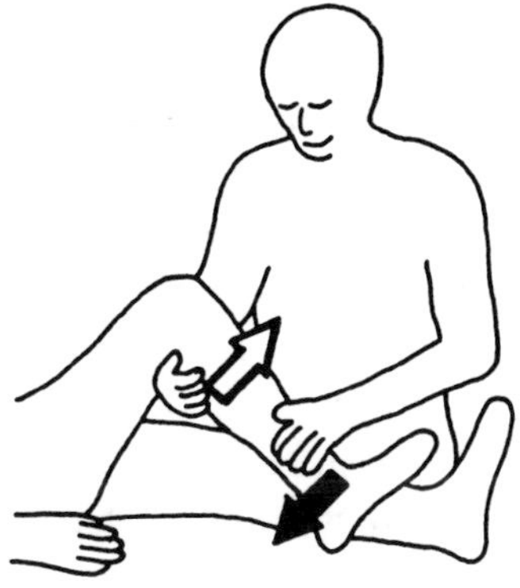

(h) Knee extension

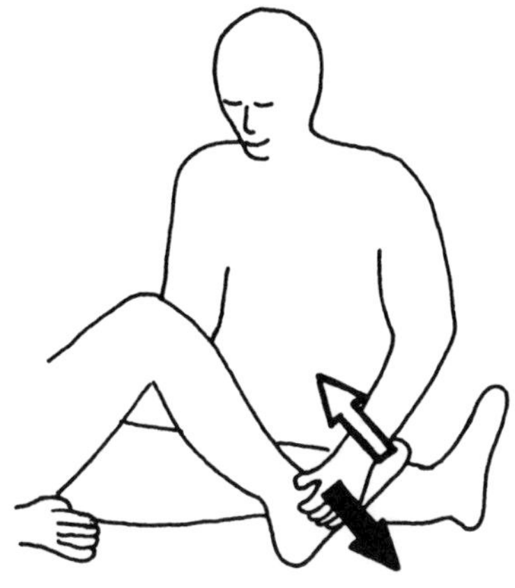

(i) Ankle dorsiflexion

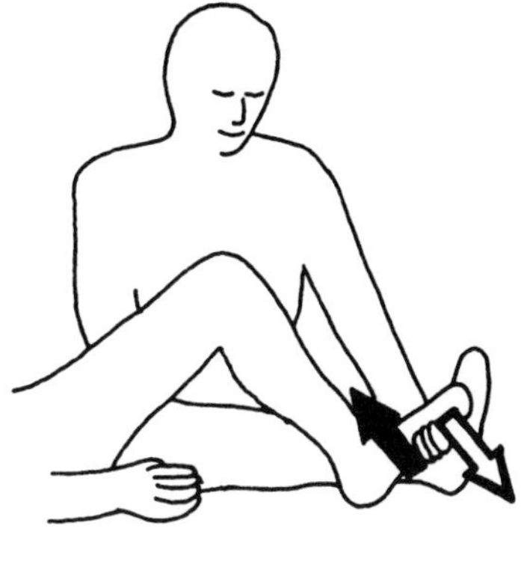

(j) Ankle plantar flexion

Figure 2.5 cont.

Table 2.4 shows the tests usually performed for each spinal nerve root level (Segatore and Villeneuve, 1988; Lindsay et al, 1991). Figure 2.5 illustrates how these are performed in practice.

Not all the muscle groups will always need to be tested, but if a deficit in a limb is detected, further investigation around that spinal level should be carried out to evaluate the extent of the problem.

In the unconscious patient, the assessment must be adapted as the patient cannot co-operate with the testing of all the muscle groups (Lindsay et al, 1991; Hickey, 1992). Any spontaneous limb movements are observed, and when a limb remains immobile to central noxious stimuli, a peripheral stimulus is used to elicit a response, using a pen or pencil to apply pressure to the side of a finger (the nail bed is not used as it can be damaged) near the cuticle or on the side of a digit. Withdrawal of the limb indicates that the motor system is intact. To test for paralysis or plegia, the patient is laid on their back if possible. To assess the upper limbs, lift and hold both of the patient's arms perpendicular to the bed. On releasing the arms simultaneously, the weaker or paralysed limb will fall more quickly and may fall at an awkward angle. To assess the lower limbs, flex the patient's knees and hold them so that the feet are flat on the bed. The weaker leg will fall more quickly, and the paralysed limb will rapidly fall in an extended position. The normal leg will hold its position briefly before gradually falling to assume a natural position (Hickey, 1992).

To assess for localising signs with intracranial pathology, it is necessary to assess general motor function. After an initial assessment of motor function, which may cover all muscle groups using

Table 2.5 General assessment of limb power

Normal power	Patient able to match resistance applied by observer to any joint movement
Mildly weak	Patient able to move against resistance but is easily overcome
Severely weak	Patient able to move limb but not against resistance
Flexion Extension No response	All tested using peripheral pain if no spontaneous movement is detected nor any with the application of central pain

When these results are recorded, any difference in sides is noted by inserting right (R) or left (L) as appropriate on the chart. When applying resistance, the nurse should allow for differences in age and build.

the MRC adapted grading scale, repeated observations can show general power in individual limbs only. Table 2.5 shows how this can be performed and documented.

Assessing sensation

Sensation passes from the peripheral nerves to the spinal cord, or via the cranial nerves to the brain stem. There are many spinal tracts running along the length of the spinal cord (see Chapter 1), so different patterns of sensory loss will result depending on the tract involved.

Spinal tract assessment includes:

- light touch;
- pain (pinprick);
- temperature;
- position sense (proprioception);
- vibration.

Nurses can readily assess and monitor the patient's response to light touch and proprioception but may feel uncomfortable at attempting other assessments, such as sensation to pain; such information is, however, of value when planning patient care. For example, patients with impaired sensation can be advised to monitor the condition of their skin and report any concerns to nursing or medical staff, as well as to avoid exposure to hot water bottles or portable heaters.

Sensation to pain is usually assessed with the patient's eyes closed to avoid visual clues. Patients are asked to say when and how they perceive the painful stimulus: is it normal (sharp), heightened (very painful), reduced (dull) or absent? The nurse should be aware of the patient's baseline sensory assessment and should base the subsequent examination around this by commencing testing at the level of 'normal' sensation. Nurses may prefer to assess the response to light touch for repeated bedside assessments, but any deterioration should be re-evaluated by assessment of the response to pinpricks. The dermatome map (see Figure 1.8) indicates nerve root distribution.

Point to note

- Initial sensory levels may improve with steroid therapy or deteriorate with oedema or a reduced blood supply. Deterioration must be reported promptly to the medical staff.

Proprioception

Proprioception/joint position sense is again tested with the patient's eyes closed. The examiner first of all demonstrates moving the patient's big toe (for lower limbs) or thumb (for upper limbs) up and then down. Movements are then repeated randomly and the patient is asked to identify the digit position. If proprioception is impaired, patients may be able to detect the movement but not the direction. In extreme cases, the whole limb can be affected, causing problems with mobilising, washing, eating and other daily activities.

Reflexes

Reflexes can be divided into stretch (deep tendon), cutaneous (superficial) and pathological reflexes (Hickey, 1992). Reflexes are documented in the following way:

Absent	0
Decreased	+ (obtainable with reinforcement)
Normal	++
Increased	+++
Hyperactive	++++ (clonus)

Deep tendon reflexes of the upper and lower limbs are assessed using a tendon hammer. If the spinal cord is damaged across its entire diameter, such reflexes will initially be absent below the level of damage during the period of spinal shock.

Cutaneous reflexes are those elicited by a stimulus in a related muscle group by a noxious stimulus, for example flexion in response to nail bed pressure, or the corneal or gag reflex.

Points to note

- In patients with urinary retention, it is important to assess the perianal reflex as an indicator of impaired sensation prior to catheterisation, particularly if the patient is not aware of any discomfort accompanying the urinary retention. Anal contraction should occur in response to light pinpricks in that region.

Pathological reflexes are those which only exist in the presence of neurological disease, for example the Babinski response (see below).

Plantar reflex

When the sole of the foot is stroked with a key or the pointed end of a tendon hammer, the big toe should flex (except in babies under 1 year of age, in whom extension is normal). If the big toe extends (upgoing plantar), this is termed a positive Babinski response and indicates a disturbance of the pyramidal tract (an upper motor neurone lesion.)

Vital signs

The control centres for the vital signs are located in the brain stem. Normal brain stem function can be affected by pressure from cerebral lesions, herniation, tumours and damage to the brain stem itself. Changes in vital signs can be caused by increased intracranial pressure in the absence of injury elsewhere in the body. The relationship between changes in vital signs and changing neurological function is based on the principle that the brain requires a constant supply of blood to maintain cerebral perfusion for cell oxygenation. When CSF pressure within the brain equals arterial pressure, the arteries are compressed and the blood supply to the brain is compromised. The central response to this is to increase the arterial blood pressure above the CSF pressure in an attempt to maintain cerebral perfusion. This is known as the Cushing's response and displays the clinical signs of increased systolic blood pressure, widening pulse pressure and bradycardia. It is recognised now that this cardiovascular response is a late finding in increased intracranial pressure, and changes in conscious level are more important indicators if intervention is to be instigated with the hope of partially reversing the situation (Hickey, 1992; Stewart, 1996).

The assessment of unconscious patients requires adaptation of the neurological examination. In such patients, the assessment of respiration and the patency of the patient's airway should also be included as these may be affected by the level of consciousness.

Conclusion

Nurses are usually the most consistent members of the multidisciplinary team for the patient and are therefore in a unique position to detect changes in neurological status and to ensure that appropriate intervention is undertaken at the earliest possible moment. Nurses do not have to rely solely on formal neurological testing: much information regarding neurological deficits can be obtained by observation during the patient's admission and routine care, such as when washing, dressing, eating and generally mobilising (Beveridge, 1995). Neurological assessment can be abbreviated for repeated use to give a quick overview of the patient's condition, one sufficient to detect important changes (Hickey, 1992).

In order to maximise inter-rater reliability, the neurological assessment must be conveyed to other members of the health care team through clear, consistent and concise documentation so that any deterioration is detected at the earliest possible moment.

Glossary

Abduction Movement of a limb or part of the body away from the body's midline.

Accommodation The adjustment of the eye to allow images of objects at various distances to be focused on the retina, a process observable as contraction of the pupil as attention is focused on near objects.

Anosmia Absence of the sense of smell.

Aphasia/dysphasia Disorders of the generation of speech. The prefix 'a' denotes absence, in this respect the absence of speech. 'Dys' denotes difficulty or impairment, in this case difficulty in generating speech, or the impaired production of speech.

Apraxia An inability accurately to perform skilled movements.

Ataxia Shaking movements and unsteady gait resulting from the brain's failure to regulate the body's posture and direction of limb movements.

Babinski response Extension of the great toe on superficial stimulation of the lateral aspect of the sole of the foot. It indicates an upper motor neurone lesion.

Consciousness A general awareness of oneself and the surrounding environment.

Cord compression The spinal cord is subjected to pressure, for example from a tumour or a herniated disc.

Diplopia Double vision.

Doll's eyes phenomenon Maintenance of a fixed forward gaze of the eyes in an unconcious patient when the head is gently rotated from side to side. Loss of this effect indicates a loss of inhibition from higher centres.

Dorsiflexion Backwards deflection (towards the upper surface) of the foot, hand or their digits.

Dysarthria Difficulty in pronouncing words because of a defect in articulation.

Dysphagia Difficulty in swallowing.

Extension The act of stretching muscles by which a limb or part of the body is straightened.

Fasciculation Brief, spontaneous contractions of a few muscle fibres, seen as a flicker of movement under the skin. It is most often associated with diseases of the motor neurones of the spinal cord.

Flexion Bending of a joint so that the bones forming that joint are brought towards each other.

Horner's syndrome Partial ptosis of the upper lid, a small pupil and anhydrosis (lack of sweating) affecting the face and neck. Results from paralysis of the cervical sympathetic nerves to the eye and face.

Hypertonia Non-voluntary increased resistance of the skeletal muscle to passive stretching.This may be rigid, indicating basal ganglion disease, or spastic indicating upper motor neurone disease.

Ipsilateral On the same side.

Kpa Kilopascals, a (metric) measure of pressure.

Lower motor neurone The anterior horn cell and cranial nerve motor cells and their axons.

mmHg Millimetres of mercury, an (Imperial) measure of pressure.

Nystagmus Repetitive rhythmical oscillation of the eyes.

$Paco_2$ Partial pressure of carbon dioxide.

Papilloedema Swelling of the optic disc.

Parosmia Alteration in the sense of smell.

Plantar flexion Movement downwards of the toes toward the sole of the foot. (Plantar refers to the sole of the foot.)

Prone/pronation Prone means lying face down. With respect to the hand, with the palm facing downwards. Pronation is, in this case, the act of turning the hand so that the palm faces downwards.

Proprioception Awareness of joint position in relation to gravity/space.

Ptosis Drooping of the eyelid.

Reflex An automatic/involuntary response to a stimulus brought about by nervous tissue circuits without consciousness necessarily being involved.

Supine/supination Supine means lying on the back with the face upwards. With respect to the hand, having the palm facing upwards. Supination is the act of, for example, turning the hand so that the palm faces upwards.

Tarsorraphy Closure of the eyelids using a suture.

Upper motor neurone Term used to describe cells of the pathway from the cerebral cortex to the lower motor neurones of the cranial nerve nuclei and anterior horn cells, including those fibres which pass directly and those which synapse on route, for example corticovestibulospinal.

Vertigo A hallucination of movement, that is, the perception of movement in the absence of any movement. This may be of the patient or the environment, and be rotatory or non-rotatory.

References

Ackerman L (1993) Alteration in level of responsiveness. A proposed nursing diagnosis. Nursing Clinics of North America 28(4): 729–45.

Barker E, Moore K (1992) Perfecting the art. Neurologic assessment. RN April: 28–35.

Bates B (1987) A Guide to Physical Examination, 4th edn. Philadelphia: JB Lippincott.

Beveridge D (1995) Back to basics. Axon 17(1): 6–8.

Butler S (1993) Functional neuroanatomy. In Morgan G, Butler S (Eds) Seminars in Basic Neurosciences. Glasgow: Royal College of Psychiatrists/Bain & Bell.

Dilorio C, Price ME (1990) Swallowing: an assessment guide. American Journal of Nursing 90: 38–41.

Ellis A, Cavanagh S (1992) Aspects of neurosurgical assessment using the Glasgow Coma Scale. Intensive and Critical Care Nursing 8: 94–9.

Evans MJ (1988) Neurologic–Neurosurgical Nursing. USA: Springhouse Clinical Rotation Guide.

Fuller G (1993) Neurological Examination Made Easy. Edinburgh: Churchill Livingstone.

Guyton AC (1992) Basic Neuroscience: Anatomy and Physiology, 2nd edn. Philadelphia: WB Saunders.

Hickey J (1992) The Clinical Practice of Neurological and Neurosurgical Nursing, 2nd Edn. Philadelphia: JB Lippincott.

Hilton G (1991) Review of neurobehavioural assessment tools. Heart and Lung 20: 436–42.

Jennett B, Teasdale G (1974) Assessment of coma and impaired consciousness. Lancet 2: 81–4.

Jennett B, Teasdale G, Murray G, Parker L (1979) Adding up the Glasgow Coma Scale. Acta Neuochirurgica 28: 13–16.

Kendall D (1916) Aids to the investigation of peripheral nerve injuries. Journal of the American Medical Association 66: 729–33.

Lindsay K, Bone I, Callander R (1991) Neurology and Neurosurgery Illustrated, 2nd edn. Edinburgh: Churchill Livingstone.

Lower J (1992) Rapid neuro assessment. American Journal of Nursing June: 38–45.

Marr J, Reid B (1988) Spinal cord testing: auditing for quality assurance. Journal of Neuroscience Nursing 23(2): 101–6.

Mitchell P, Ozuna J, Cammermeyer M, Fugate Woods N (1984) Neurologic Assessment for Nursing Practice. Reston, Virginia: Reston Publishing Company.

Pressman E, Zeidman S, Summers L (1995) Primary care for women. Comprehensive assessment of the neurologic system. Journal of Nurse-Midwifery 40(2): 163–71.

Segatore M, Villeneuve M (1988) Spinal cord testing: development of a screening tool. Journal of Neuroscience Nursing 20(1): 30–3.

Shpritz D (1994) Neurological aspects of critical care. Emergency neurologic assessment. Critical Care Nurse 5(5): 66–8.

Stenger K (1993) Surveillance of spinal cord motor and sensory function. Nursing Clinics of North America 28(4): 783–92.
Stevens S, Becker K (1988) A simple, step-by-step approach to neurologic assessment parts 1 and 2. Nursing 18(9): 53–61; 18(10): 51–8.
Stewart N (1996) Neurological observations. Professional Nurse 11(6): 377–8.
Sullivan J (1990) Neurologic assessment. Nursing Clinics of North America 25(4): 795–809.

Further reading

Wilson-Pauwels L, Akesson E, Stewart P (1988) Cranial Nerves: Anatomy and Clinical Comments. Philadelphia: BC Decker.

Chapter 3 Pathological and clinical aspects of CNS tumours

Geoffrey Sharpe

Introduction

The clinical manifestations of tumours depend largely upon the pathological nature of the lesion and its position within the CNS. This chapter will outline the basic pathological and clinical aspects of CNS tumours and discuss these with respect to the more common tumour types.

Pathology of CNS tumours

Whilst the brain and spinal cord are a frequent site of metastatic disease, primary tumours arising within the CNS are uncommon, with an age-adjusted incidence of 6–12 per 100 000 population per year. They occur more frequently in adults than children, although in this latter group they comprise the most common non-haematological tumours. Childhood tumours arise most frequently in the posterior cranial fossa, whereas the cerebral hemispheres are the site of most adult tumours.

The aetiology of brain tumours remains largely unknown, although genetic predisposition (Table 3.1) or exposure to environmental factors such as radiation or chemical carcinogens may be implicated in a small proportion of cases. Primary CNS lymphoma is associated with immune deficiency states such as that following organ transplantation or with HIV infection.

Primary glial tumours of the CNS have been subject to various classification systems including those of Kernohan et al (1949) and Daumas-Duport et al (1988), which involve a four-tier grading system. More recently, tumours of the CNS have been classified

Table 3.1 Familial conditions associated with a higher risk of primary CNS tumours

Familial predisposition	Associated CNS tumour
Peripheral neurofibromatosis (von Recklinghausen's disease, NF-1)	Optic nerve glioma, astrocytoma
Central neurofibromatosis (NF-2)	Bilateral acoustic neuroma, meningioma
Tuberous sclerosis	Giant cell astrocytoma
von Hippel–Lindau syndrome	Haemangioblastoma
Gorlin's syndrome	Medulloblastoma
Turcot's syndrome (familial adenomatous polyposis and brain tumour)	Astrocytoma

according to the putative cell of origin, the stage of development and the grade of the tumour. This is the basis of the current World Health Organisation (WHO) classification (Kleihues et al, 1993), which is outlined in Table 3.2. The apparent complexity of this classification is due to the inclusion of many rare tumours and their variants.

Table 3.2 Pathological classification of CNS tumours

Neuroepithelial tumours of the CNS

1. Astrocytic tumours
   a. Astrocytoma (WHO grade II) – variants: protoplasmic, gemistocytic, fibrillary, mixed
   b. Anaplastic (malignant) astrocytoma (WHO grade III)
   c. Glioblastoma multiforme (WHO grade IV) – variants: giant cell glioblastoma, gliosarcoma
   d. Pilocytic astrocytoma (non-invasive, WHO grade I)
   e. Subependymal giant cell astrocytoma
   f. Pleomorphic xanthoastrocytoma
2. Oligodendroglial tumours
   a. Oligodendroglioma (WHO grade II)
   b. Anaplastic (malignant) oligodendroglioma (WHO grade III)
3. Ependymal cell tumours
   a. Ependymoma (WHO grade II)
   b. Anaplastic ependymoma (WHO grade III)
   c. Myxopapillary ependymoma
   d. Subependymoma
4. Mixed gliomas
   a. Mixed oligoastrocytomas (WHO grade II)
   b. Anaplastic (malignant) oligoastrocytoma (WHO grade III)
   c. Others

5. Neuroepithelial tumours of uncertain origin
    a Polar spongioblastoma
    b. Astroblastoma
    c. Gliomatosis cerebri
6. Tumours of the choroid plexus
    a. Choroid plexus papilloma
    b. Choroid plexus carcinoma
7. Neuronal and mixed neuronal-glial tumours
    a. Gangliocytoma
    b. Dysplastic gangliglioma of cerebellum
    c. Ganglioglioma
    d. Anaplastic (malignant) ganglioglioma
    e. Desmoplastic infantile ganglioglioma
    f. Central neurocytoma
    g. Dysembryoplastic neuroepithelial tumour
    h. Olfactory neuroblastoma
8. Pineal parenchymal tumours
    a. Pineocytoma
    b. Pineoblastoma
    c. Mixed pineocytoma/pineoblastoma
9. Embryonal tumours
    a. Medulloepithelioma
    b. Primitive neuroectodermal tumours with multipotent differentiation
        i. Medulloblastoma
        ii. Cerebral primitive neuroectodermal tumour
    c. Neuroblastoma
    d. Retinoblastoma
    e. Ependymoblastoma

Other CNS neoplasms

1. Tumours of the sellar region
    a. Pituitary adenoma
    b. Pituitary carcinoma
    c. Craniopharyngioma
2. Haemopoietic tumours
    a. Primary malignant lymphoma
    b. Plasmacytoma
    c. Granulocytic sarcoma
    d. Others
3. Germ cell tumours
    a. Germinoma
    b. Embryonal carcinoma
    c. Yolk sac tumour
    d. Choriocarcinoma
    e. Teratoma
    f. Mixed germ cell tumours
4. Tumours of the meninges
    a. Meningioma – variants: meningothelial, fibrous, transitional, psammomatous, angiomatous, microcystic, secretory, clear cell, chordoid, metaplastic

   - b. Atypical meningioma
   - c. Anaplastic (malignant) meningioma
5. Non-meningothelial tumours of the meninges
   - a. Benign mesenchymal
   - b. Malignant mesenchymal
   - c. Primary melanocytic lesions
   - d. Haemopoietic neoplasms
   - e. Tumours of uncertain histogenesis
6. Tumours of cranial and spinal nerves
   - a. Schwannoma
   - b. Neurofibroma
   - c. Malignant peripheral nerve sheath tumour (malignant schwannoma)
7. Local extensions from regional tumours
   - a. Paraganglioma
   - b. Chordoma
   - c. Chondroma
   - d. Chondrosarcoma
   - e. Carcinoma
8. Metastatic tumours
9. Unclassified tumours
10. Cysts and tumour-like lesions

The separation of primary CNS tumours into benign and malignant neoplasms is, however, not as clear as that with tumours arising elsewhere in the body. Even tumours that appear to be histologically 'benign' may be locally invasive or prove fatal purely because of their size or position. Conversely, the majority of high-grade 'malignant' tumours will not metastasise outside the CNS, although such spread may occasionally be observed with medulloblastoma, primary cerebral lymphoma or with germ cell tumours, which may disseminate via surgical shunting of the CSF.

Clinical manifestations of CNS tumours

The presenting symptoms and signs are due to a combination of focal or global neurological deficits, epilepsy or raised intracranial pressure.

Neurological deficits

The presence of focal neurological symptoms or signs is strong clinical evidence of a structural brain lesion and specific clinical syndromes are well recognised.

Cerebral hemisphere tumours

Frontal lobe tumours are often initially clinically silent, but as the tumour progresses, the features of impaired higher mental function, change in personality and epilepsy may develop. Urinary incontinence may indicate involvement of the corpus callosum. Deeper lesions may also be associated with expressive dysphasia if the dominant hemisphere is affected, contralateral hemiparesis or gait disturbances. On examination, abnormal grasp reflexes may be demonstrable.

Temporal lobe tumours are typically associated with hemiparesis, homonymous hemianopia (or upper quadrantinopia) and epilepsy. Tumours involving the dominant hemisphere may cause expressive or receptive dysphasia.

Parietal lobe lesions may be associated with hemiparesis, neglect of the contralateral side of the body and inattention, together with a homonymous hemianopia (or lower quadrantinopia). Involvement of the dominant hemisphere may affect both receptive and expressive language, whilst the non-dominant hemisphere may affect left/right discrimination and the interpretation of body image. Dyspraxia, that is, the inability to formulate and carry out complex co-ordinated sequences of movement, may also be observed.

Primary occipital tumours are uncommon but may present with homonymous hemianopia or visual misinterpretation.

Posterior cranial fossa tumours

Tumours of the cerebellar hemispheres give rise to ataxia of the ipsilateral limbs, and nystagmus is often present. Midline tumours cause trunkal ataxia. Hydrocephalus is common and may be associated with neck stiffness.

Tumours of the brain stem present with progressive but sometimes intermittent lower cranial nerve palsies and long tract signs. In younger children, behavioural disturbances are not uncommon, although hydrocephalus is rare.

Midline tumours

Non-functioning tumours of the pituitary gland may present either with visual symptoms from compression of the optic pathways (typically a bitemporal hemianopia), pituitary dysfunction or a combination of the two. More rarely, pituitary apoplexy as a result of infarction or haemorrhage can present acutely with impaired consciousness, acute visual disturbance and severe headache. Functioning pituitary adenomas present with specific endocrine disturbances rather than focal deficits.

Suprasellar tumours may present in a similar manner to non-functioning pituitary adenomas, together with symptoms of hypothalamic dysfunction or hydrocephalus.

Tumours of the optic chiasm or of the hypothalamus are seen most commonly in children or adolescents and may present with disturbances of growth and puberty as well as with visual failure. Hydrocephalus is not infrequently associated with these tumours.

Tumours of the posterior third ventricle or of the pineal region may present with Parinaud's syndrome (failure of upward gaze, ptosis and dilatation of the pupils) and hydrocephalus.

Tumours of the spinal cord

Primary tumours of the spinal cord are relatively uncommon the main symptoms being local pain at the level of the lesion and neurological dysfunction at and below that level. In adults, the spinal cord terminates as the conus medullaris at the level of the first and second lumbar vertebrae. Tumours arising above this level therefore lead to a spinal cord syndrome with both cord and nerve root damage, whereas those arising below this level will involve the lumbar and sacral nerve roots only and result in a cauda equina syndrome.

In spinal cord lesions, the clinical findings are of upper motor neurone type with typically upgoing plantar responses, hyperreflexia and increased tone. In contrast, cauda equina lesions present with local pain, loss of sphincter tone and function and perianal 'saddle' anaesthesia. Flaccid lower limb paralysis may soon follow. Lesions affecting the region of the conus medullaris have effects intermediate between these two syndromes.

Extradural spinal cord tumours lie outside the spinal theca and are frequently metastatic in origin. They present with local pain and predominantly motor impairment with sphincter disturbances. Intradural tumours may arise either in the subarachnoid space as extramedullary tumours such as neurofibromas or meningiomas, or as intrinsic intramedullary tumours such as gliomas. Intradural extramedullary tumours present with spinal nerve root compression, local pain and spinal cord compression. There may be a large extraspinal component. Intradural intramedullary tumours arise within the substance of the cord and may involve it diffusely over several segments. They may also be associated with the development of a syrynx. Laterally placed lesions may also lead to a

Brown–Séquard-type syndrome (ipsilateral flaccid paralysis and loss of proprioception/touch with contralateral loss of pain and temperature sensation).

Epilepsy

Epilepsy is a common feature of brain tumours as well as of other organic brain damage. 'Late-onset' epilepsy, that is, focal or generalised seizures occurring for the first time after the age of 25 years, is indicative of a structural lesion and requires further investigation. Epilepsy may be the first or only presenting symptom of a brain tumour.

An epileptic attack (also known as a fit or a seizure) is the clinical manifestation of an abnormal episodic discharge of neurones. A convulsion describes the tonic and/or clonic accompaniment of an attack, whilst an aura or warning is the manifestation of focal epileptic activity that occurs before an attack.Epilepsy may be classified upon the type of attack (Table 3.3).

Table 3.3 Classification of epilepsy

1. Partial seizures (i.e. seizures beginning locally)
   a. Simple partial seizures (no impairment of consciousness)
   b. Complex partial seizures (with impairment of consciousness)
      i. Progressing from simple partial seizure *or*
      ii. With impaired consciousness at onset
   c.Partial seizures which become secondarily generalised
2. Generalised seizures (i.e. bilateral and without local onset)
   a. Absence seizures
   b. Myoclonic seizures
   c. Clonic seizures
   d. Tonic seizures
   e. Tonic-clonic seizures
   f. Atonic seizures
3. Unclassified (i.e. inadequate or incomplete data)

Partial seizures always imply focal cerebral pathology and may give clues to the location of a lesion. Tumours arising in the motor strip area can give rise to the so-called 'Jacksonian march' in which the primary focus causes a specific localised convulsion that 'marches' to other areas as the seizure discharge spreads to contiguous areas of the motor cortex. Partial seizures arising within the temporal lobes can give rise to a variety of seizures with either olfactory or gustatory phenomena, feelings of *déjà vu* or complex automatic behaviour such as chewing and lip-licking.

Post-ictal manifestations include marked tiredness/sleepiness, confusion, headache and even a transient hemiparesis (Todd's paralysis).

Raised intracranial pressure

The classical clinical triad associated with raised intracranial pressure is headache, vomiting and papilloedema. The headache is typically described as frontal and 'behind the eyes' or occasionally occipital or localised to the area of the tumour. It is often worse in the morning, is exacerbated by coughing or stooping and may be associated with vomiting. Impending visual failure as a result of raised intracranial pressure may be heralded by transient visual obscurations.

Raised intracranial pressure may result directly from the space-occupying effect of the tumour and any surrounding oedema or may arise from the obstruction of the CSF pathways with consequent obstructive (non-communicating) hydrocephalus. Epilepsy may also result as a secondary effect of hydrocephalus.

Clinical and pathological aspects of the more common tumour types

For the more common tumour types, it is possible to distinguish several characteristic clinical patterns depending upon the natural history of the tumour together with its location.

Gliomas

Gliomas are neuroepithelial tumours and constitute the largest histological group of primary CNS tumours.

High-grade gliomas

Glioblastoma multiforme represents the most common and most malignant end of the glioma spectrum. It may arise *de novo* or from a pre-existing low-grade glioma. When there is histological evidence of astrocytic origins, it may correctly be referred to as a grade IV astrocytoma, or if purely undifferentiated as glioblastoma multiforme. The two terms are, however, often used interchangeably.

The peak incidence is in the late fifth and sixth decades, although it may be seen at any age including childhood, where the outlook may not be so poor as in later life. It typically presents as a large mass within the cerebral hemispheres with associated oedema. It spreads readily along white matter pathways and also by ependymal routes to give multiple intraventricular seedings. 'Multifocal' glioblastoma, in which there is no obvious connection between tumour masses, is also occasionally seen. Microscopically, the tumour cells are often of bizarre appearance with a wide variation in their size and shape. Evidence of their malignant behaviour is reflected in the marked mitoses, extensive necrosis and vascular endothelial hyperplasia. The endothelium itself may undergo neoplastic change resulting in the very aggressive gliosarcoma. The clinical history at presentation is short, often with only a few weeks' history of headaches and progressive neurological impairment. The anaplastic (grade III) astrocytoma does not show necrosis and vascular hyperplasia but remains a highly aggressive tumour.

The median prognosis of patients with high-grade gliomas is less than 1 year from diagnosis. Clinical studies have identified prognostic factors associated with better survival, including grade III rather than grade IV histology, age less than 60 years and a good performance status (Salcman, 1990). The length of the history, presentation with fits and the ability to debulk the tumour surgically may also be of some prognostic importance (Figure 3.1).

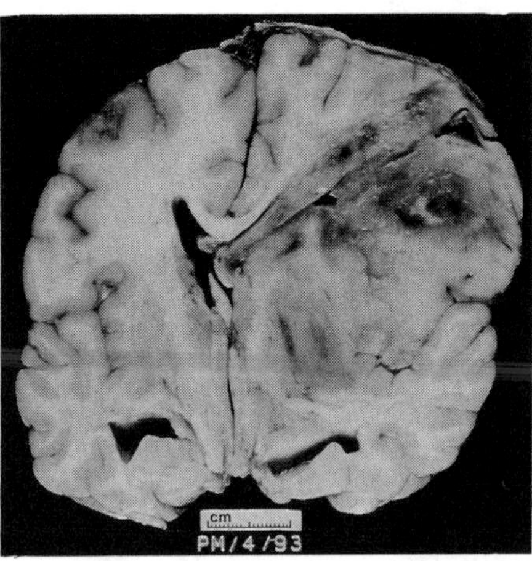

Figure 3.1 High grade glioma of left cerebral hemisphere showing necrosis and mass effect.

Low-grade gliomas

The low-grade gliomas (grades I and II) are a diverse group of tumours whose clinical behaviour is influenced by both the pathological subtype and their anatomical position.

Pilocytic ('hair-like') grade I astrocytomas are observed most commonly in children, with a peak incidence at around 10 years of age. They comprise the majority of the cystic cerebellar astrocytomas and are also found in association with the optic chiasm, brain stem and hypothalamus as well as in the cerebral hemispheres. Histologically, they appear relatively 'benign' with Rosenthal fibres (thick fibrils) and granular bodies implying a protracted gliotic process. These tumours do not readily infiltrate local brain and may be amenable to total resection, although in certain sites this is not possible and here the tumour behaviour may not always be so benign. Frank anaplastic change is uncommon.

The other low-grade gliomas, including the fibrillary, protoplasmic and gemistocytic types, are generally classified as Grade II tumours, although the gemistocytic variant seldom behaves benignly and commonly shows evidence of focal high-grade characteristics. Such tumours may be large at presentation and associated with little or no oedema.

Gliomas at special sites

Special mention should be made of optic nerve/chiasmatic gliomas and of brain stem gliomas as these tumours are often treated without histological verification.

The majority of optic gliomas involve the optic chiasm and present in young children with visual failure that may be accompanied by endocrine disturbances or symptoms of raised intracranial pressure. There is an association with neurofibromatosis type 1 (NF-1; see Table 3.1). The majority of such tumours are not amenable to surgery, and the need for biopsy, especially in children, is debated. The majority of such lesions are believed to be low-grade gliomas, although a spectrum of tumours ranging from simple hamartomas to high-grade lesions has been described. The need for treatment is often based upon the clinical behaviour of the lesion and also the age of the child.

Likewise, the diffuse gliomas involving the brain stem and pons may also be treated without histological confirmation as a biopsy may be inadvisable, the diagnosis being based upon the clinical and radiological findings. The data that are available suggest that the majority are astrocytic in nature and predominantly of low grade.

Oligodendroglioma

These represent only 6% of all gliomas and typically occur in the frontal lobes of adults in the fourth and fifth decades. They generally behave in an indolent fashion and often present with a short history of raised intracranial pressure superimposed on a background of epilepsy. They are thought to arise primarily from an oligodendrocytic rather than from an astrocytic lineage, although mixed tumours 'oligoastrocytomas' are not uncommon. Histologically, they are characterised by cells with large round nuclei surrounded by a 'halo' of clear cytoplasm, giving rise to the typical 'honeycomb' appearance. Calcification is a common finding and is often observed on a plain X-ray. They are generally regarded as low-grade (grade II) tumours, although high-grade anaplastic variants occur. Oligodendrogliomas can display a tendency to CSF seeding in up to 5% of cases.

Ependymoma

These tumours represent 5% of all intracranial gliomas but are the most common primary intraspinal tumour. They arise within the ependymal cells lining the ventricular system and central canal, and are most commonly observed in association with the fourth ventricle, although they can occasionally arise within the brain parenchymal tissue. Histologically, the tumour cells retain many of the epithelial features of normal ependymal cells and have a tendency towards CSF seeding. Several variants are described (see Table 3.2) with the ependymoblastoma now categorised along with the primitive neuroectodermal tumours.

Medulloblastoma

The primitive neuroectodermal tumours (PNETs) are a group of tumours that may arise throughout the CNS but most commonly occur within the posterior cranial fossa, where the tumour is usually referred to as a medulloblastoma. Histologically, they have a common appearance as dense cellular masses of uniform small oval or round cells. They have a tendency to disseminate early and extensively via the CSF pathways and occasionally metastasise outside the CNS to involve bone/bone marrow. The presence of metastases adversely affects the prognosis and surgical CSF shunting is generally avoided if possible because of a potential risk of systemic dissemination.

Medulloblastoma typically presents between the ages of 5 and 15 with signs of cerebellar infiltration and raised intracranial pressure. Although CT and MRI can usually suggest the nature of such lesions, histological confirmation is necessary and usually awaits definitive surgery. The outlook for children with a localised medulloblastoma who receive craniospinal axis radiotherapy is relatively good, with a 5 year disease-free survival of around 60%. The prognosis in patients who (i) are less than 3 years of age (who may present with more aggressive disease and who may not be able to receive full therapy because of the potentially severe late effects of radiation), (ii) have supratentorial PNETs, or (iii) have dissemination at presentation may be worse. The prognosis in adult patients is less clear but may be similar to that observed in children.

Pituitary tumours

Tumours of the anterior pituitary gland are usually slow-growing adenomas that are often described as 'microadenomas' when less than 1 cm in size and confined to the pituitary fossa, and as 'macroadenomas' when they exceed this size. 'Functional' tumours are often microadenomas and present with the clinical manifestations of the hypersecretion of hormones such as prolactin, growth hormone, adrenocorticotrophic hormone (ACTH) or more rarely gonadotrophins or thyroid stimulating hormone (TSH). 'Non-functional' adenomas are often larger and cause local mass effects resulting in headache, visual field defects and cranial nerve palsies if the cavernous sinus is compressed. They may also be accompanied by hormone deficiencies due to compression of the adjacent normal gland, although a moderate rise in serum prolactin may be seen if the pituitary stalk is compressed sufficiently to reduce the inhibitory control from the hypothalamus. Histologically, they have traditionally been classified according to the light microscope appearances of the tumour cells as eosinophilic, basophilic or chromophobe adenomas. Immunochemical staining techniques have led to a more practical classification based upon the hormone type secreted, for example prolactinoma. True pituitary carcinomas do occur but are rare.

Craniopharyngioma

Craniopharyngiomas are histologically benign tumours arising from epithelial rests in the suprasellar region associated with Rathke's pouch. They account for 3% of all intracranial tumours and are seen most commonly in late childhood or early adolescence. They are partly solid and partly cystic neoplasms that may compress and adhere to adjacent structures, including the optic nerves and chiasm, the hypothalamus, the pituitary gland and the third ventricle. Presenting features depend upon the structures affected and include endocrine or visual dysfunction, mental deterioration or hydrocephalus.

Primary cerebral lymphoma

Primary cerebral lymphoma is a non-Hodgkin's lymphoma localised to the CNS and is usually of a high grade B-cell type. It is seen with increased frequency in situations of immune deficiency such as that following organ transplantation or associated with HIV infection. It is also seen in a sporadic form in which the incidence increases with age.

The clinical manifestations of primary cerebral lymphoma are variable and are indistinguishable from those of other brain tumours. They typically present with a rapidly progressive syndrome and usually show a dramatic response both clinically and radiologically to corticosteroid therapy. The tumours may appear as single or multiple masses in periventricular areas and with evidence of subependymal spread. Surgery is normally limited to a biopsy. The lymphoma also has the capacity to disseminate widely within the CNS, and radiological examination of the spine, together with CSF cytology and ophthalmic assessment, are essential.

Radiotherapy often results in a rapid physical and radiological improvement but without any long-term survivors, the majority relapsing locally within 18 months. Intensive chemoradiotherapy may result in a long-term survival rate of up to 40% in those patients able to tolerate such therapy.

The prognosis for patients with HIV-related primary cerebral lymphoma depends upon the extent of the underlying disease, with poor radiation tolerance and compromised bone marrow reserves often making intensive therapy impossible or inappropriate.

Germ cell tumours

These relatively rare tumours arise most frequently in association with the pineal gland but may also be found in the suprasellar region. The majority are germinomas and are histologically indistinguishable from the more common testicular seminoma or ovarian dysgerminoma. Both benign and malignant forms of teratoma (or non-germinoma) are also occasionally encountered. Like their systemic counterparts, they may secrete alphafetoprotein (AFP) or the beta subunit of human chorionic gonadotrophin (β-HCG) which may be detectable in the CSF or in serum. The presence of AFP is specific for non-germinoma whilst the β-HCG level may be raised in either. The diagnosis may therefore be made on radiological and tumour marker assay, thus avoiding the need for biopsy. Surgical excision plays no useful role in germinoma as these tumours are exquisitely sensitive to radiation and chemotherapy, although it may be useful in the removal of differentiated teratoma following successful primary therapy.

These tumours may also seed throughout the CSF and may disseminate more widely via surgical shunts, which should be avoided if possible. The cure rate for small, localised germinomas approaches 100%, although the prognosis for patients with non-germinoma or with metastatic disease is less good.

Meningioma

Meningiomas constitute about 15% of all intracranial tumours, are found most commonly in the middle and older age groups, and may be more common in females. They arise from dural sites and are typically solitary lobulated masses, although large plaques or multiple tumours are well described. The vast majority are histologically benign and appear as sheets of polygonal cells with oval nuclei. Several histological subtypes are recognised (see Table 3.2) but may not be of any major prognostic significance. True malignant or anaplastic meningiomas are less common but are associated with a greater chance of recurrence, invasion of brain substance and tendency to metastasise.

Benign meningiomas do not usually directly invade brain parenchyma but instead exert their symptoms by local pressure effects, the clinical syndromes reflecting the position of the tumours. An osteoblastic change in adjacent bone, known as hyperostosis, may be seen.

Anterior cranial vault and parasagittal meningiomas may be associated with a long history of slow mental and personality changes prior to clinical presentation, with focal deficits, epilepsy or raised intracranial pressure. More posterior tumours affecting the middle third of the sagittal sinus or the frontotemporal region typically present early with focal epilepsy, whilst posterior hemispheric lesions are usually silent until they cause raised intracranial pressure or hemianopia.

Basal meningiomas include those of the olfactory groove, sphenoid wing and suprasellar region. Olfactory groove tumours give rise to anosmia and may later cause Foster–Kennedy syndrome (ipsilateral optic atrophy and contralateral papilloedema) in addition to raised intracranial pressure. Sphenoid wing meningiomas are frequently of the *en plaque* type and medially placed tumours may be associated with proptosis and cranial nerve involvement, leading to diplopia, ophthalmoplegia and visual failure. Tumours of the outer third of the sphenoid wing may cause hemiparesis or epilepsy. Suprasellar meningiomas cause optic chiasmatic compression and bitemporal hemianopia.

The prognosis for meningiomas is determined by the histology, extent of surgery and performance status. The outcome for patients with malignant meningiomas is poor, with a median survival of less than 3 years.

Metastatic disease

Secondary involvement of the CNS is more common in incidence than are primary tumours. It frequently occurs in the setting of advanced disease, so is often not reflected in neurosurgical series.

Tumours with a particularly high risk of CNS metastases include small cell lung cancer, melanoma, lymphoblastic and Burkitt's lymphomas and acute lymphoblastic leukaemia. Such tumours are relatively rare, and the majority of metastases seen are from breast and non-small cell lung cancers.

The cerebral hemispheres are the favoured site, being involved in over 75% of cases, although multiple metastases are seen in about 50%. The clinical presentation is similar to that of a primary brain or spinal tumour.

Leptomeningeal disease or 'carcinomatous meningitis' may present with a short, non-specific illness prior to the more classical symptoms of cranial nerve palsies, visual failure, pain and raised intracranial pressure. The diagnosis is normally confirmed by the finding of tumour cells in the CSF.

Malignant disease may also be associated with non-metastatic manifestations in the CNS. These are rare and ill understood but include cerebellar degeneration, encephalitis and myelitis. Similar syndromes also involve the peripheral nervous system and the skeletal muscles.

Conclusion

The CNS may be involved by a wide spectrum of tumours, both primary and secondary. These exhibit a wide spectrum of clinical and pathological features and are associated with varying prognoses. This chapter has attempted to outline the basic clinical and pathological aspects of diagnosis, together with the typical natural history of some of the more common tumour types.

References

Daumas-Duport C, Scheithauer BW, O'Fallon J, Kelly P (1988) Grading of astrocytomas. A simple and reproducible method. Cancer 62: 2152–65.

Kernohan JW, Mahon KF, Svien HJ, Adson AW (1949) A simplified classification of gliomas. Proceedings of the Staff Meetings of the Mayo Clinic 24: 71–5

Kleihues P, Burger PC, Scheithauer BW (1993) The new WHO classification of brain tumours. Brain Pathology 3(3): 255–68.

Salcman M (1990) Epidemiology and factors affecting survival. In Apuzzo MLJ (Ed.) Malignant Cerebral Gliomas. Park Ridge, IL: American Association of Neurological Surgeons, 95–109.

Chapter 4
Clinical neuro – imaging

Juliet Britton and Virginia Ng

Introduction

Neuroradiological investigation's main value is in assessing the correct anatomical site of the tumour and assisting in determining the neurosurgical approach. Intracranial neoplasms may, for all practical purposes, be divided into two clinical groups: those which are theoretically resectable and therefore potentially curable, and those which are not. Neuroradiological assessment needs to help in the evaluation of a tumour's resectability, for although computed tomography (CT) and magnetic resonance imaging (MRI) appearances may be able to suggest the type of tumour present, histological diagnosis requires a biopsy.

Tumours that are not resectable may be surgically debulked to help relieve patients' symptoms. Removed tissue will then be examined histologically to provide the diagnosis. Alternatively, only a small sample of tissue may be taken. CT or MRI will be used to localise the area of tissue that is most likely to provide the correct histological diagnosis. CT and MRI play an important role in following up patients with CNS tumours. Both techniques may be used to detect recurrence and monitor the response of tumours to radiotherapy and chemotherapy.

Techniques

The techniques employed are:

- plain films;
- cerebral angiography;
- CT scanning;
- MRI;

- nuclear medicine: conventional brain scan, simple photon emission computed tomography (SPECT) and positron emission tomography (PET);
- myelography.

Plain films

Before the advent of newer imaging techniques such as CT and MRI, skull X-rays were important in the management of neuro-oncology patients. Elaborate machines were used to immobilise the patient's head to obtain high-quality films without any movement artefact. The detection of midline shift (for example, the displacement of pineal calcification) and bony erosion gave an indication of the underlying abnormality. The use of skull X-rays in such a context is now largely obsolete owing to their replacement by CT and MRI.

Cerebral angiography

Cerebral angiography used to be a valuable technique in the detection and delineation of intracranial tumours, relying on the demonstration of new vessels and tumour blushes. Displacement of the normal vessels was used to locate avascular masses. The practice of cerebral angiography has also changed over the past 20 years as more sophisticated equipment has become available. Nowadays, this procedure is performed in an angiography suite containing a floating-top table, upon which the patient lies, and a rotating C-arm that houses the X-ray tube (Figure 4.1). This enables X-ray pictures

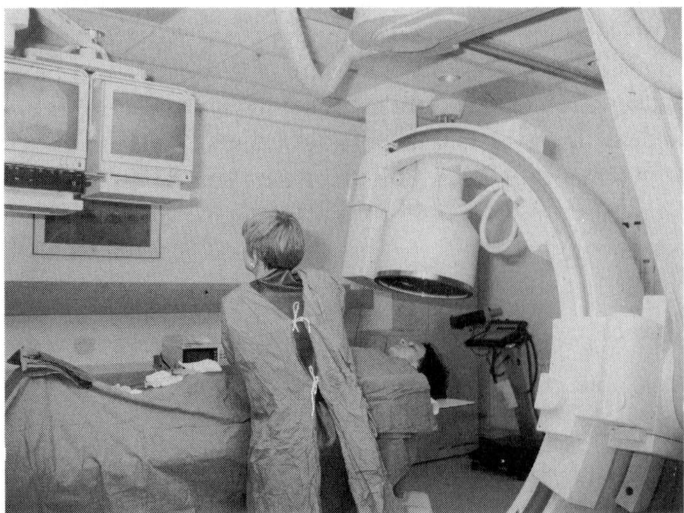

Figure 4.1 Angiograph suite. Patient lies supine on the moveable table, the x-ray tube rotates around the patient to obtain views in different directions. The patient is draped with green towels to ensure sterile conditions.

to be obtained from many different directions without the patient needing to move. Preparation of the patient begins once the patient is selected for angiography. A full blood count and clotting screen are performed, and a full drug and allergy history is taken . The patient is consented prior to the procedure, and risks such as cerebrovascular accidents are explained. In a neuroscience unit, the risk of stroke and permanent disability should be less than 1%.

Once the patient is on the table, the skin over both groins is shaved and sterilised. Sterile drapes are placed over the patient exposing an area of skin, usually the right groin. In some units, patients, particularly children, will receive a general anaesthetic, but in many departments the normal practice is to perform angiography following local anaesthetic to the skin and underlying structures. Following the local anaesthetic a needle is introduced into the femoral artery, through it, a wire and catheter are advanced up to the arch of the aorta, and selective catheterisation of the cerebral vessels is then performed. During the injection of contrast medium, images of the patient's vessels are obtained. (Figure 4.2). The procedure is not particularly painful, but when contrast is injected the patient may experience a feeling of warmth and see flashing lights.

Should embolisation of a tumour be necessary, the procedure is the same as for a diagnostic angiogram except that different catheters are used; these are placed further intracranially, and occlusive devices such as acrylate compounds ('glue') or coils are deployed through these fine-bore catheters. Embolisation can be carried out

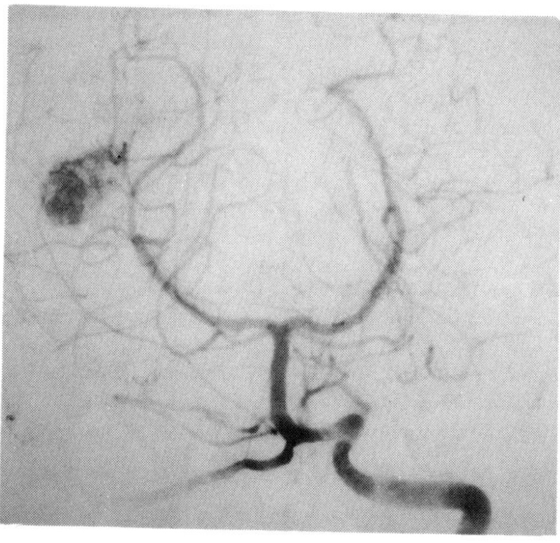

Figure 4.2 Angiogram. Injection of contrast has shown the intracerebral blood vessels, the rounded area of increased vascularity demonstrates the presence of a tumor.

under local anaesthetic with sedation or under general anaesthesia. The latter is sometimes necessary because of pain induced by vasospasm at the time of embolisation.

Computed tomography

This technique, together with MRI, remains the workhorse of diagnostic neuro-oncology. CT was invented by Sir Godfrey Hounsfield, and he installed the prototype machine at Atkinson Morley's Hospital, London, in 1972. The early scanners were relatively slow. Newer-generation scanners have scan times of less than 2 seconds per slice.

CT uses X-rays to obtain a cross-sectional image of the patient. The scanner consists of a moveable table on which the patient is placed, and the scanner gantry, which contains the X-ray source and an array of detectors that rotate around the patient during each scan. The patient remains stationary during the scan (Figure 4.3). The bore through which the patient is fed in the gantry has a length of about 20 cm and a diameter of 75 cm. Thus only a small proportion of the patient is within the bore of the gantry at any time, and there is no sense of being enclosed in a confined space. Because acquisition of images with CT (unlike MRI) is relatively quick, restless patients do not pose a particular problem.

CT is particularly useful for the demonstration of calcification and bony abnormality such as erosion by tumours. The image is displayed on a monitor and is composed of small squares called pixels. Each pixel is depicted as a shade of grey, black or white to

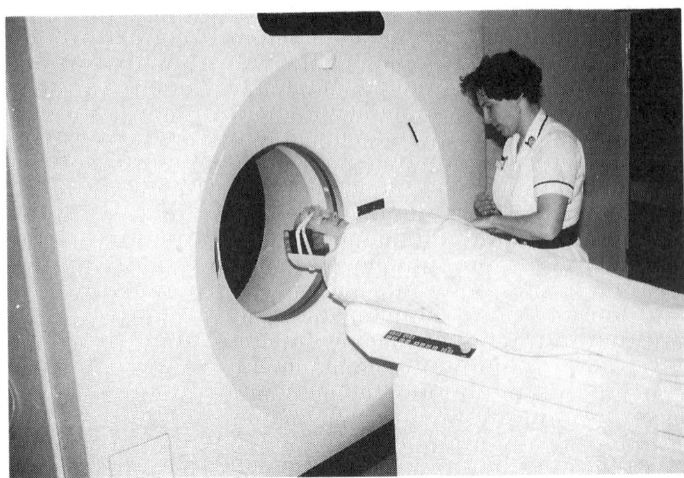

Figure 4.3 CT scanner. This shows the diameter of the gantry relative to the patient's head size.

indicate the density of the tissue that lies in the path of the X-ray beam. Bone, which is dense, absorbs X-rays and therefore attenuates (reduces) the beam strength reading in the detector; bone is displayed as white. Air does not absorb the X-ray beam and is depicted as black. Fluid such as CSF absorbs very few of the X-rays and is therefore relatively black. Brain is displayed as shades of grey (Figure 4.4).

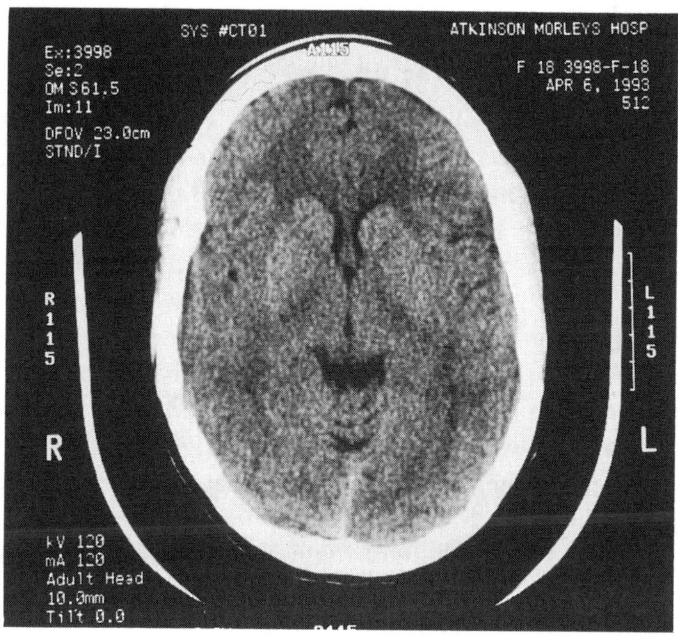

Figure 4.4 Axial CT of normal adult head. Note that the different tissues of the brain are depicted as various shades of grey.

Intravascular contrast medium utilises the element iodine to block the passage of X-rays and attenuate the beam (it appears white). This performs the role of opacifying vascular structures or structures where there is a breakdown of the blood–brain barrier. Most contrast media used nowadays are of the non-ionic, water-soluble low-osmolar type, which are safer and more comfortable for the patient. In hospitals where ionic contrast is still used, patients may be asked to be nil by mouth prior to the investigation because of the risk of vomiting.

A routine examination of the head for tumours entails a set of images being obtained pre- and post-intravenous contrast medium administration. The examination usually takes 10–15 minutes. If contrast is given, the examination time will double. In the paediatric population, it may be necessary to anaesthetise the skin prior to the procedure; this is usually in the form of a topical application of an anaesthetic cream. Recognised common side-effects of contrast include a feeling of generalised warmth, a metallic taste in the tongue, unusual sensations in the perineum and occasionally a feeling of urinary incontinence. More serious events such as urticaria are less common. The incidence of major side-effects such as anaphylaxis is 1 in 10 000. Because of this, there should be resuscitation facilities to hand.

Magnetic resonance imaging

Unlike CT, which uses ionising radiation, MRI uses radiowaves and a powerful magnet to detect the nuclear magnetic resonance signal from protons in the human body. The patient is metal-checked prior to this examination. This involves a list of exclusion criteria, such as a permanent cardiac pacemaker and ferromagnetic vascular clips (Figure 4.5). Prior to entering the scanning room, all ferromagnetic objects such as coins, pens with clips, and credit cards, are removed. Staff accompanying the patient into the examination room will have to go through the same procedure. The patient, dressed in his or her own clothing, lies on the table in the scanning room. The head is placed within the head coil, with padding on either side of the temporal region. The patient is fed into the centre of the magnet; compared with CT, the bore of the magnet is smaller and longer, which may give the patient the sensation of being buried in a tunnel (Figure 4.6). However, there are magnets on the market that try to address the problem of claustrophobia by producing a larger bore and shorter tunnel.

The field strength of most magnets in current use varies from 0.5 T (Tesla) to 1.5 T. Lower field strength magnets are also used in some units. The duration of a sequence, that is, a set of images generated, varies, and in a high field strength magnet it may be as short as 3 minutes. Most MRI examinations of the head take 20–30 minutes, during which time several different sequences are obtained. Patients find the examination less acceptable than CT because it is noisy and the environment is enclosed.

Claustrophobic patients can be sedated, usually in the form of intravenous diazepam. An MR-compatible pulse oximeter is usually employed under such circumstances for respiratory and cardiac monitoring. In addition, an observer is usually placed inside the scanning room, near the patient, as an added precaution.

Anaesthesia can be performed using MR-compatible equipment and piped gases.

Please tick appropriate box	YES	NO
Do you have a Pacemaker or artificial heart valves?		
Have you **EVER** had any metal fragments in your eye(s) or worked with high speed metal machining tools?		
Have you ever had a brain haemorrhage?		
Have you **EVER** had any surgery to your head or neck?		
Have you had **ANY** operations in the last year?		
Do you have any joint/limb replacements or metal implants?		
Have you any shrapnel, war or bomb blast injuries?		
Do you have a false limb, calliper or brace?		
Have you ever had cosmetic surgery or tattoos?		
Are you epileptic? Have you ever had a fit?		
Are you wearing a hearing aid?		
Are you wearing removable metal dentures?		
Are you wearing any patches (HRT, nicotine, etc.)?		
Have you had an MRI scan at this Centre before? If yes please give date (approx).		
Have you a follow up consultation arranged? If yes, please give date, time and place.		
For women of child-bearing age: could you be pregnant?		

Articles to be secured in lockers outside the Scanning Room: Hearing aids, keys, money, credit cards, watches, pagers, scissors, hair clips, jewellery etc. All articles are left entirely at the owner's risk. Lodestone cannot be held responsible for any loss or damage to any items.

I confirm that I have read the above and that it is correct to the best of my knowledge and belief.

Signature: .... (patient/parent/guardian) Date: ....

Figure 4.5 Checklist for MRI.

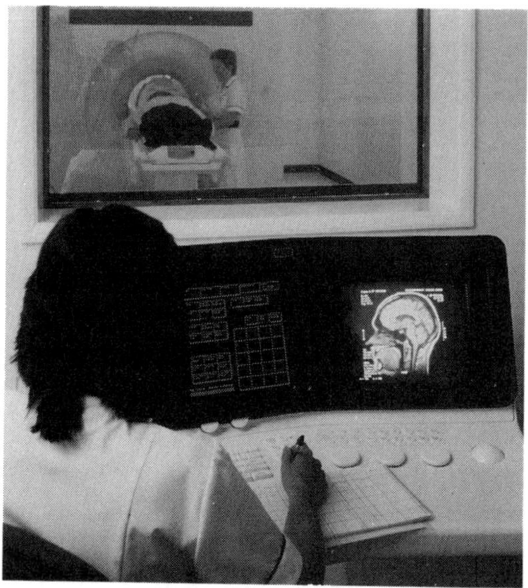

Figure 4.6 The radiographer seated at the control console is able to monitor the patient on the examination table. Patients requiring additional care will have a member of staff in the room with them.

Because of the noise generated by the magnet, ear plugs or headphones are usually worn inside the scanning room to comply with Health and Safety rules. The radiographer controls the examination from a separate room where the computer console is situated.

There are many ways of obtaining an image using MRI. An individual set of pictures is obtained by a particular pulse sequence. They all relate to three 'weightings' (W): T1, T2 and proton density (PD). As a rough guide, fluid is black on T1W and white on T2W images. Brain is depicted as various shades of grey. T1W images are used for anatomy; T2W images detect even minor changes in the water content of soft tissues and are the more sensitive sequences. When scans are described in a report, tissues that look white are said to have high signal intensity, and tissues that look relatively black are said to have low signal intensity (Figure 4.7).

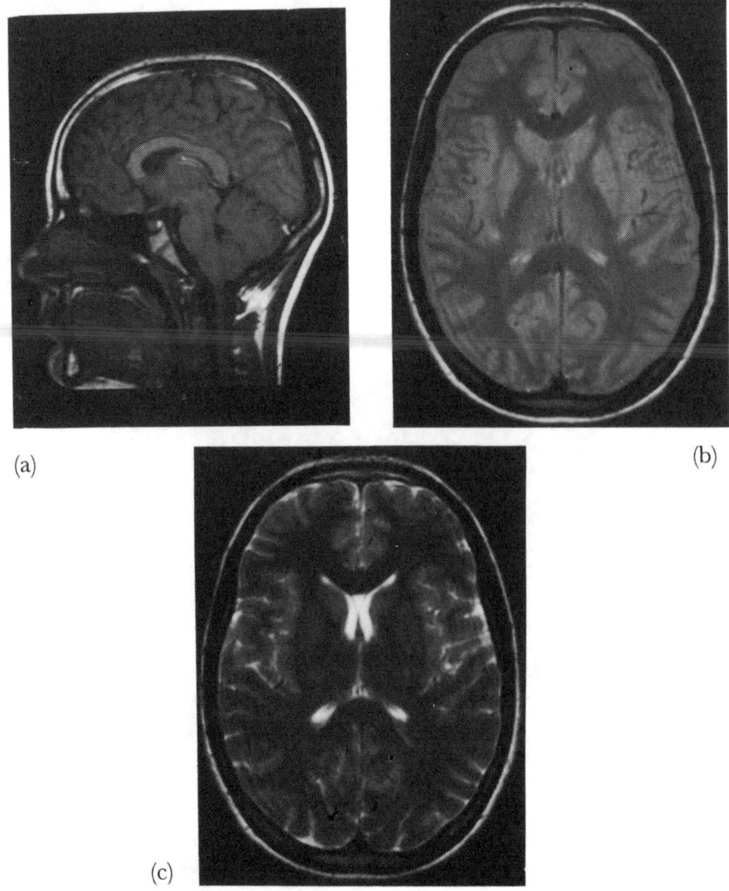

Figure 4.7 Normal MRI of adult head a) Sagittal T1W image showing CSF as black (b) Axial PD image showing CSF as grey (c) Axial T2W image showing CSF as white.

Contrast medium is also employed, the compounds being entirely different from those employed in CT. However, both types show vascularity and breakdown of the blood–brain barrier. A paramagnetic substance such as Gadolinium-DTPA (Gd-DTPA) is currently approved for use intravenously in both adults and children. Gd-DTPA does not have side-effects (see CT contrast agents). Following the administration of contrast, T1W images are obtained as contrast enhancement is not detected on T2-weighted sequences.

In specialised centres, a technique known as magnetic resonance spectroscopy (MRS) is used as an adjunct to routine MRI in an attempt to delineate further the components of tumour tissue and in some cases to differentiate radiation necrosis from tumour recurrence. The examination is no different from a normal MRI in terms of the procedure undergone by the patient.

Apart from the lack of ionising radiation, the advantages of MRI are primarily in the display of soft tissue detail and in the technique being truly three-dimensional. On CT, bone obscures certain areas of the brain such as the posterior fossa. MRI does not have this problem and is therefore the investigation of choice.

Contrast between different tissues can be altered by acquiring images on different sequences, in order to highlight pathological changes.

Nuclear Medicine

Conventional brain scan

For a conventional brain scan, radiopharmaceuticals are given intravenously to the patient, which accumulate in lesions with neovascularity or an altered blood-brain barrier. Various agents are employed that usually contain ^{99m}Technetium. The patient is scanned in the dynamic (straight after the injection) and static (between 1 and 2 hours after the injection) phases. The scan occasionally needs to be repeated at 3–4 hourly intervals if the results are equivocal. Conventional brain scanning has little use in a purely neuroradiological setting but may still be used to look for brain metastases.

The procedure is undertaken by sitting the patient in front of the gamma camera whilst the data are collected and images are obtained in various projections such as anterior-posterior (AP) and lateral.

Single photon emission computed tomography

SPECT is similar to conventional brain scanning except that data are collected by a rotating gamma camera. The patient is supine rather than seated. There has been an increase in the use of this technique with new applications being found. It can discriminate between tumour recurrence and radiation necrosis; CT and MRI images cannot distinguish between the two.

Positron emission tomography

A number of positron-emitting agents have been used to study regional cerebral blood flow. An expensive cyclotron unit is needed to create the short-lived radionuclides required for this investigation, and there are hence very few centres that offer PET. There has been a decline in the use of PET because of the relatively poor anatomical resolution. However, newer functional radiopharmaceuticals outlining tumour physiology have rejuvenated the role of PET in clinical oncology. The cost of the units will also hopefully decrease in the next few years, making this technique more commonly available.

Current scanners take an hour for data acquisition. Blood samples are taken from either the radial artery or a heated hand vein to measure the input curve for the conversion of cerebral activity detected by the scanner to absolute metabolic rates.

The theoretical radiation hazards for the patient chiefly concern the lenses of the eyes. There is almost no risk to medical personnel in close proximity to the patient.

Myelography

Myelography is mainly used in units where MRI is not freely available, particularly outside routine screening times or in patients in whom MRI is contraindicated. In exceptional circumstances, it is employed to differentiate between leptomeningeal metastases and abnormal vessels on the spinal cord surface. Myelography is usually followed by CT in the region of interest.

In adults, this procedure is performed under local anaesthetic. A small spinal needle is inserted in the lumbar region, and water-soluble contrast medium such as that employed in CT is introduced into the thecal sac. In children, this procedure is usually performed under general anaesthesia. The duration of the procedure varies according to the ease of the lumbar puncture and, in experienced hands, can be as short as 20 minutes. However, if followed by CT, the whole procedure usually lasts for 1 hour. Following the introduction of contrast into the subarachnoid space, plain X-rays are taken with the patient viewed in different directions (Figure 4.8).

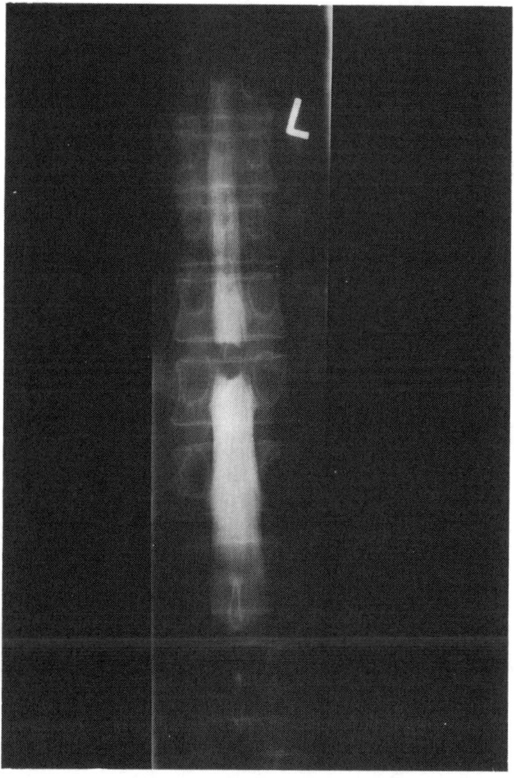

Figure 4.8 Myelogram demonstrating intradural extramedullary tumour as a round area outlined by the white of the contrast in the CSF.

Post-myelography, the patient is nursed with the head elevated at 45 degrees for 8 hours to try to reduce the incidence of headache. Rehydration is also useful. Occasional chronic CSF leak may necessitate an epidural blood patch. Other complications are rare but can include bleeding, infection, damage to nerves, paralysis, bladder, bowel and muscle dysfunction and allergic reaction to the contrast medium.

CNS tumours

Tumours of the CNS will be appreciated on imaging because they displace and alter the shape of normal anatomical structures. They are also seen because they display a different density on CT or signal intensity on MRI in comparison to normal brain. Some tumours also become more evident (enhance) following an intravenous injection of contrast medium. Different tumours have different density or signal intensity characteristics on imaging, but these are not the most important factors in reaching a diagnosis. Knowledge of the age of the patient and location of the tumour are just as, if not more, important in suggesting the diagnosis. The types of brain tumour found in childhood are different from those found in adults.

Although radiotherapy and chemotherapy have, in certain selective groups, led to some prolongation of life (see Chapters 6 and 7), the tumours with the best prognosis are still those which have well-defined margins and can be completely removed. This must also mean that they involve areas of brain that are relatively 'neurologically silent' and do not involve adjacent important anatomical structures such as major arteries or veins.

The relationship to adjacent vascular structures is best assessed on MRI and may be supplemented either by MRI angiography or conventional angiography. Newer techniques, such as functional imaging, may also assist in determining the relationship of the tumour to various areas of the cerebral cortex, in particular the motor strip and visual cortex. Imaging may also be used to predict tumour type and therefore prognosis prior to surgery, but in reality many intracranial tumours resemble each other radiologically, and a minimum of stereotactic biopsy is going to be necessary to establish the diagnosis.

Common intracranial malignancies in adults

Intracranial tumours are derived either from cells that are usually found within the brain or its covering (the dura), or from secondary malignancies arising from cells elsewhere in the body. The former group are termed primary neoplasms and account for two-thirds of intracranial tumours; metastases account for the remaining third.

Primary intracranial neoplasms may be further subdivided into those of neuroglial origin, otherwise called gliomas, and a second group of non-glial tumours that comprise a large group of histologically and biologically different tumours. Gliomas account for approximately half of all primary intracranial tumours. Of the non-glial tumours, meningiomas, pituitary adenomas, acoustic neuromas and lymphomas are relatively common. The types of tumour seen in children are different, with the involvement of different sites, and will be considered separately.

1. Tumours occurring in the brain in adults:
- gliomas of grades II, III and IV;
- primary intracerebral lymphoma;
- intracranial metastases.
2. Tumours arising outside the brain but within the cranial cavity:
- meningioma;
- pituitary adenomas;
- acoustic schwannomas.

Glial tumours

Gliomas make up to 45–50% of primary intracranial tumours. The vast majority of these are infiltrating tumours that are usually well demonstrated on imaging, particularly MRI. By their very nature, they cannot be completely resected.

Glial tumours may originate from astrocytes, oligodendrocytes or ependymal cells. By far the most common are astrocytomas. Astrocytomas can be further subdivided by their resectability and biological activity into the relatively benign, which include the pilocytic astrocytoma, the subependymal giant cell astrocytoma of tuberous sclerosis and the newly described pleomorphic xanthoastrocytoma (all of which are paediatric tumours), or the more malignant infiltrating group that is mainly made up of the fibrillary astrocytomas. The difference in biological activity of these two groups is now recognised in the new WHO grading, which grades astrocytomas as I–IV with increasing malignancy. Grade I astrocytomas are the pilocytic astrocytomas usually found in childhood (see Chapter 3).

Fibrillary astrocytomas

These account for the vast majority of intracranial tumours in adults. They vary in malignancy from the relatively benign WHO grade II fibrillary astrocytoma to the highly malignant WHO grade IV glioblastoma multiforme. The most frequent is glioblastoma multiforme, the most malignant, which has a peak incidence in the seventh decade of life. Together with the grade III anaplastic astrocytoma, they account for over 70% of all astrocytomas. The most usual site for these tumours is in the cerebral hemispheres. It is rare to find primary gliomas in adults in the posterior fossa, where metastases, haemorrhage and infarction are the main causes of mass lesions within the cerebellar hemispheres.

Grade II fibrillary astrocytomas

Peak incidence is in the fourth and fifth decades of life. These tumours appear as low-density, poorly defined lesions involving large areas of the cerebral hemisphere with relatively little mass effect on CT (Figure 4.9a).Intravenous contrast medium is usually given as part of the procedure, but these tumours rarely enhance, and the pre- and post-contrast images therefore look virtually identical (Figure 4.9b). Some low-grade astrocytomas may be missed by the inexperienced eye on CT because of the relative lack of mass effect and the subtle difference in density. Subtle change may not be seen when the tumour lies close to the skull because of the artefact that bone generates on CT. This may be compounded by the fact that because the tumour infiltrates along the white matter tracts, and does not destroy brain, the patients may have relatively few symptoms, leading to a false sense of security. The main message here is that not all tumours enhance and lack of enhancement therefore does not exclude a tumour. The converse is also true: other diseases affecting the brain may enhance.

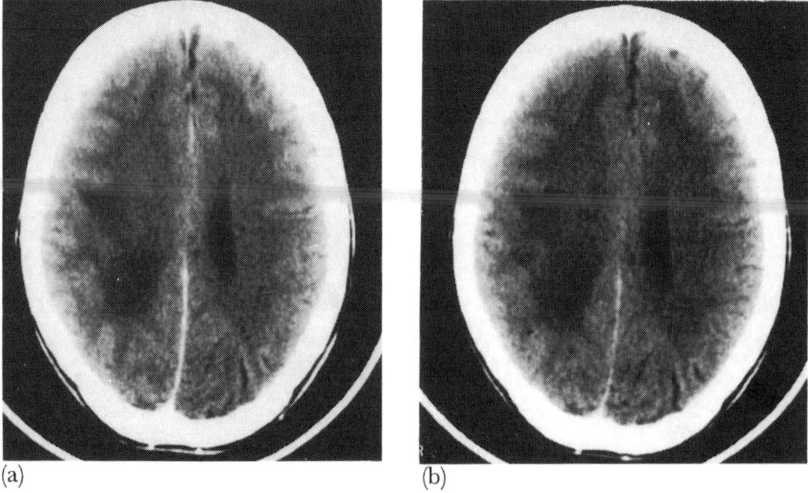

(a) (b)

Figure 4.9 Fibrillary astrocytoma – grade II (CT) (a) unenhanced (b) enhanced.

Cerebral infarction and encephalitis may give a very similar appearance on CT, with a low-density, non-enhancing mass. The differential diagnosis is made by knowledge of the mode of presentation and distribution of the abnormal appearance; for example low-density change associated with an infarct should conform to a known vascular territory (Figure 4.10). It is sometimes very difficult to differentiate infarcts from tumours, and in this situation a follow-up

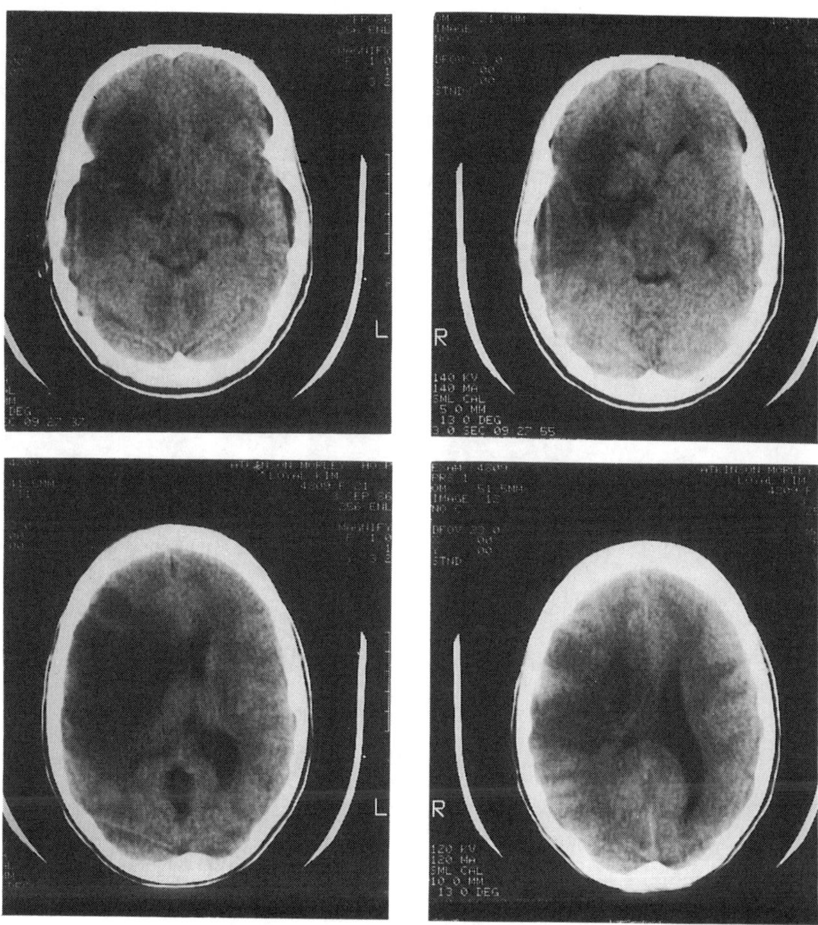

Figure 4.10 CT right middle cerebral artery infarct.

scan at 6–8 weeks may be suggested. At this stage, any mass effect from an infarct should have resolved, and mass effect from a low-grade tumour will persist or might even progress.

MRI is technically superior to CT because of its increased sensitivity to any alteration in water content in the brain, and there is no bone artefact to degrade the image. It is therefore better at showing the extent of the tumour. Low-grade gliomas are usually seen as areas of low signal intensity (relatively dark) on T1W and high signal intensity (white) on T2W images (Figure 4.11 a, b). Contrast enhancement following intravenous Gd-DTPA does not usually occur. By scanning in multiple planes, the neuroradiologist is able to demonstrate the extent of the tumour involvement, and the infiltrative nature of the lesion can be more fully appreciated. These tumours do not have surrounding oedema, and any signal change

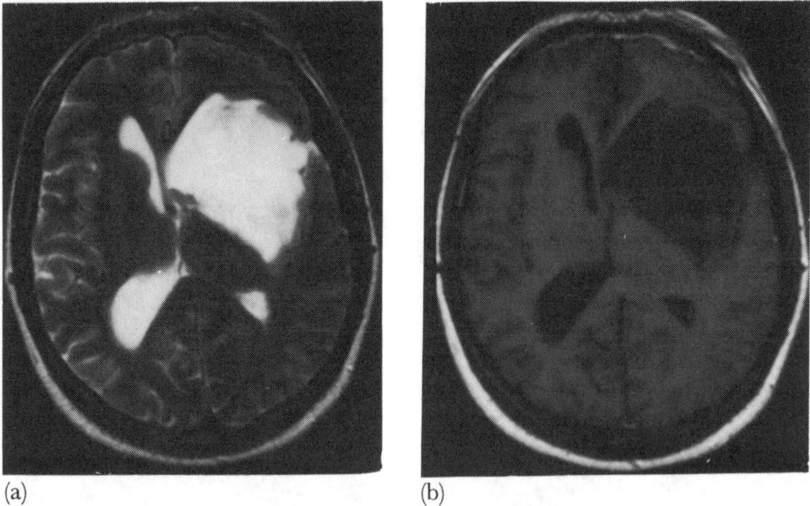

(a) (b)

Figure 4.11 Grade II fibrillary astrocytoma, (a) T_2W, left (b) T_1W, right.

therefore indicates active disease. Unfortunately, even with tumours that appear to have relatively well-defined margins, malignant cells may be found in areas of brain outside the area of signal change seen on MRI.

Whilst attempts may be made at total surgical resection, the long-term survival time has not yet been shown to be dramatically altered by such radical surgery. As already stated, because these tumours infiltrate along white matter tracts, neurological deficit may be minimal. Extensive resection can therefore leave these patients with a much greater neurological deficit after surgery than they had before. In addition, not all tumours are suitable for such surgery because of their anatomical sites of involvement, for example the motor cortex.

All low-grade fibrillary astrocytomas and intermediate grades show a tendency to progress with time to higher grades of malignancy. Although a tumour may initially be diagnosed as grade II, it will eventually transform to grade III and grade IV. When following up these patients on imaging, the neuroradiologist is looking not only for extension of disease, but also for possible progression to a higher grade.

Anaplastic astrocytomas and glioblastoma multiforme

These tumours (WHO grade III and grade IV) may arise *de novo* or in pre-existing low-grade astrocytomas. The peak incidence is at a slightly older age, being in the sixth decade in anaplastic astrocytomas and the seventh decade in glioblastoma multiforme.

With increasing malignancy, the imaging findings may change. However, this is not universal, and imaging characteristics alone can not be used to accurately predict tumour grade or even type.

Anaplastic astrocytomas

Mass effect is usually more obvious with the higher-grade malignancies. Anaplastic astrocytomas (WHO grade III) are usually associated with low-density change on CT, with areas of irregular or ring enhancement following intravenous contrast medium. On MRI, an area of low signal is seen on T1W and a high signal on T2W images, with areas of irregular enhancement following Gd-DTPA (Figure 4.12). These tumours may rarely haemorrhage but do not show necrosis.

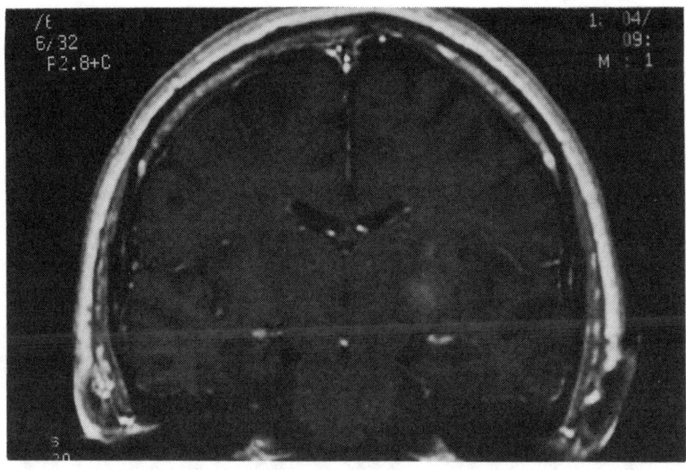

Figure 4.12 Grade III fibrillary astrocytoma, MRI T1W enhanced image. Irregular enhancement is seen in and adjacent to the left internal capsule.

Glioblastoma multiforme

As the name glioblastoma multiforme suggests, the appearances of these tumours (WHO grade IV), even within the same patient, can be very variable. The most common finding on CT is an irregular area of high density that shows a thick rim of shaggy enhancement following intravenous contrast medium, with surrounding low-density change consistent with vasogenic oedema (Figure 4.13). The area of relative non-enhancement within the centre of the tumour represents necrosis, which may or may not be haemorrhagic. Although the surrounding low-density change is usually described as oedema, tumour cells will in reality be found infiltrating through this area. Enhancement is only seen where there are sufficient numbers of cells to result in alteration of the blood–brain barrier and neovascularity. With progression of the disease, areas of irregular enhancement are seen separate from the original main area. These tumours invade white matter tracts and are commonly seen to cross the corpus callosum in a butterfly distribution.

On MRI, the central area of the tumour shows a mixed signal and, following contrast, there is usually enhancement. The central areas of necrosis do not enhance. High-grade gliomas may metastasise either around the ventricular margins or in the subarachnoid space; these are better identified on MRI (Figure 4.14). Areas of brain that looked normal on CT will also be shown to be abnormal on MRI.

Oligodendroglioma

Oligodendrogliomas (WHO grades II–IV) are gliomas that, instead of arising from astrocytes, arise from oligodendrocytes. However, many of these have mixed cellular origins and are therefore termed

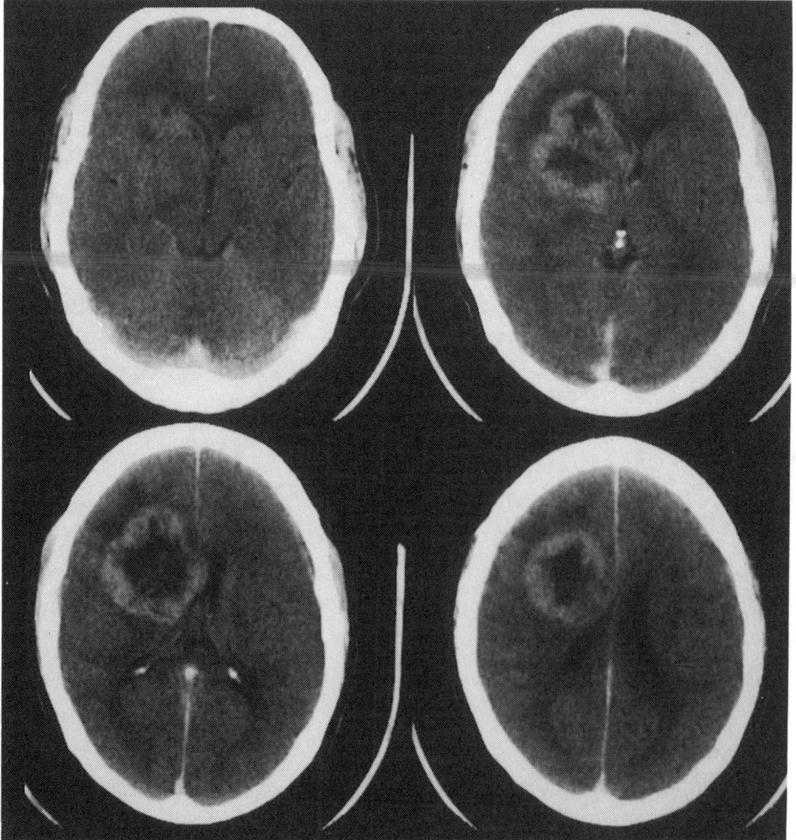

Figure 4.13 Contrast enhanced axial CT – glioblastoma multiforme, note irregular ring of enhancement in right frontal lobe.

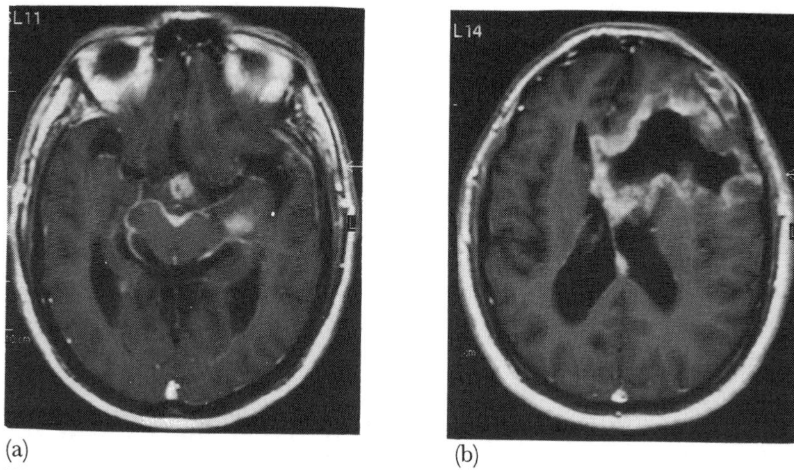

(a) (b)

Figure 4.14 Glioblastoma metastasising through CSF pathways. (a) Areas of abnormal enhancement are seen lining the surface of the midbrain, the pituitary stalk and medial temporal lobe. (b) Enhancement is seen around the resection site, this may be due to surgery but the enhancement of the ventricular walls equals metastatic disease.

oligodendroastrocytomas. They are relatively uncommon tumours, comprising only 2–5% of primary intracranial tumours. Similar to the more common astrocytomas, oligodendrogliomas range in malignancy from WHO grades II to IV. Imaging does not usually help in the grading of these tumours.

The characteristic finding of oligodendrogliomas is a mass lesion that is at least partly densely calcified lying in a relatively peripheral position within the cerebral hemisphere (Figure 4.15). It may have associated cysts and show enhancement at a lower grade of malignancy than do astrocytomas. The presence of calcification alone

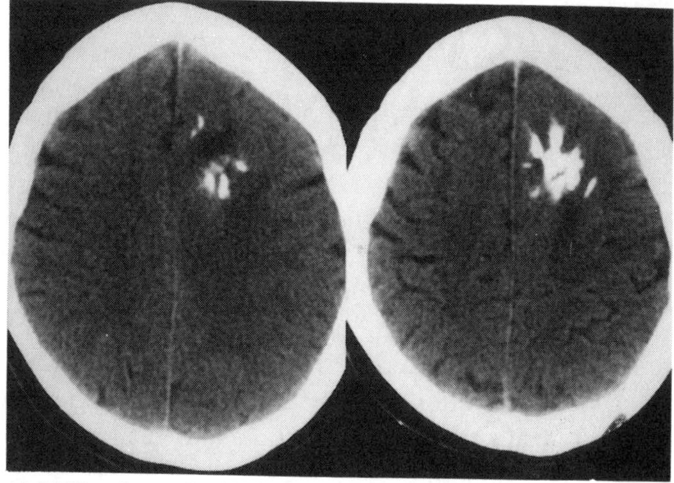

Figure 4.15 Unenhanced axial CT - oligodendroglioma, note the calcification.

cannot differentiate oligodendrogliomas from astrocytomas as low-grade astrocytomas may also show calcification. As astrocytomas are statistically more common, one is more likely to see a calcified astrocytoma than a typical oligodendroglioma.

Primary intracerebral lymphoma

Intracerebral lymphoma may be either primary or secondary. Primary intracerebral lymphoma occurs in three major clinical settings. The first is in the immune-compromised patient with AIDS, the second is in patients who are immune compromised secondary to organ transplants, and the third covers a group of patients who are not immune compromised. In the latter group, the patients are generally elderly, with a peak incidence in the sixth decade of life. Immune-compromised patients tend to present in their thirties.

Intracerebral lymphoma may be a solitary mass or multiple lesions. The lesions are classically found adjacent to the ventricles (periventricular) and commonly involve the basal ganglia. On CT, they are most commonly hyperdense and uniformly enhancing, with surrounding oedema (Figure 4.16 a, b). On MRI, the enhancement is easier to see, and the relationship of the tumour to the ventricular system is better delineated (Figure 4.17). On the T2W scan, the central mass is of relatively low signal intensity. Although the mass appears well defined, lymphomas are, like high-grade gliomas, not encapsulated masses and diffusely invade adjacent brain. If steroids are given, the mass may rapidly decrease in size. The tumours also tend to be sensitive to radiotherapy and a combination of radiotherapy and chemotherapy. However, despite these newer treatment regimens, the prognosis is still poor, with early recurrence of disease.

Intracranial metastases

Secondary brain tumours are common, representing, depending on the reported series, between 33% and 40% of intracranial tumours in adults. Although all ages may be affected, secondary malignancy in the brain is most common in the fourth to seventh decades of life. In up to 30% of patients with carcinoma, metastatic brain disease is the first manifestation, and unfortunately the prognosis is usually poor. In untreated cases, life expectancy is between 1 and 3 months, and radiotherapy alone increases this to only 6 months. The tumours that most commonly metastasise to brain are lung, breast and malignant melanoma. Gastrointestinal and genitourinary tract tumours are less common, accounting for only 10% of cases. The

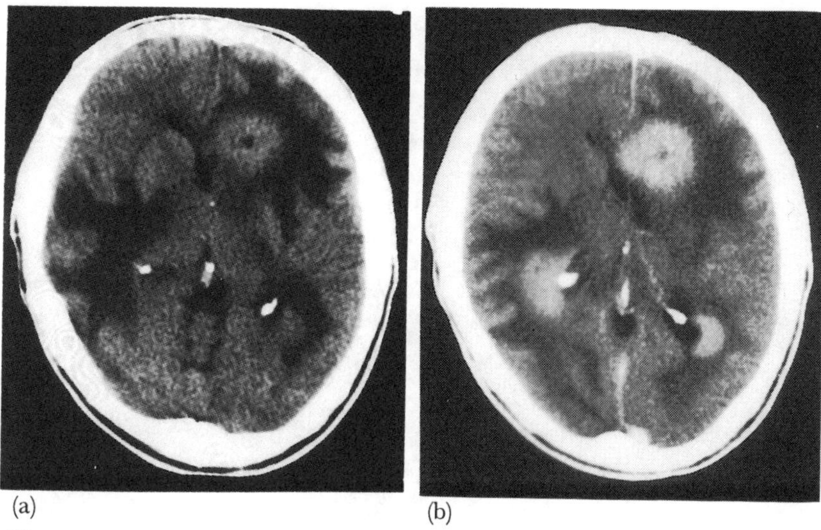

(a) (b)

Figure 4.16 Primary intracerebral lymphoma (a) Unenhanced axial CT demonstrating the hyperdense lesion in the typical periventricular site (b) Uniform enhancement after intravenous contrast injection.

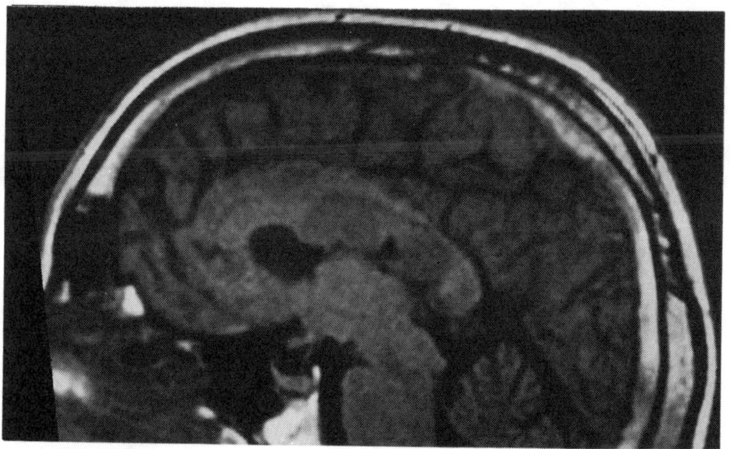

Figure 4.17 MRI lymphoma showing relationship of tumour to the ventricular walls.

majority of metastases (80%) are supratentorial; however, gastrointestinal and genitourinary tumours are more common in the posterior fossa (Figure 4.18)

There is another group of tumours that spread to the intracranial compartment but not primarily to the brain itself; that is, they are extra-axial. Carcinoma of the prostate involves the bone and adjacent dura and may create relatively large masses that compress the adjacent brain. Secondary lymphoma and leukaemia usually involve the meninges and only very rarely the brain itself. Skull metastases

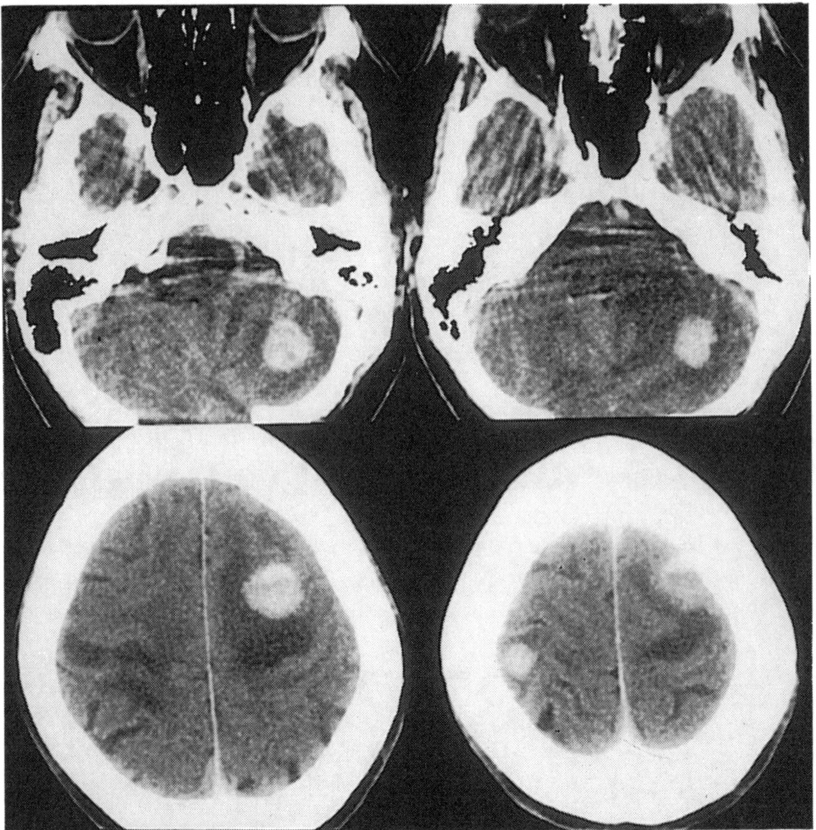

Figure 4.18 CT of multiple metastases, enhancing rounded masses with adjacent oedema.

from breast, bronchus, kidney and thyroid can spread inward to involve the dura. Diffuse spread along the leptomeninges in the subarachnoid space is called carcinomatous meningitis and occurs mainly with adenocarcinomas from the lung, stomach, breast and ovaries, although also occurring with melanoma.

Radiologically, the clue to making the diagnosis of metastatic disease is the presence of multiple lesions; solitary brain metastases are, however, common, and in some series 50% of intracranial metastases have been reported as solitary. With increasing sensitivity in imaging, particularly in contrast-enhanced MRI, the incidence of reported solitary lesions is falling. This concurs with the post-mortem findings that 85% of metastases are multiple.

Because of its availability, CT is still the usual primary investigation in these patients. Metastases are often seen as multiple rounded lesions found in the cerebral hemispheres, commonly at the grey/white matter junction (Figure 4.18). They may be hypo-, iso- or hyperdense in relationship to the adjacent brain, but following contrast medium administration, there is usually rim or nodular enhancement. Rim enhancement is due to the fact that the centre of the lesion is necrotic and no longer perfused with blood and therefore does not enhance. Melanoma metastases are typically hyperdense secondary to the presence of melanin or haemorrhage. Adenocarcinoma from the gut or osteogenic sarcomatous metastases may calcify. The majority of tumours have adjacent oedema, which may be minimal or extensive. Metastases occurring within grey matter usually have relatively little oedema. Unfortunately, on CT scans relatively small metastases, particularly if they are peripheral, may be missed, even following contrast enhancement.

The signal characteristics on MRI will vary on both T1W and T2W images, particularly if haemorrhage has occurred. In melanoma metastases, there is a characteristic signal change on MRI secondary to the presence of melanin. Peritumoural oedema is readily detected on the T2W images. Contrast-enhanced MRI is significantly more sensitive in detecting multiple lesions than is CT. Some centres in the USA will even use triple-dose gadolinium to try to increase the detection rate. Patients who have had a solitary lesion demonstrated on CT warrant an MRI to look for other lesions, partly to help to confirm the diagnosis and also because the presence of multiple lesions may alter the clinical management. Solitary metastases are amenable to surgery.

Carcinomatous meningitis is best demonstrated on MRI with enhancement of the meninges, which may be diffuse or irregular and lumpy. There may be spinal, as well as intracranial, involvement.

Multiple enhancing lesions may be seen in diseases other than metastases. Pyogenic abscesses also tend to form at the grey/white matter junction. Multiple sclerosis may give a similar appearance. A solitary metastasis may be difficult to differentiate from glioblastoma multiforme.

Meningioma

Meningiomas arise from the cells of the arachnoid granulations found in the dura mater, the membrane that encases the brain. They can potentially arise from anywhere on the surface of the intracranial cavity but are usually parafalcine and adjacent to suture lines. They are relatively common tumours, accounting for 15–20% of all intracranial tumours, with a preponderance in females. Peak incidence is in the fifth and sixth decades of life. They can rarely be found in children.

Meningiomas vary in their histological classification and biological propensity to recur. Recurrence depends mainly on resectability, and this in turn depends on the site of the tumour and the involvement of adjacent structures. There is little correlation between the histological type or the MRI appearances and early recurrence.

On CT, meningiomas are usually broad-based, hyperdense, well-circumscribed, uniformly enhancing mass lesions arising from the cerebral convexity. They may show calcification (Figure 4.19). It is common to see oedema (low-density change) involving the white matter of the adjacent hemisphere.

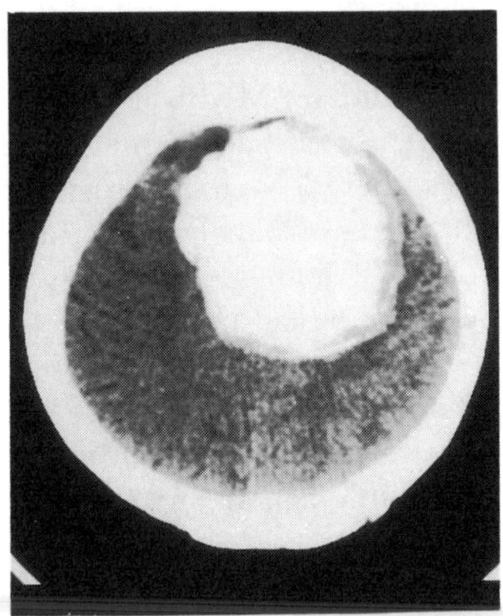

Figure 4.19 CT: Meningioma arising from the falx.

On MRI, meningiomas are of similar signal intensity to grey matter on both T1W and T2W images, and enhancement is seen with Gd-DTPA (Figure 4.20 a, b). There is usually a well-defined plane of cleavage between the tumour and the adjacent brain. MRI has the advantage over CT of being able to assess more fully the involvement of adjacent structures. For example, at the most common site, that is, parafalcine, 50% of tumours will invade the adjacent superior sagittal sinus. If a tumour is found in this site, the superior sagittal sinus needs to be fully evaluated with conventional MRI, supplemented by MRI venography (Figure 4.21 a, b) and in certain circumstances conventional cerebral angiography. The extent of involvement is important in planning surgery; total occlusion of the middle third of the superior sagittal sinus by the tumour at the time of presentation means that the tumour and involved sinus may be safely removed. Paradoxically, partial occlusion necessitates that a portion of the tumour will be left behind as an acute oblitera-

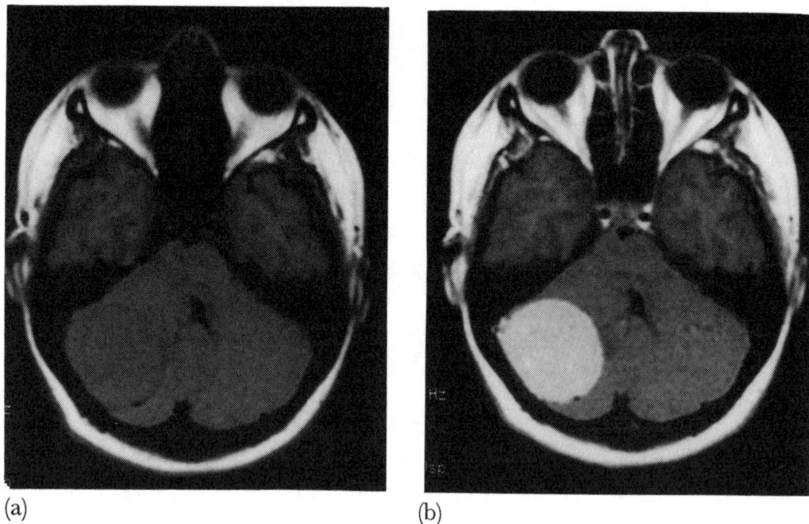

(a) (b)

Figure 4.20 MRI of posterior fossa meningioma, T1W (a) Pre-contrast (b) Post contrast.

tion of the middle third of the sinus during surgery will usually result in death secondary to cerebral venous sinus thrombosis.

Conventional cerebral angiography may also have a place in the treatment of meningiomas. These tumours tend to be highly vascular and are supplied by branches of the external carotid artery. Preoperative embolisation (see the section on cerebral angiography p. 82) of tumour circulation can be performed to minimise intraoperative blood loss.

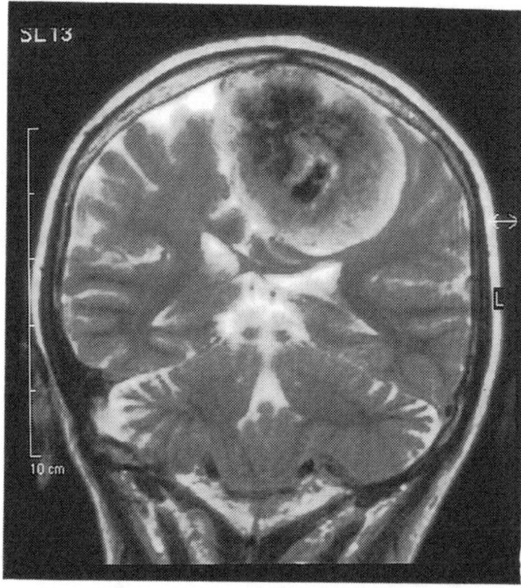

Figure 4.21 (**a**) Meningioma occluding the superior sagittal sinus conventional T2 coronal view.

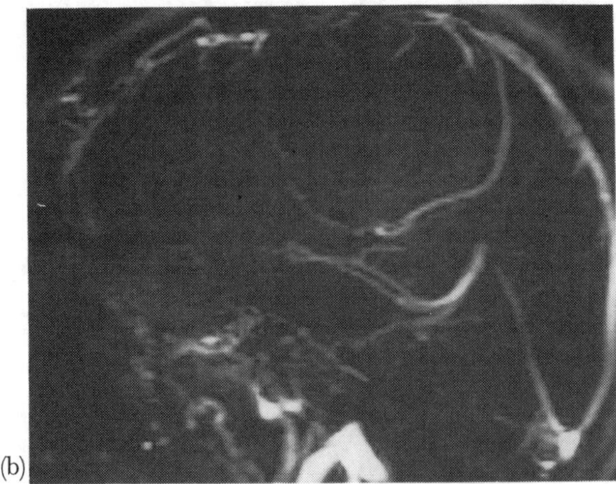

(b)

Figure 4.21 (b) MR venogram, middle third of superior sagittal sinus not visualised due to occlusion.

Meningiomas may also be found arising from other sites, for example the sphenoid wing (where they may invade the orbit), adjacent to the pituitary either above it and abutting the gland or lateral to it and involving the cavernous sinus. In certain sites, the tumour will be harder to resect, and the prognosis will be affected. Some of these patients will be referred for radiotherapy following surgery, and others will have radiotherapy when recurrence is demonstrated. Although the imaging appearances of a meningioma are fairly characteristic, similar findings may be seen in other tumours, for example metastases, schwannomas and even glioblastomas. An excision biopsy provides the histology.

Pituitary adenomas and acoustic schwannomas

There are two other relatively common tumours found in adults that may arise in structures adjacent to the brain and compress it when they enlarge. Pituitary adenomas account for between 6% and 10% of intracranial malignancy, and schwannomas, of which the acoustic neuroma is by far the most frequent type, another 6%. Both of these tumours are very rare in childhood. The diagnosis rests on the typical site in which these tumours arise.

Pituitary adenomas

There are two basic types of pituitary adenoma, the first being the microadenoma, which is by definition less than 10 mm in diameter. Patients with microadenomas present with endocrine dysfunction. The second type, macroadenomas, expand the sella turcica and then extend superiorly to compress the optic chiasm and other structures in the base of the brain. This group of patients therefore present with visual field abnormalities and may or may not have abnormal hormone levels.

Both CT and MRI may be used to make the diagnosis, but MRI is better at delineating the relationship between the tumour and the adjacent structures (Figure 4.22). The sella turcica is usually enlarged and, on CT, will be seen to contain a mass that is isodense to brain and then enhances uniformly with contrast. The patient may be scanned in the routine axial position but may also be asked to position his or her head so that direct coronal scans may be obtained. This positioning may be very uncomfortable for the patient but is of value in reducing artefact from bone and demonstrating the relationship of the tumour to the optic chiasm. The direction in which the tumour extends can be variable; however, one of the most common appearances is of a 'cottage loaf' configuration (Fig 4.22) when the mass extends into the chiasmatic cistern. Only about 5% of these tumours are shown to calcify on CT.

On MRI the tumour has similar signal intensity to grey matter on both T1W and T2W scans, and enhances uniformly. These tumours not infrequently haemorrhage or form cysts; this will alter the signal characteristics and MRI appearances.

In the adult population, pituitary adenomas need to be differentiated from meningiomas, craniopharyngiomas, aneurysms,

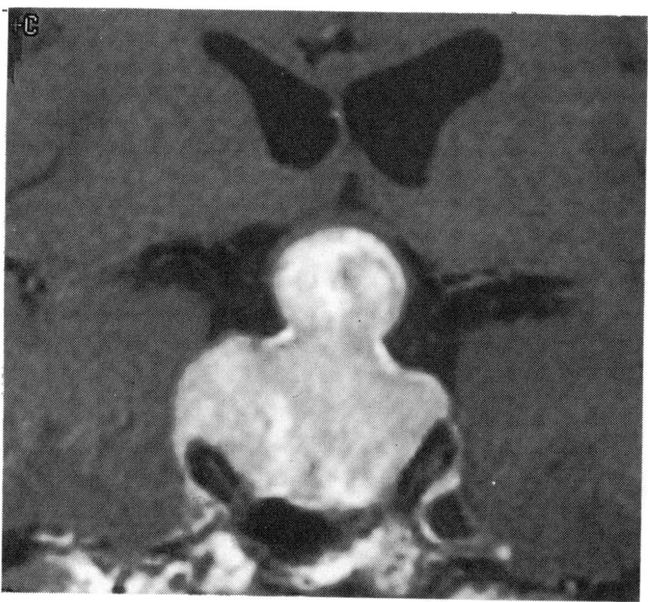

Figure 4.22 MRI of pituitary adenoma, coronal T1 contrast enhanced view.

secondary malignancies and tumours arising from the bone of the skull base.

Acoustic schwannomas

Acoustic schwannomas are slow-growing, benign tumours that arise from the vestibular division of the VIIIth cranial nerve. Recurrence is due to residual tumour left behind at original surgery as complete resection may not be possible. The most common mode of presentation is unilateral hearing loss, but some patients may have symptoms secondary to compression of the adjacent brain or cranial nerves.

Small acoustic tumours may be missed on CT, but larger ones occupying the cerebellopontine angle cistern may distort the brain stem and enlarge the internal auditory canal. This latter feature is well seen on CT, particularly if bone windows are used. Following intravenous contrast, there is intense enhancement which, particularly in large tumours, may be inhomogeneous.

Acoustic schwannomas are best demonstrated by MRI. This is now the investigation of choice in a suspected acoustic neuroma as it is the most sensitive test for displaying a small tumour. When used with larger tumours, MRI demonstrates the relationship between the tumours and the adjacent brain (Figure 4.23 a, b).

The second most common tumour to arise from the cerebellopontine angle cistern is the meningioma. Both meningiomas and acoustic schwannomas enhance with contrast, and their signal characteristics on MRI may not help in telling the two apart. The shape

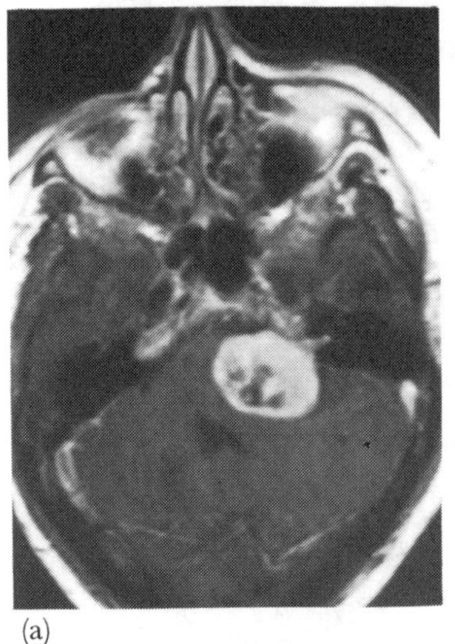

(a)

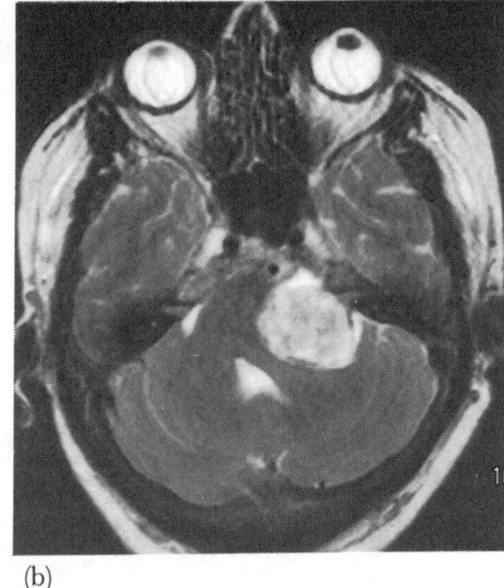

(b)

Figure 4.23 MRI of acoustic neuroma (a) Enhanced T1, note how enhancement extends down the VIIIth cranial nerve within the internal auditory meatus. (b) T2W scan demonstrating distortion of the adjacent pons.

of the two tumours is, however, different. The meningioma characteristically has a broad base spreading along the petrous bone. The acoustic neuroma resembles an ice cream on a cone, with a rounded lesion projecting into the cistern, forming an acute triangle with the petrous bone and extending in a triangular fashion down the internal auditory meatus.

Common paediatric tumours

Posterior fossa
- Pilocytic astrocytoma
- Medulloblastoma
- Ependymoma
- Brain stem glioma

Pineal
- Germinoma
- Teratoma
- Pineoblastoma

Cerebral hemisphere
- Pilocytic astrocytoma
- Fibrillary astrocytoma
- Primitive neuro–ectodermal tumour (PNET)
- Ependymoma
- Ganglioglioma, etc.

Suprasellar
- Optic pathway glioma
- Craniopharyngioma

Intraventricular
- Choroid plexus papilloma

Between 15% and 20% of all primary CNS tumours are found in the paediatric age group. After leukaemia, CNS tumours are the second most common malignancy in children. The types of tumour and where they are sited vary from those in the adult population. Primary tumours in the posterior fossa are particularly common in children between the ages of 4 and 11. Supratentorial tumours are more common in the very young (under 2), and over 12 years of age the incidence of supratentorial tumours begins to equate with that in adults. In children, the lower-grade tumours such as the grade I pilocytic astrocytomas occur relatively frequently, and conversely highly malignant PNETs are also found. Supratentorial masses are more commonly found in the midline than in the cerebral hemispheres.

Posterior fossa tumours

Tumours within the posterior fossa usually present with raised intracranial pressure and hydrocephalus secondary to compression of the fourth ventricle. Radiologically, an attempt is made to differentiate between the relatively benign pilocytic astrocytomas and the malignant medulloblastomas that arise within the cerebellar hemispheres and the intraventricular ependymoma. Gliomas may also arise within the brain stem; these patients present with cranial nerve palsies and long track signs, hydrocephalus only occurring later in the course of the disease.

Pilocytic astrocytoma

Pilocytic astrocytomas (WHO grade I) account for approximately 33% of paediatric infratentorial tumours. The peak incidence is at around 10 years of age, the majority of children affected being between 5 and 15 years old. On CT, the solid component of the tumour (the mural nodule) is hypodense, whilst on MRI it is of low signal intensity on T1W and high signal intensity on T2W images. The mural nodule itself intensely enhances with contrast. The cyst wall does not usually enhance, indicating that it is not lined with tumour cells and represents compressed brain that does not require excision at surgery. Although these tumours are not encapsulated, they do not infiltrate adjacent brain, and the long-term prognosis is therefore excellent.

The most common site for pilocytic astrocytomas is the cerebellar hemispheres, but they may be found elsewhere, where they have a similar radiological appearance. The second most common site is the optic chiasm and hypothalamus, but they may also be found within the brain stem and cerebral hemispheres. The characteristic appearance of these tumours is a cyst with a nodule of enhancing tissue in the wall (Figure 4.24), but some tumours are completely solid.

Medulloblastoma

Medulloblastomas belong to a group of tumours, known as primitive neuro-ectodermal tumours (PNETs). Medulloblastomas are nearly always found in children and are highly malignant, with a WHO grade IV classification.

Cerebellar medulloblastomas are found mainly in children between the ages of 5 and 15. They arise within the roof of the fourth ventricle and classically lie in the midline, compressing the fourth ventricle. The tumour may also be found in early adult life, when it more commonly lies eccentrically within the cerebellar hemisphere.

On CT, these tumours are commonly hyperdense prior to contrast enhancement and show either uniform or irregular

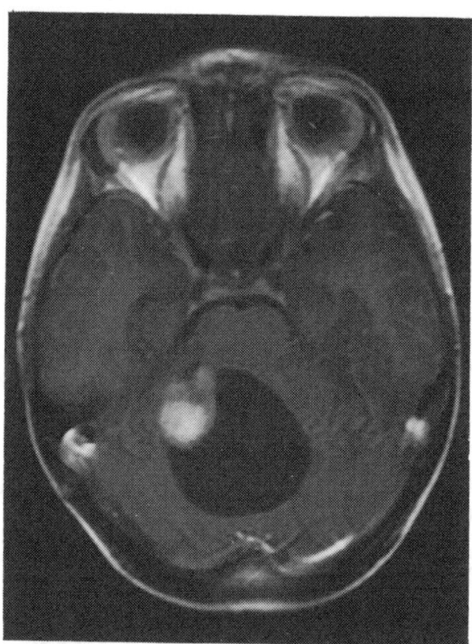

Figure 4.24 Grade I pilocytic astrocytoma. MRI T1 with contrast, note the typical appearance of a cystic lesion with a mural nodule.

enhancement. The latter appearance is partly due to necrosis and cyst formation. There is usually significant peritumoural oedema.

MRI demonstrates the relationship of the tumour to the fourth ventricle better than CT and might help in discriminating between the medulloblastoma and the rare paediatric ependymoma. The tumour is of low signal intensity in relationship to adjacent brain on T1W images and, unusually for a tumour, is of low signal intensity in relationship to CSF on Proton density (PD) and T2W images (Figure 4.25), most other tumours being hyperintense on T2W images. The combination of features, hyperdensity on CT and hypointensity on T2W images can help in discriminating the medulloblastoma from the other common paediatric tumour found in the posterior fossa, the cerebellar astrocytoma.

Supratentorial PNETs are rare and may be found in the cerebral hemispheres or the pineal gland, where they are known as pineoblastomas. They show similar imaging to medulloblastomas on CT and MRI.

CSF seeding

This group of tumours seed early and extensively through the CSF pathways. The presence of metastatic disease alters the prognosis and also the treatment given to the child. Unfortunately, although there has been improvement in life expectancy in this group of

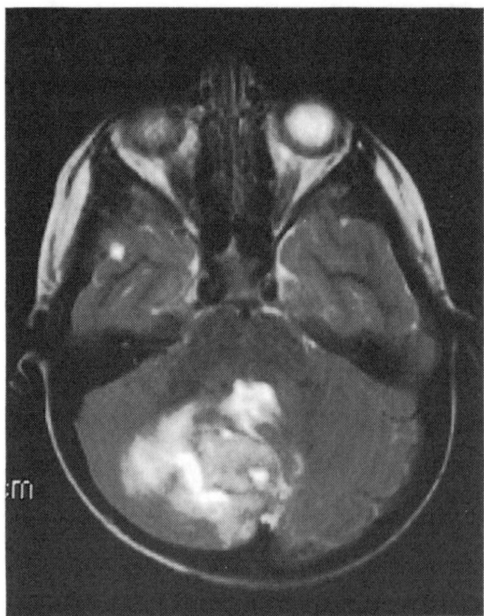

Figure 4.25 Medulloblastoma, T2 showing relatively low signal intensity within the tumour which lies posterior to the fourth ventricle.

patients, the treatment itself may have devastating consequences, particularly upon intellectual development. For this reason, it is imperative that the tumour is staged correctly. This should ideally be done prior to surgery, but adequate imaging is a lengthy procedure. There is usually a rush to get the child to theatre; many children are unable to co-operate for any period of time, let alone for a lengthy investigation, so there are many potential difficulties. A general anaesthetic is usually necessary to perform an MRI of the whole head and spine. T1W images pre- and post-Gd-DTPA administration demonstrate metastatic seeding as fine nodular enhancement over the surface of the brain or spinal cord (Figure 4.26) or within the subarachnoid space in the lumbosacral spine.

Ependymoma

Fourth ventricular ependymomas

These tumours are relatively rare but need to be considered in the differential diagnosis of a child with a posterior fossa mass. They have a relatively low histological grading at presentation. However, because they unfortunately commonly arise from the floor of the fourth ventricle, it is difficult to effect a complete resection, and recurrence at the primary site is therefore relatively common.

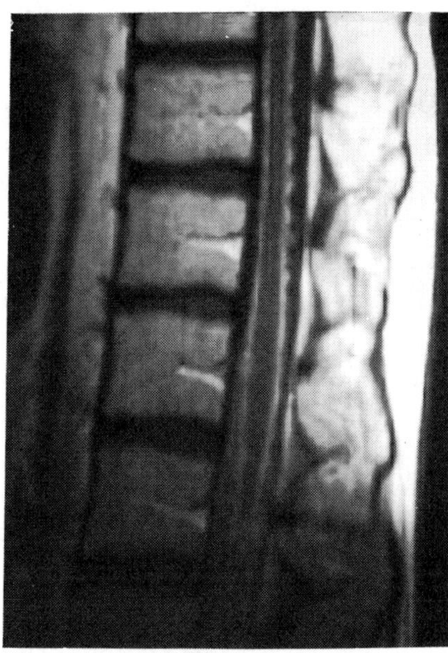

Figure 4.26 Nodular enhancing metastases coating the spinal cord. On this sequence the CSF should be black, the abnormal enhancement has made it white.

On CT, a mass lesion is usually detectable within the posterior fossa in the position of the fourth ventricle, which is partially obstructed, leading to obstructive hydrocephalus of the other three ventricles. The lesion is commonly hyperdense and partly calcified (Figure 4.27). Differentiation from the other two common posterior fossa tumours of childhood, the medulloblastoma and cerebellar astrocytoma, is often difficult.

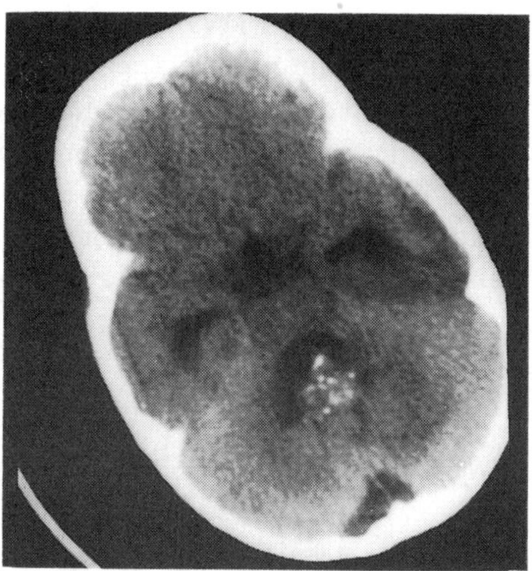

Figure 4.27 CT of ependymoma, patchy calcified mass within the fourth ventricle.

On MRI, the relationship of the tumour to the fourth ventricle is better demonstrated, and this may help in differentiating ependymoma from medulloblastoma. Ependymomas show mixed signal intensity on both T1W and T2W images. This is partly due to the propensity of the tumour to contain small haemorrhages and cysts. Following the administration of intravenous contrast medium, there is irregular and inhomogeneous enhancement.

Ependymomas may also occur in the cerebral hemispheres. Contrary to what one expects, they do not always arise within the ventricle but are commonly found in the cerebral substance itself. A fairly well-defined lesion of mixed attenuation is usually demonstrated on CT, with patchy calcification. The administration of contrast medium shows irregular or rim enhancement. On MRI, the relationship to the ventricular wall is better defined.

Brain stem gliomas

Both the benign pilocytic astrocytoma and the more malignant fibrillary astrocytoma may involve the brain stem.

The histology of the classical pontine glioma is mostly of the fibrillary type. The tumour is usually large at the time of diagnosis but may be difficult to appreciate on CT, where, secondary to bone artefact, the visibility of structures is particularly poor within the posterior fossa. The tumour infiltrates through the pons, causing expansion of this structure, and may only show as slightly lower density on CT in comparison with adjacent brain.

The MRI appearance is diagnostic, making biopsy unnecessary prior to starting treatment with radiotherapy. The tumour is demonstrated as low signal intensity on T1W (Figure 4.28a) and high signal intensity on T2W images (Figure 4.28b). The dramatic expansion of the pons is fully appreciated on MRI. These tumours rarely enhance on CT or MRI unless they have undergone more malignant change. The initial response of the tumours to radiotherapy is usually good, with a reduction in size of the mass and some return of the signal change to normal. They usually rapidly recur within 18 months to 2 years, and at that time enhancement may be seen.

Pilocytic astrocytomas are also found in the brain stem, although not commonly within the pons. The more usual site is in the medulla or midbrain, where an area of intense enhancement is suggestive of the diagnosis. In this situation, an attempt at surgical removal is worthwhile.

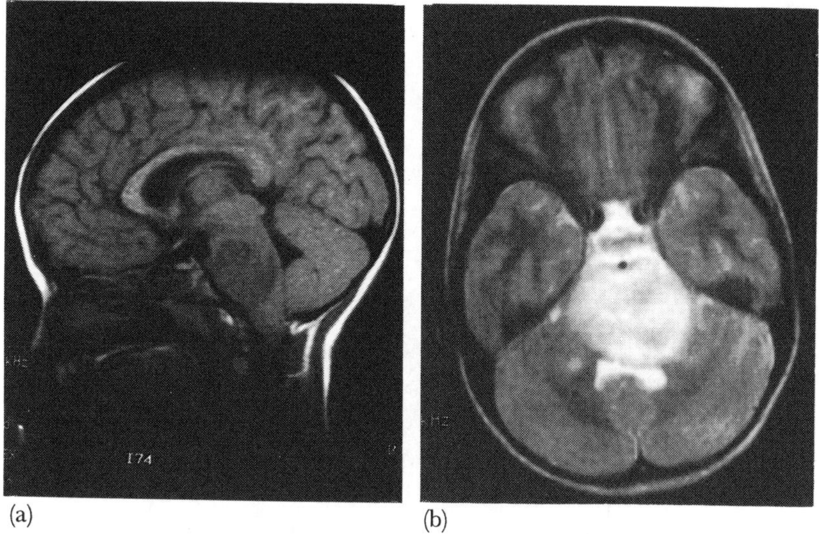

(a) (b)

Figure 4.28 Brain stem glioma, shows altered signal intensity on (a)T1 (b) T2 with expansion of the pons.

Supratentorial tumours in childhood

Primary tumours may arise in the cerebral hemispheres in children, but many supratentorial tumours are midline. These are the optic pathway gliomas, craniopharyngiomas and tumours arising in the pineal gland. Tumours found in the cerebral hemispheres include astrocytomas, ependymomas, PNETs and a group of relatively benign but very rare tumours that arise from neuronal rather than glial cells. All of these supratentorial masses can be difficult to differentiate radiologically, but they may have some radiological features that help in suggesting the diagnosis. Choroid plexus papillomas, which are another paediatric tumour, may, however, be identified by their site of origin within the ventricles and their associated non-obstructive hydrocephalus.

Optic chiasm and hypothalamic gliomas

These are childhood tumours, and if the cell type is pilocytic, they tend to be relatively indolent. There is a genetic predisposition associated with neurofibromatosis type 1. Because of their involvement with the optic pathways and the floor of the third ventricle, total surgical excision is usually hazardous. Like pilocytic astrocytomas elsewhere, they usually enhance intensely. If the tumour is primarily sited within the optic chiasm, spread occurs along the optic nerves and optic tracts (Figure 4.29). Cyst formation occurs, but this is less common than in cerebellar astrocytomas. There may be trapped collections of CSF adjacent to the tumours, which are sometimes named arachnoid cysts. Unfortunately, the more aggressive fibrillary astrocytomas may also occur at this site. Although enhancement is less common with this group and usually not so uniformly intense, there is an overlap in the radiological appearances, making it difficult to differentiate between these two groups radiologically.

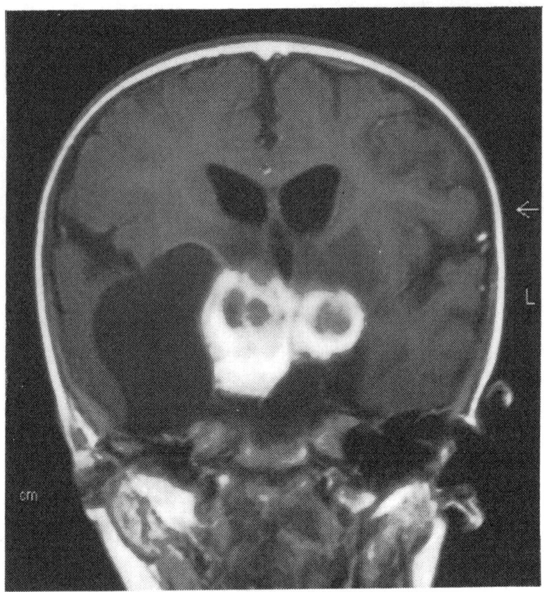

Figure 4.29 Optic chiasm glioma, coronal view.

Craniopharyngioma

Craniopharyngiomas arise within the suprasellar cistern and most commonly occur in children between the ages of 8 and 12. They account for 50% of paediatric suprasellar masses. Radiologically, they have a characteristic appearance on CT. Ninety per cent will be partly calcified, 90% are cystic (Figure 4.30) and they have a solid component that usually enhances. The cystic component is readily identified on MRI but because calcification is poorly identified using this modality, CT scanning may be of value in confirming the diagnosis.

Pineal gland tumours

Pineal tumours are relatively common in children but still only account for 3–8% of intracranial masses in this age group. Two-thirds of tumours are germ cell in origin, the majority of patients being male.

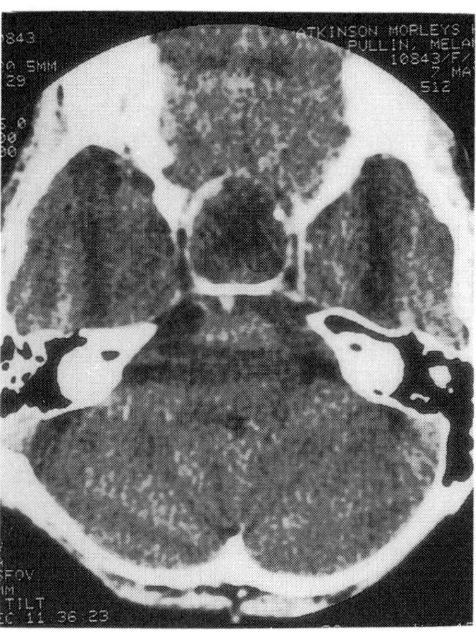

Figure 4.30 Craniopharyngioma, CT. Partly calcified, and cyst mass.

On CT and MRI, these tumours are characterised by their strong enhancement with contrast (Figure 4.31). They commonly spread through the CSF, and the enhancing metastases need to be sought for throughout the intracranial and spinal subarachnoid spaces at the time of diagnosis.

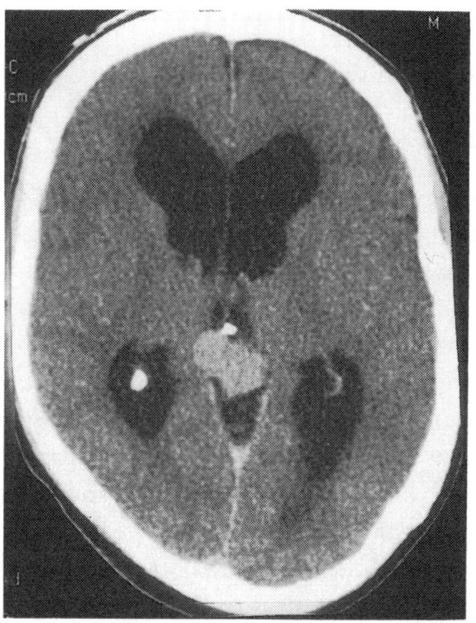

Figure 4.31 Pineal tumour MRI intensely enhancing, well defined mass arising in the pineal gland.

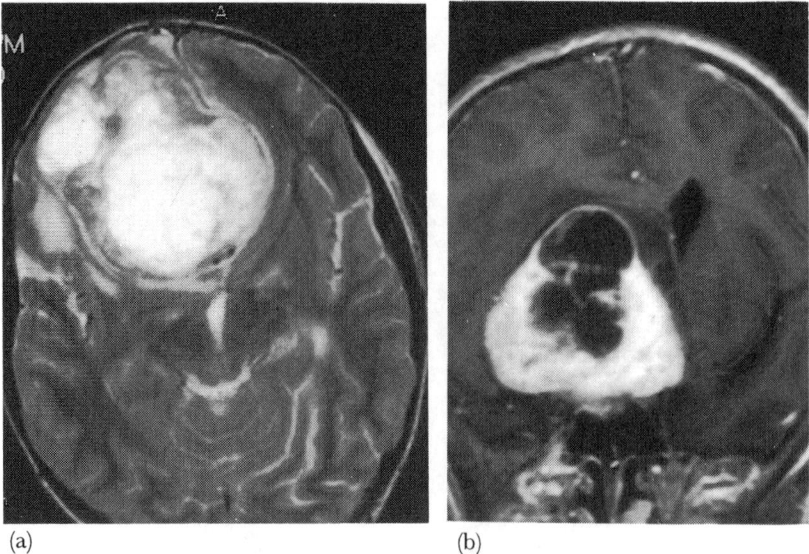

(a) (b)

Figure 4.32 Ganglioneuroma: (a, b) large mass arising in the inferior frontal lobe. Note the asymmetry of the skull vault secondary to remodelling and indicative that the tumour has been present some time.

Teratomas are the second most common pineal tumour and are again more common in male patients. The diagnosis may be suggested if the mass appears partly fatty and heavily calcified on CT (Figure 4.32a).

Primitive neuroectodermal tumours rarely occur in the pineal gland, and if they arise they are known as pineoblastomas. On MRI and CT, they show signal characteristics and attenuation values similar to those of medulloblastomas within the posterior fossa.

Tumours of neuronal origin

Neuronal tumours are exceedingly rare and are outnumbered by tumours of glial cell origin by a factor of 100. Ganglioneuromas and gangliocytomas tend to be peripheral in position and have signal intensities very similar to those of other tumours; in other words, on T1W images they are of low signal intensity, and on T2W images they are of high signal intensity. Some of these tumours enhance, some are cystic and some calcify. In reality, it can be very difficult to differentiate these from the more malignant intrinsic tumours, and biopsy is necessary. Features supporting a more benign histology include the tumour being peripheral in position and expansion of the adjacent skull vault (Figure 4.32a). The patients tend to be in a younger age group. The central neurocytoma has a classical site of origin. It arises from the septum pellucidum and extends into the adjacent lateral ventricles. It is commonly calcified and partly cystic.

Choroid plexus papilloma

Choroid plexus papillomas are found in children under the age of 5, the classical site being the trigone of the lateral ventricle. These are very vascular tumours and are commonly associated with four-ventricular hydrocephalus. The hydrocephalus is not due to obstruction of the ventricular system but is thought to be due to a combination of overproduction of CSF and impaired absorption. If resected, these tumours are potentially curable, but even the more benign ones may recur or seed through the CSF. On both CT and MRI, they are recognised by their ability to enhance with contrast intensely and uniformly. Choroid plexus papillomas are usually surrounded by CSF, and the surface of the tumour has a slightly irregular, frond-like appearance (Figure 4.33). These tumours may rarely be found in young adults, when they are more commonly sited within the fourth ventricle extending laterally through the foramen of Luschka into the adjacent basal cisterns. When they occur in this site, they are generally smaller and less commonly associated with hydrocephalus.

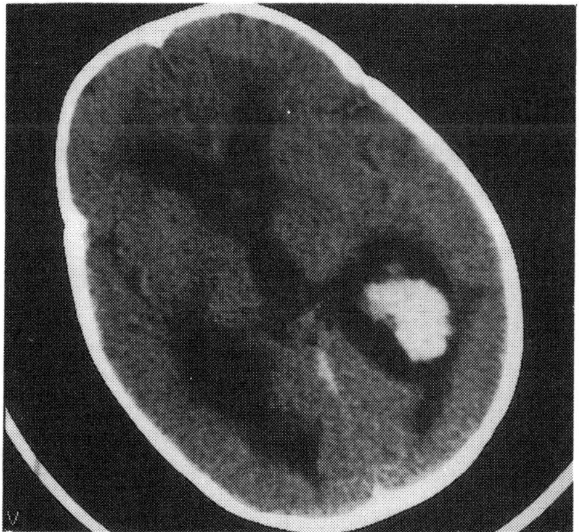

Figure 4.33 Choroid plexus papilloma CT with enhancing mass in the trigone of the lateral ventricle and hydrocephalus.

Tumours of the spine and spinal cord

Spinal cord tumours are classified according to their relationship to the spinal cord and meninges. They fall into three categories:

1. extradural lesions, that is, lesions of the osseous spine, epidural space and paraspinal soft tissues; these tumours compress the dura and spinal cord;

2. intradural extramedullary lesions, which are inside the dura but outside the spinal cord;
3. intramedullary lesions, which are within the spinal cord itself.

MRI is the investigation of choice, myelography being used only in exceptional circumstances.

Extradural lesions

The most frequently encountered neuro-oncological lesion in this category is the metastasis. Primary extradural neoplasms are uncommon and include chordoma, lymphoma and sarcomas.

In the adult population, approximately 50% of all metastases in the spine causing epidural spinal cord compression arise from breast, lung or prostate carcinoma. In children, the primary pathology is usually Ewing's sarcoma, neuroblastoma, osteogenic sarcoma or rhabdomyosarcoma.

In adults, the location of the red bone marrow dictates the site of metastases, and although all vertebral levels can be involved, the lower thoracic and lumbar spine are the most frequently affected sites. The diagnosis of cord compression can be established by MRI, or by myelography when MRI is not available.

The pattern is slightly different in the paediatric population, with metastatic tumour typically invading the spinal canal through the neuroforamen and encasing the spinal cord, causing circumferential cord compression.

On T1W scans, the metastasis replaces fatty marrow, and the metastasis therefore appears as a dark area surrounded by normal high-signal marrow (Figure 4.34a). The T2W scan shows the CSF as white and demonstrates the displacement and compression of the cord (Figure 4.34b).

Intradural extramedullary tumours

Between 80% and 90% of all tumours in this group are nerve sheath tumours and meningiomas (Figure 4.35). This group of tumours are not likely to be encountered in the neuro-oncology setting and will not be discussed further. However, metastases both from CNS tumours and primary tumours elsewhere in the body may occur in this space. They may be demonstrated on myelography, but MRI is the investigation of choice using Gd-DTPA to demonstrate multiple enhancing masses.

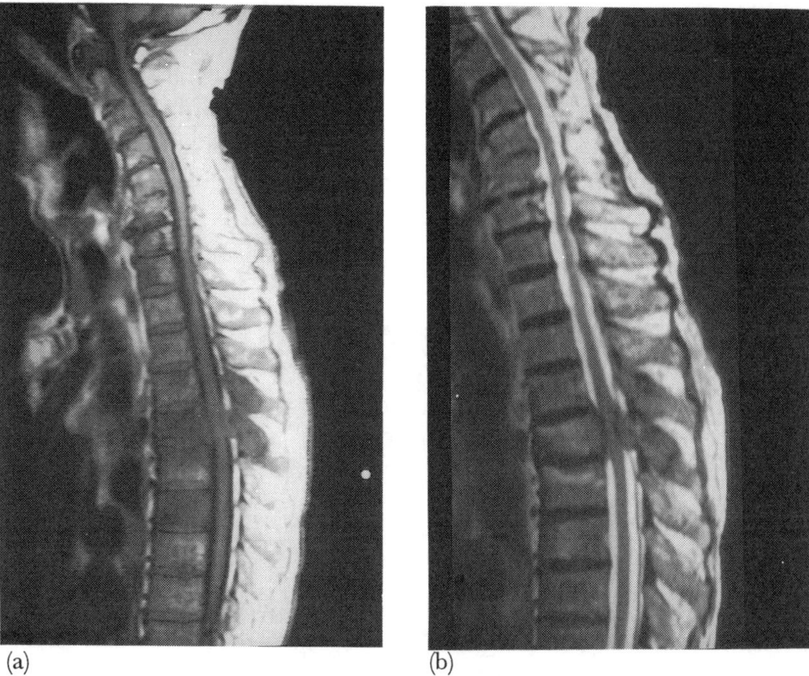

(a) (b)

Figure 4.34 Spinal MR (a) T1W normal marrow is white secondary to fat, when replaced by tumour the marrow appears black (b) T2W, the metastases in the bone are not so clearly seen but the compression of the cord, outlined by white CSF, is better appreciated.

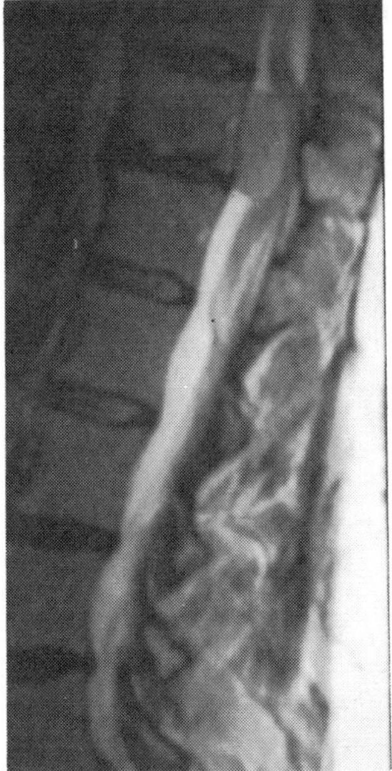

Figure 4.35 Spinal MR, a tumour outlined by CSF is seen displacing and compressing the spinal cord.

Intramedullary tumours

Tumours of the spinal cord are usually malignant, 90–95% being gliomas. Ependymomas and low-grade astrocytomas account for over 95% of spinal cord gliomas. These tumours expand the cord and commonly enhance with contrast (Figure 4.36). Cystic cavities and syrinx may be associated with the solid component of the tumour. Non-enhancement of the cavity walls usually indicates that there is no tumour involvement.

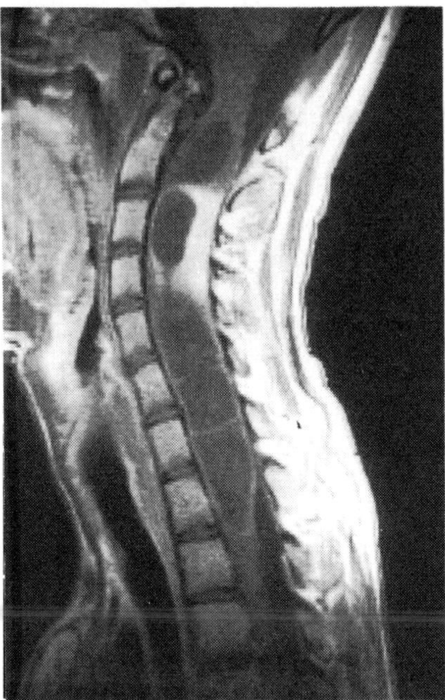

Figure 4.36 Enhancing intramedullary tumour with associated cyst formation leading to expansion of the whole cervical cord.

Ependymomas are usually found in the conus medullaris and filum terminale. Because these tumours are usually slow growing, there is often a long history. The bone adjacent to the tumour may be eroded and seen on plain films and CT as a widened spinal canal with scalloped posterior vertebral bodies and neuroforaminal enlargement with large lesions.

Further reading

The descriptions of tumours in this text are of necessity somewhat limited, and it has been impossible to cover all the complex tumours that involve the central nervous system. There are many good neuroradiology text books, the two listed below both being comprehensive texts.

Osborn A (Ed.) (1994) Diagnostic Neuroradiology. St Louis: Mosby.
Atlas S (Ed.) (1991) Magnetic Resonance Imaging of the Brain and Spine. New York: Raven Press.

Chapter 5
Neurosurgery

Clare Addison and Sarah Shah

Introduction

The diagnosis of a CNS tumour forms the beginning of the next road for patients and their families. Consideration must now be given to the exact location of this lesion and its possible type before further plans can be made. Tumour typing is only accurately achieved by surgery, enabling tissue to be excised and analysed in the laboratory. For many, the prospect of hospitalisation is itself enough without the additional worry of pending brain or spinal surgery and uncertainty over the future (Markin, 1986).

Surgery is offered with three principal aims:

1. to make an accurate diagnosis;
2. to relieve symptoms of raised intracranial pressure;
3. to reduce tumour mass prior to further adjuvant treatment.

The exact nature of the operation on offer will largely be determined by the location of the lesion and the patient's clinical status. In the majority of cases, safe radical excision will be attempted, via a craniotomy that provides the best possible access to the area concerned.

Neurosurgery carries with it a significant risk to the patient of stroke, haemorrhage, neurological impairment and even death, so the decision to go ahead with any neurosurgical option is, unlike the case in more routine surgery, not to be taken lightly. Whilst the collection of a small biopsy sample for analysis can be achieved with relatively minimal risk to the patient, the surgeon may in some cases feel that the location of the tumour lends itself well to a removal attempt or debulking. Understandably, if the tumour can be safely removed, either substantially or even in part, this will be of benefit to the individual, offering in most cases extended life expectancy. A radical excision is likely to achieve no more than a 95% reduction in tumour size because of the inaccessibility of infiltrating cells that peripherally invade normal brain (Kaye, 1997). In situations where the tumour is small and deep seated, very diffuse or located in vital brain (for example, the speech centre), a biopsy sample can be accurately obtained stereotactically (see p. 131).

Nursing staff should be involved in all discussions with patients and carers during this time to ensure continuity and consistency of information, with the aim of avoiding unnecessary misunderstanding and confusion. Medical staff will take time to explain the situation, options and possible risks to the patient, and the nurse must be able to reinforce this accurately if needed. Ultimately, where possible, the decision to proceed surgically must be made by patients themselves, and it is therefore the team's responsibility to ensure that they have received all the necessary information to make this decision in an informed way. If the patient, however, has difficulties with cognition, the next of kin will need to take a more active role, in the best interest of that person.

Preoperative care

> Hospitalisation regardless of disease provokes anxiety, and more so in patients undergoing surgery than in medical patients (Cochran, 1984)

Current extensive nursing literature supports the provision of preoperative information aimed at reducing anxiety levels in the patient (Caunt, 1992; Webb, 1995; Depuis et al, 1996; Martin 1996). Similarly, preoperative visits by theatre nurses have been widely advocated to allay patient anxiety (Carter and Evans, 1996). This information has been shown to have significant positive effect on the level of postoperative pain and the speed of recovery (Radcliffe, 1993). With this in mind, nurses must assess the preoperative needs of each individual patient and family. Major concern for the patient booked for neurosurgery is based around fears of loss of function, the level of current disability, the abilities of the surgeon, the operation itself and the diagnosis (Markin, 1986). There may also be a fear of loss of mental ability, self-control and those characteristics that makes someone a unique individual. Nurses, however, often focus on the specifics of the operation itself, that is, the length of surgery and who will greet the patient in the anaesthetic room, as these queries are more easily discussed and answered (Markin, 1986).

As with all types of surgery, routine patient preparation will be required with respect to medical history, documentation, consent, patient identification, record of allergies, weight and blood testing for standard blood chemistry, haemoglobin level and cross-match. In addition, a baseline neurological assessment must be documented. In some cases, there may be grounds for chest X-ray and electrocardiographic reports. Patients will usually be fasted for a minimum of 4 hours prior to surgery and intravenous fluid replacement considered if this period is to be extended.

Up until the late 1970s, skin preparation for cranial surgery involved total head shaving. Head shaving is now minimal, involving only the immediate area, and is in some cases not performed at all (Braun and Richter, 1995). However, the psychological implications for the patient needing even a small quantity of hair shaved for a procedure is not to be underestimated. Nurses must show sensitivity to this issue when preparing patients for cranial surgery and allow them time to express their concerns and fears; this will often be the beginning of a progressive alteration in their body image (see Chapter 10). It is important preoperatively, where possible, for the patient to wash his or her hair and have a bath or shower. Once anaesthetised, the patient's skin will be prepared further.

Routine dress code includes theatre gown, name bands, anti-embolus stockings (McConnell, 1990) and an absence of jewellery, make-up and nail varnish. It is the nurse's responsibility to ensure that all the preoperative requirements have been met and verified as correct before administering any premedication.

It is customary for the anaesthetist to visit patients preoperatively to assess their suitability for anaesthesia and prescribe the relevant premedication. Premedication in the field of neuroanaesthesia is rarely sedative, in order to avoid masking neurological change. Anecdotally, however, patients expect a premedication to make them feel sleepy and relaxed. The nurse must therefore ensure that patients are aware of the expected effects of their medication. Patients will in most cases have been commenced on oral steroid therapy (for example, dexamethasone) which acts by suppressing cerebral oedema (see Chapter 8). Dexamethasone will be administered through to the postoperative phase where, after a few days, it is usually reduced. Prophylactic antibiotics such as cefuroxime may be used either intraoperatively as a single dose or postoperatively as a short course (Holloway et al, 1996).

Where appropriate, partners or other family/friends should be involved throughout the preoperative phase. Patients themselves will often be reassured by their presence, and the carer will also feel included and supported (Raleigh et al, 1990). It has been suggested that educating significant others may help to relieve anxiety, enabling them first to cope with all that is going on, and second to provide the necessary support when the patient is discharged home or moves on for further treatment (Webb, 1995). A partnership between patient and nurse often develops when the patient is allowed to manage his or her own anxiety by adopting an active role in the preparation for surgery and recovery (Salmon, 1992). It might be that a visit to the operating theatre or recovery room is appropriate, as may be a meeting with the nurse who will be caring for them in recovery. It should, however, be noted that some patients because of fear, cognitive difficulties or personality, may not express any interest in what is to happen to them, and this must be understood and respected.

The trip to the operating theatre can be a frightening one for many patients. In some cases, it may therefore be appropriate for a calming family member or friend to accompany them to the anaesthetic room as a support and encouragement. Where this is not possible, the nurse must fulfil this role as well as ensuring a detailed hand-over to theatre staff.

With the majority of neurosurgical procedures lasting in excess of 2 hours, particular care and attention must be paid to the positioning of the patient and protection of pressure areas. For supratentorial and anterior fossa surgery, the patient will usually be placed in the supine position, whereas for occipital or posterior fossa surgery, either the prone or the sitting position will be used, allowing access to the back of the head. Spinal access will be achieved with the patient in the prone position. Positioning can be time-consuming but is essential before the surgeon can proceed with the actual surgery.

Neurosurgical techniques

Surgical intervention is considered to be the first step in the treatment of a brain tumour (Broderson, 1995). As already discussed, surgery cannot always result in a total removal of the tumour microscopically, but it can accomplish a removal of all the visible tumour (Broderson, 1995).

The surgical technique offered depends on the type and location of the tumour. A provisional diagnosis of the type and precise location of the tumour is obtained through a detailed patient history and diagnostic radiology in the form of CT and MRI scans (see Chapter 4). However, a precise diagnosis of the type of tumour can only be made through an analysis of tissue samples, which can only be obtained through surgery.

Advances in medical technology, particularly in the case of diagnostic radiology, have enabled surgeons accurately to locate brain tumours, separating them from oedematous surrounding tissue. As a result, the surgeon is able to make smaller bone flaps to access the tumour, resulting in less exposure of normal brain (Conie, 1991).

Surgical techniques in the treatment of brain tumours can be divided into:

- open surgical techniques;
- minimally invasive techniques.

Open surgical techniques

Surgery for brain tumours using open techniques is dependent on the location of the tumour. Open techniques are divided into the:

- supratentorial approach;
- infratentorial approach;
- trans-sphenoidal approach;
- skull base approach.

Supratentorial approach

Supratentorial approaches are used to treat brain tumours above the tentorium, in the frontal, temporal, parietal and sometimes occipital lobes of the brain, as well as tumours within the lateral and third ventricles. The supratentorial approach is often performed through a craniotomy.

Craniotomy

A craniotomy can be performed in the area of the frontal, temporal, parietal or occipital bones, or a combination of any of these areas, in order to reach the area of the brain where the tumour is situated (Kane, 1991). A craniotomy, performed for tumours located above the tentorium, that is, supratentorial tumours, is an opening through the skull to expose the underlying structures. The surgeon makes holes (burr holes) in the skull over the area of brain where the tumour is located and then cuts between these burr holes to form a bone flap. The bone flap is either a free flap that is removed during the course of the operation and replaced at the end of the procedure, or a flap that is not completely removed but remains secured to an adjacent muscle; this is known as an osteoplastic flap. The use of an osteoplastic flap is preferable because it still has an intact blood supply, which supplies the bone flap with the nutrients essential for wound healing. A free flap is used when the brain is very oedematous, allowing for additional postoperative swelling to take place without detriment to the patient (Kane, 1991). If the tumour involves the bone, the bone flap may be removed altogether and may be replaced at a later stage with an artificial flap made of titanium.

Infratentorial approach

Infratentorial approaches are used to treat brain tumours located below the tentorium in the region of the brain known as the posterior fossa. These tumours can be found in structures such as the cerebellum, brain stem, fourth ventricle and cerebellopontine region.

The infratentorial approach is often performed through a craniectomy.

Craniectomy

A craniectomy is performed to access tumours that are located below the tentorium, that is, infratentorial tumours. A craniectomy involves the surgeon making a burr hole in the skull over the area of brain where the tumour is located. The bone adjacent to the burr hole is then removed in small pieces. This technique enables the surgeon to remove the thick bone that lies over the posterior fossa region and prevent injury to the underlying venous sinuses. At the end of the procedure, the removed bone can be replaced with autologous bone graft chips (Broderson, 1995). Other surgeons prefer not to replace the removed bone chips but instead believe that effective wound closure is gained by closure of the dura, being maintained by the strong muscles of the neck.

Some surgeons, however, prefer to remove posterior fossa tumours via a craniotomy approach, replacing the bone flap, instead of a craniectomy approach.

There are other surgical approaches to remove tumours located in areas of the brain that are not accessible through craniotomy or craniectomy.

Trans-sphenoidal approach

Trans-sphenoidal approach enables the excision of pituitary gland tumours, located deep in the structure of the brain. This approach is generally preferred to craniotomy unless there is a large expansive lesion, as a craniotomy approach necessitates the need for significant frontal lobe retraction to access the area. The trans-sphenoidal approach is via the nose, involving a submucosal dissection along the nasal septum; then, by removing part of the wall of the sphenoid sinus, the bony floor of the sella turcica, which houses the pituitary gland, is reached. The bony floor of the sella turcica is then opened and the tumour can be removed. Nasal packs are placed postoperatively to prevent haemorrhage and to realign the nasal mucosa to the septum. These packs are removed after 48–72 hours.

Skull base approaches

Rare tumours of the base of the brain are difficult to access and excise, so surgical techniques devised to reach these tumours are very intricate and painstaking. These surgical techniques are often performed in conjunction with ear, nose and throat or occasionally maxillary facial surgeons. Because of the limited view associated with surgery for skull base tumours, it is necessary for the surgeon to use a surgical microscope in order to avoid damage to vital structures (Broderson, 1995). There are many possible approaches for the excision of skull base tumours. Examples of surgery to remove skull base tumours are given below.

Transoral approach

The transoral route enables accessibility to tumours including rare tumours such as clival chordomas that are situated anterior to the base of the brain and at the cervicomedullary junction. This approach involves removal of the arch of the first cervical vertebra C1 (otherwise known as the 'atlas'), the odontoid peg and the clivus, providing access to the front part of the brain stem.

Le Forte maxillotomy

The Le Forte maxillotomy is a modification of the transoral approach. This approach uses the knowledge of facial fractures known as 'Le Forte', in particular the Le Forte I fracture. The Le Forte I fracture occurs horizontally in the area of maxilla just above the teeth. A maxillotomy is made along the line of the Le Forte I fracture in this area of thinner facial skeleton. It gives a greater exposure to skull base tumours in a longitudinal plane but does not increase exposure of the tumour in a lateral plane.

Other skull base techniques involve combined supra- and infratentorial approaches with removal of the mastoid and/or petrous bone.

Minimally invasive techniques

As stated earlier, one of the main aims of surgery is to establish an accurate diagnosis of the tumour. This can only be achieved through removal of tumour tissue samples for analysis. Removal of tumour for diagnosis can be made through the open surgical techniques that have been already discussed or through closed surgical techniques.

Minimally invasive techniques include:

- burr hole for biopsy (stereotactic and freehand);
- image-guided craniotomy using a frameless stereotactic technique;
- endoscopic techniques.

A burr hole is described as ‘a hole made in the cranium using a special drill’ (Hickey, 1996). The use of a burr hole technique to obtain a tissue sample for histology enables the surgeon to make a surgical incision that is smaller in comparison with that of a craniotomy. As a result, manipulation of the brain is minimised and post-operative cerebral oedema is reduced (League, 1995).

Burr hole for biopsy

Stereotactic technique

Obtaining tumour tissue samples via a burr hole technique requires precise and accurate location of the tumour itself. This can be achieved with the use of CT scans and MRI, a computer programme and a stereotactic system, which together provide precise information on the co-ordinates of the tumour.

The stereotactic system comprises a frame that is fixed onto the patient’s head with pins that are screwed into the skull (see Figure 5.1). The frame has visible markings or calibrations on its structure. The stereotactic frame, along with the CT and MRI scans and the computer programme, generates three-dimensional coordinates of a specific point, enabling the surgeon to remove a sample of tumour with minimal damage to the surrounding brain tissue.

Stereotaxy has enabled surgeons to obtain samples from areas of the brain that were previously considered inaccessible and too dangerous to biopsy using a freehand technique. Stereotactic biopsy is performed for multiple lesion tumours, tumours lying deep within the brain and tumours located in the brain stem, thalamus and cerebellum (Broderson, 1995).

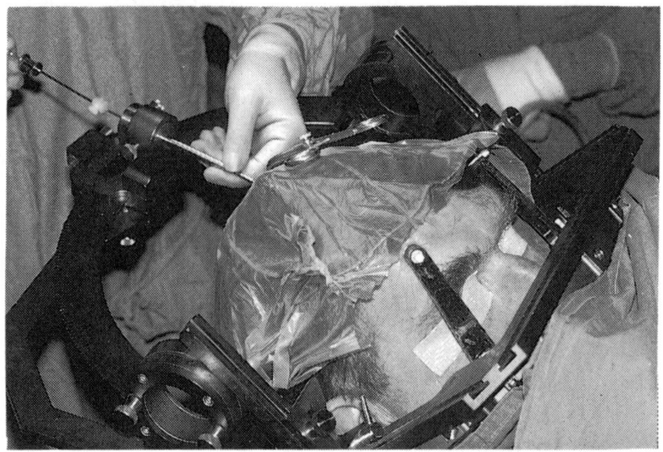

Figure 5.1 Stereotactic frame being utilised to undertake stereotactic guided biopsy.

Freehand technique

For superficial tumours lying close to the surface of the brain, particularly in areas of the brain that are easily accessible, a biopsy can be obtained through a burr hole using what is termed a 'freehand technique'. This freehand technique uses information from the CT or MRI. Freehand technique is not as accurate as stereotactic biopsy, and its use is dependent on the location of the tumour and the skill of the surgeon. For example, superficial tumours located in the non-dominant hemisphere can be biopsied using the freehand technique.

Image-guided craniotomy using a frameless stereotactic technique

Recent advances in stereotaxy have produced a technique called frameless stereotaxy. The technique follows the same principles as the conventional stereotactic technique, but the stereotactic frame is replaced by skin markers such as vitamin E capsules or lead discs. These markers produce high signals when imaged with CT or MRI and provide the computer with accurate information to form a three-dimensional image of the head.

Frameless stereotaxy dispenses with the cumbersome, restrictive frame of conventional stereotaxy, enabling modified craniotomies to be performed for the resection of small superficial tumours and ensuring minimal damage to the surrounding brain tissue (Thomas and Kitchen, 1994; Broderson, 1995).

Endoscopic techniques

Endoscopy is also used as a surgical technique in neurosurgery. Endoscopic techniques are currently used to treat hydrocephalus resulting from aqueduct stenosis and to remove colloid cysts. Endoscopic techniques may in future play a greater role in the removal of tumours such as ependymomas.

Stereotactic radiosurgery

Stereotactic radiosurgery is a relatively new approach used to treat primary malignant brain tumours (Ward-Smith, 1997). It involves closed skull destruction of a defined intracranial tumour using radiation in a single session (Kondzidka and Dade-Lunsford, 1993). It is a closed, bloodless operation using neuroradiological and computer technology to define and locate the tumour. Then instead of a scalpel, high-dose radiation is used to halt tumour growth (Ward-Smith, 1997). The tumour is not completely destroyed or removed but instead undergoes necrosis over a period of time. The patient is awake for the procedure and does not need to have a general anaesthetic, which itself carries risks (see Chapter 6).

Surgery of tumour types

Astrocytoma and glioblastoma

Astrocytomas, including glioblastomas, which are the most malignant type, can occur anywhere in the CNS. If located in the cerebral hemispheres, they can be reached through frontal, parietal, temporal or occipital craniotomy. However, surgery for these tumours is limited to the fact that they are rarely encapsulated and may not be restricted to one area of the brain. Posterior fossa astrocytomas are common in children.

Oligodendroglioma

These tumours occur mainly in the frontal lobe of the brain, so excision is via a frontal or frontoparietal craniotomy.

Meningioma

Meningiomas arise from the dura and are most commonly found along the falx cerebri or the sphenoid wing. These tumours can be excised via a frontal or frontotemporal craniotomy. Petroclival meningiomas sometimes require a combined supratentorial and infratentorial approach.

Ependymoma

These tumours are more common in children but can be found in adults. They are commonly found in the fourth ventricle and are accessed via a posterior fossa craniectomy.

Brain stem glioma

These are excised via a posterior fossa craniectomy.

Medulloblastoma

Medulloblastoma is the most common type of solid tumour in children. It is rare in adults, accounting for only 1% of CNS tumours (Grossman, 1991). As it is a tumour that arises in the cerebellum, it is excised via a posterior fossa craniectomy.

Haemangioblastoma

This benign tumour is found in the cerebellum and is excised via a posterior fossa craniectomy.

Acoustic neuroma

This benign tumour is accessed via a retromastoid craniectomy.

Surgery for spinal tumours

Surgery on the spine can be performed to remove or debulk spinal tumours. Tumours of the spine are classified according to their relationship to the dura and the spinal cord itself. The tumour can be either extradural or intradural, that is, located outside or inside the dura. Intradural tumours can be further divided into intramedullary or extramedullary, that is, within or outside the spinal cord. The majority of spinal tumours are extradural (78%), only 4% being located within the spinal cord itself (intramedullary tumours). Primary spinal tumours are very rare, the majority being metastatic tumours. The common primary sites for metastatic spinal tumours are the breast, lung, prostate and kidney (Lindsay et al, 1991). The thoracic region of the spine is the most common place for metastatic spinal tumours.

Surgery, which is the common form of treatment for spinal tumours, aims to remove the tumour and thus relieve the symptoms of spinal cord compression. The surgical approach for spinal tumours depends on whether the tumour is extradural, intradural or intramedullary. For metastatic tumours, a laminectomy approach is not appropriate as metastatic tumours often involve the vertebral body. The approach therefore involves spinal decompression via an anterior vertebral approach. The vertebral body is removed and then, by using a bone graft or metal fixators, the vertebral column is fused and supported. For intradural tumours, a laminectomy approach can be used to excise the tumour (Lindsay et al, 1991).

Other perioperative techniques

Cavitron ultrasonic surgical aspirator

An ultrasonic aspirator uses ultrasonic energy to break up and remove tumour tissue without unnecessary damage to the surrounding brain tissue. The surgeon uses the cavitron ultrasonic surgical aspirator (CUSA) in conjunction with a surgical microscope. The CUSA is a valuable technique, rapidly removing large amounts of most types of brain tumour and resulting in a reduction in operating time (Grossman, 1991; Broderson, 1995).

Cortical mapping

Cortical mapping is an intraoperative technique used in the resection of tumours that are located in, or adjacent to, the motor, sensory and language areas of the cerebral cortex.

The patient remains awake during the procedure if cortical mapping involves the dominant hemisphere, enabling any alterations in the patient's speech and/or motor movement to be detected. The aim is to remove the maximum amount of tumour with the least damage to these vital areas, thereby minimising postoperative deficits.

If the non-dominant hemisphere is being mapped, the patient can be observed while sedated, but not paralysed under a general anaesthetic (Broderson, 1995).

Electrophysiological monitoring

If the tumour arises from or involves a cranial nerve, intraoperative monitoring of the function of this cranial nerve can limit intraoperative damage and preserve postoperative cranial nerve function. The best example of electrophysiological monitoring is in surgery to remove an acoustic neuroma where cranial nerves V, VII, VIII and IX are involved in the dissection of the tumour and are at risk of damage (Broderson, 1995).

Preoperative embolisation of tumour

Preoperative embolisation has been found to be useful in the resection of vascular tumours such as meningiomas. Preoperative embolisation reduces the blood flow to one or more of the arteries that supply the tumour. As a result, intraoperative bleeding is greatly reduced, thus facilitating tumour resection (Broderson, 1995).

Postoperative management

The aims of postoperative care of patients undergoing surgery for brain tumours are:

- to ensure a safe recovery from a general anaesthetic;
- to detect complications that can arise as a result of intracranial surgery;
- to prevent secondary damage to the brain that can result from intracranial surgery.

Postoperative management of neurosurgical patients is a continual process that begins in the intensive care unit (ICU) or recovery area and continues during their stay on the surgical ward until they are ready for discharge.

Postoperative management for the first 12–24 hours

Following intracranial surgery, the patient spends the first 6–24 hours in the ICU or high-dependency unit (HDU). This is to ensure close monitoring and the detection of any complications, as well as a quick post surgical recovery.

Specialist knowledge of the functions of the CNS assists the nurse to perform an accurate assessment of the neurological status of the patient and facilitates the early detection of postoperative deficits and complications (Kane, 1991). However, patient care needs the co-operation of the whole multidisciplinary team (see Chapter 9). The early detection and prevention of complications necessitates the possession of both assessment skills and teamwork. Combined multidisciplinary teamwork will maximise the patient's recovery from intracranial surgery (Arsenault, 1985).

The postoperative care of patients following surgery for brain tumours is based on the potential problems and complications that may arise as result of the surgery. Planning and implementing the nursing care for these patients should be individual and can take the form of a nursing care plan. The following discussion of postoperative care will look at potential problems that can arise, but it is important to remember that each patient is an individual and therefore not every patient will develop all of these problems. Postoperative care will be discussed in terms of the potential problems and complications that can arise following neurosurgery.

Neurological deterioration

Following intracranial surgery, the patient is at risk of raised intracranial pressure, which is reflected in an altered conscious level. Raised intracranial pressure results from the development of postoperative cerebral oedema, haematoma, infarction, tension pneumocephalus or hydrocephalus (more common following posterior fossa surgery). Although cerebral oedema normally occurs at 24–96 hours post-surgery, the patient may already have preoperative oedema, which is exacerbated by manipulation of the brain during surgery (Arsenault, 1985).

Depending upon the site and nature of the operation, bleeding post-surgery may be intracerebral, intraventricular, subarachnoid, sub- or extradural. Pre-existent coagulopathies from underlying liver disease or drug therapy such as warfarin will enhance bleeding potential. Disturbance of the cranial contents during tumour excision may lead to the rupture of tiny bridging vessels or small arterioles in the tumour bed, which may gradually ooze as the patient's systemic blood pressure increases postoperatively. Intracranial bleeding is clinically manifested by progressive vomiting, increased drowsiness and developing or worsening focal deficits. Clinical findings are confirmed by urgent CT scan and may result in the patient's rapid return to theatre.

Hydrocephalus occurs as a result of a disruption of the CSF flow through the ventricular system and subarachnoid space. It may already be present preoperatively in the presence of fourth ventricular compression from tumour, or as a result of surgery causing aseptic meningitis in the posterior fossa region (Kauffman and Carmel 1978). Hydrocephalus is clinically manifested as a gradual progressive deterioration of conscious level, confirmed by the presence of enlarged ventricles on CT scan. Some patients will need the surgical insertion of an external ventricular drain or ventricular peritoneal shunting device to relieve this pressure.

The risk of cerebral infarction depends on the location and nature of tumour. There is always a small chance of surgical trauma to blood vessels within the operative field, which could result in an area of ischaemia. This risk could be enhanced if the tumour is very vascular or encasing a blood vessel. The occurrence of an infarct can be seen in either a gradual or a sudden deterioration in neurological status. As infarction takes several hours to develop, confirmation on CT scan is only after a period of time where there is visual evidence of microscopic necrosis.

Tension pneumocephalus occurs when air enters the head during neurosurgical procedure or through a CSF leak. The air can collect in the tissue itself or be trapped in the dural layers during surgical closing. As the air warms from room to body temperature, the gases expand, acting as any intracerebral mass does by increasing intracranial pressure. The presence of air is confirmed on CT, and treatment might involve needle aspiration or repair of the CSF leak. The inspiration of high-concentration oxygen can be beneficial in treating pneumocephalus. High-concentration oxygen displaces soluble gases such as nitrogen from the intracranial space. The oxygen is then reabsorbed and utilised.

The aim of nursing care is to monitor the patient's neurological function in order to detect any change and ensure prompt management. Assessment of the patient's neurological function is therefore carried out half-hourly for the first 6 hours post-surgery, reducing in frequency as the patient's condition dictates. Once the patient has returned to the ward, neurological assessment is performed every 2–4 hours. Following the removal of supratentorial tumours, patients are nursed with the head of the bed elevated at between 30 and 45 degrees (Kane, 1991). This aids venous drainage from the head, thus reducing intracranial pressure.

The patient can potentially develop seizures as a result of manipulation of the brain during surgery. This aspect of postoperative nursing care will be discussed below.

In cases where spinal surgery is indicated, the postoperative complications of haemorrhage and oedema remain, but the clinical indications would involve deterioration in spinal motor and/or sensory function. With this in mind, nurses will assess each limb's motor and sensory function regularly, reporting changes in levels of sensation and movement as appropriate (see Chapter 2). There may also be interference with bowel, bladder and respiratory function, depending on the spinal level involved (see Chapter 1).

The location of the tumour and the subsequent surgery may result in cranial nerve dysfunction. Cranial nerve dysfunction can lead to problems such as facial palsy, swallowing impairment, a reduced gag reflex or a depressed corneal reflex. The aims of nursing care are to help patients to understand the implications of cranial nerve dysfunction, to enable them to optimise function and achieve independence in activities of daily living, and to ensure patient safety. Patients with a facial palsy that affects closure of the eyelid may require regular eye care to prevent infection and corneal damage. Patients who have swallowing difficulties are in danger of aspirating food and fluids. They may require an assessment of their swallowing function to be performed by a speech therapist and may require supervision with eating and drinking.

Respiratory depression

The neurosurgical patient is at risk of developing potential respiratory depression primarily as a result of the general anaesthetic but also potentially because of raised intracranial pressure. The location of some tumours, particularly those in the posterior fossa region, may result in postoperative respiratory depression. The aims of nursing care following intracranial surgery are thus to ensure a safe recovery from the anaesthetic, to maintain a patent airway and to prevent hypoxia. Assessment of respiratory function is carried out half-hourly for the first 6 hours post-surgery, reducing the frequency to hourly for the next 6 hours. The assessment of respiratory function, including the rate, depth and pattern of respiration, is an important indicator of raised intracranial pressure.

During the immediate postoperative period, analysis of the patient's blood gases can be performed to determine the levels of carbon dioxide and oxygen. Serum oxygen levels should be maintained above 10 kPa (kilopascals) in order to ensure that the brain is provided with sufficient levels of oxygen essential for normal cellular metabolism. The brain normally has a high metabolic rate, requiring oxygen and glucose for normal function. The brain uses 20% of the total oxygen used by the body (Tortora and Anagnostakos, 1987). The serum carbon dioxide partial pressure should be kept below 6.5 kPa. High levels of carbon dioxide act as a cerebral vasodilator, accentuating any pre-existing cerebral oedema. Respiratory assessment is particularly important for patients following surgery for the removal of a posterior fossa tumour as the respiratory centre is located in the posterior fossa region. Surgery within this area can cause respiratory problems as a result of oedema or haematoma.

After the immediate post-surgical period, optimal respiratory function and maintaining a patent airway is a multidisciplinary team approach involving nursing staff and physiotherapists. Correct positioning of the patient, physiotherapy and suctioning all contribute to maintaining a patent airway.

Cardiovascular instability and arrhythmias

The patient who has just undergone intracranial surgery is potentially at risk of cardiac instability as a result of the general anaesthetic, the surgical technique itself and postoperatively raised intracranial pressure. Cardiac instability can also arise as a result of surgery for tumours within the posterior fossa region as this is in close proximity to the vasomotor centre. Surgery within this region can cause oedema or a haematoma and subsequent cardiac problems.

A patient undergoing neurosurgery may develop cardiac arrhythmias associated with the presence of blood in the CSF (Hickey,

1996). Raised intracranial pressure has itself been shown to cause ECG changes. The changes that have been identified are T wave inversion, S–T depression and S–T elevation (Syverud, 1991). However the dramatic changes to blood pressure and pulse rate, namely, an increase in blood pressure and bradycardia, known as the Cushing response, are only seen with severe and often irreversible intracranial pressure (Lindsay et al, 1991).

The aim of nursing care is to ensure a safe recovery from surgery and to monitor and detect any cardiac arrhythmias or instability. Assessment of cardiac function, which includes the monitoring of blood pressure, heart rate and rhythm, is initially performed half-hourly for the first 6 hours post-surgery, reducing in frequency to hourly for the subsequent 6 hours.

Pain

Pain is often experienced following many surgical techniques, not least neurosurgery, although pain following craniotomy is generally thought to be minimal (Quiney et al, 1996). Pain following craniotomy can result from the stretching of the falx, dura or blood vessels within the cranial vault (Schofield, 1995). Stretching of these structures can occur during surgery and also postoperatively as a result of raised intracranial pressure due to cerebral oedema or haematoma.

The aim of nursing care is to ensure that the patient is comfortable and pain-free. An assessment of the patient's pain, taking note of the location, duration and severity, is a vital aspect of nursing care. The use of a pain tool is important in assessing a patient's pain, gives the patient more control over its management and can also be used to evaluate the effectiveness of analgesia. The use of a pain tool provides consistency in the management of pain, which is important for all patients (Schofield, 1995).

Administering analgesics is the prime method of pain relief to ensure patient comfort, but it is not the only method. Other techniques, such as relaxation, correct positioning, providing a restful environment and communication to reduce anxiety, should be considered. In order to maintain patient comfort, analgesia must be administered regularly to avoid peak and trough pain. Traditionally, patients undergoing neurosurgery are not given an opioid analgesic for fear of the depressant effect on their conscious level; however, some authors feel that it is appropriate to administer opioid analgesics in order to achieve effective pain relief (Stoneham and Walters, 1995). Pain management is important not only to maintain patient comfort, but also to prevent increases in intracranial pressure. Ineffective pain management can potentially contribute to raised intracranial pressure through increased cerebral blood flow as a result of stress and anxiety.

Dehydration and poor nutrition

Following neurosurgery, the patient is at risk of dehydration as a result of a number of factors. The patient may have a depressed conscious level post-surgery. The location of the tumour can affect the patient's ability to eat and drink; that is, tumours in the posterior fossa region can result in damage to the cranial nerves that are responsible for swallowing and hence affect the patient's ability to swallow. The patient may feel also nauseous as a result of the anaesthetic. These will all affect the patient's ability to eat and drink normally. Surgery to remove tumours in the frontotemporal region can cause pain and oedema of the temporomandibular joint and impede the patient's ability to eat and drink.

Fluid and electrolyte imbalances are not uncommon following intracranial surgery (Arsenault, 1985). Severe disturbances in electrolyte balance can occur with diabetes insipidus. This is a condition that can often occur following surgery near or to the pituitary gland and results in the production of very dilute urine and high serum sodium levels. Diabetes insipidus must be treated to prevent dehydration. It is important to maintain adequate hydration for neurosurgical patients as dehydration can reduce the blood flow to the brain and thereby reduce the supply of essential oxygen and nutrients required for cellular rejuvenation and repair following surgery.

The aim of nursing care is to ensure that the patient maintains an accurate and adequate fluid balance. This includes monitoring both fluid intake and urine output. Following a general anaesthetic, patients are also at risk of urinary retention. Urinary output is an important indication of the fluid status of a patient. Monitoring the urinary output can indicate whether the patient is dehydrated or is developing diabetes insipidus. The urinary output should be greater than or equal to 0.5 ml/kg body weight per hour. In order to achieve adequate fluid intake, oral fluids should be supplemented with intravenous fluids until the patient is able to drink. Anti-emetics should be administered to treat postoperative nausea and vomiting.

The post-surgery patient requires adequate nutrients to promote wound healing and cellular repair. Therefore encouraging the patient to commence oral nutrition as soon as possible is important. If the patient cannot eat normally, nasogastric enteral feeding may be needed.

Wound care

As with any surgical wound, the immediate post-operative period requires close observation of the wound for signs of oozing, swelling, redness and tenderness. Following cranial surgery, patients may have a head bandage covering the site, making close inspection difficult. In this case, the dressing must be closely observed for staining, which should be marked and monitored. There may in some cases be a wound drain in place, which should remain patent for 24–48 hours. Spinal wounds are often only covered with a light dressing, making observation easier, although early movement of the patient to make this possible will require effective analgesic cover.

After 48 hours, the risk of secondary haemorrhage decreases, but the risk of infection remains until the wound is properly healed. Any interference with dressings should be aseptic and kept to a minimum. Intraoperative antibiotics may have been administered as they have been shown to reduce the incidence of postoperative wound infection (Holloway et al, 1996). Suspected infection should be reported immediately and wound swabs sent for culture.

Neurosurgery for tumour will usually require the opening of the dura, leaving a small risk of a CSF leak. Any leaks must be investigated promptly as they could potentially result in bacteria entering through the dura and leading to meningitis. It may be that the leak resolves itself, although more commonly the siting of a lumbar drain is needed to ease the pressure. If the leak is persistent, there may be no option other than to take the patient back to theatre for dural repair. A suspected CSF leak can be confirmed by testing for the presence of glucose in the discharged fluid.

Any sutures or wound clips are generally removed after 5–7 days providing the wound is dry. However, because of head movement, wounds in the posterior fossa region require 7–10 days healing.

It should not be forgotten that efficient wound healing is aided by good nutritional status.

Seizures

Seizures, be they focal or generalised, can occur in patients with a brain tumour (see Chapter 3). This is due to altered neuronal excitability, which leads to abnormal electrical discharges from the brain cells themselves. For many of these patients, it is their presenting symptom; for others, it comes as a complication of the neurosurgery that they have endured, especially from tumours in the parasagittal and parietal regions. Postoperative seizures may also result from underlying intracerebral haemorrhage so CT scanning would be considered. The nature of the seizures themselves is variable and dependent upon the extent of the abnormal electrical discharge.

In the event of this being limited to a single area of one hemisphere, the seizure will be localised in nature with little effect on conscious level (simple partial). If this should spread to the other hemisphere, impaired consciousness is often a feature (complex partial). Clinical features of these seizures are related to the area of the brain involved. For example, frontal lobe epilepsy involving the motor cortex might cause jerking in one part of the body, indicating a focus in the contralateral motor cortex. If this spreads along a motor pathway, for example from thumb to hand to arm, it is described as a 'Jacksonian march' after the 19th-century neurologist John Hughlings Jackson.

Generalised seizures involve extensive parts of both hemispheres and are manifested in absence attacks, myoclonic jerks, and tonic-clonic, tonic or clonic seizures. In absence seizures, there is an abrupt cessation of activity during which the patient is unresponsive to the external environment.

Tonic-clonic seizures begin with a loss of consciousness, although some people do experience some warning signs or an aura. There is often a cry or grunt as air is forced through the closed vocal cords as the thoracic muscles initially contract on the commencement of the tonic (rigid) phase, the person may bite down on his or her tongue or lip, causing bleeding, breathing ceases during this stage and cyanosis with pupil dilatation often occurs. The bladder and less commonly the bowel may also empty at this point. In the clonic (jerking) phase that follows, violent rhythmic jerking of face and limbs is seen. Profuse sweating, hypertension and tachycardia also occur. Breathing is irregular and often stertorous, with excessive salivation. Postictally, stupor and confusion are common, and the person may sleep for several hours (Gumnit, 1995; Hickey, 1986).

Tonic seizures display a loss of consciousness and subsequent rigidity, which may result in severe injuries, whereas clonic seizures are characterised by abrupt jerking movements without a preceding tonic phase.

Principles of management during a generalised seizure are to protect the patient from accidental injury and to maintain a patent airway. If it is possible to turn the patient onto his or her side during the seizure, this should be done. A pillow may be placed under the patient's head, and all obstacles should be removed from the area to prevent accidental injury, but no attempt to restrain the patient should be made as clonic seizures can be so violent that fractures can result if restraint is applied.

The nurse should stay with the patient and provide reassurance. Where possible the area should be cleared of non-essential personnel and the patient's privacy maintained. No attempt to insert oral airways or mouth guards should be made during the seizure. If possible, oxygen should be given. As the observation of seizures provides vital information the nurse should record a full account of any witnessed seizure to include information such as whether the patient experienced an aura or warning, how the seizure began and proceeded, what part of the body was involved, whether there were any changes in pupil size or reactivity, whether any incontinence occurred, whether loss of consciousness was evident and how long each phase lasted. The post-ictal (after the seizure) stage is also important: did the patient sleep, was there any other behavioural change, did any weakness persist after the seizure (Todd's paralysis), and if so, how long did this last? The patient should always be placed in the recovery position after the seizure stage has finished, and patency of the airway remains the nurse's priority. Any medication given and its effect should also be recorded.

A generalised seizure lasting for longer than 3 minutes or a sequence of seizures with no recovery noted is termed 'status epilepticus' and constitutes a medical emergency that requires medical assistance to prevent brain damage secondary to hypoxia, oedema or metabolic effects such as acidosis. If the patient's airway is compromised, a cardiac arrest call is indicated. Excessive seizures produce extremely elevated levels of creatine kinase, which may result in renal failure. Hypoglycaemia should also be avoided by careful monitoring. The administration of first-line anticonvulsants such as rectal diazepam or intravenous diazemuls may be required in doses titrated to the seizure response. Benzodiazepines will depress respiration, and this should be closely monitored.

The long-term management of seizures is achieved ideally by mono-anticonvulsant drug therapy and aims to render the patient fit-free. The drugs most commonly used are phenytoin and sodium valporate, but in the event of poor control a combination of drugs may be required. Therapeutic drug levels may need monitoring to achieve the optimum anticonvulsant effect (see Chapter 8).

As with all aspects of care for neuro-oncology patients, the emphasis is on symptom control and quality of life. The nurse must fully appreciate the additional social implications that seizures create and instigate the necessary support for these patients. The social stigma associated with epilepsy is well documented, also affecting the individual's ability to drive and in some cases to continue in employment (Jacoby 1993). This enforced change in lifestyle, stigmatisation, altered body image and anxiety for the future may have a profound negative effect on motivation and coping strategies.

Impaired mobility

A reduction in the level of independence because of cerebral oedema or underlying cranial or spinal pathology can leave the patient exposed to the risk of constipation, deep vein thrombosis, pressure areas, muscle wasting and stiffness. There are many preventative nursing measures that can be offered to reduce this risk and aim to promote independence and maintain safety. An assessment tool, for example the Waterlow score (Waterlow, 1991), can be used to establish a patient's vulnerability to the complications of immobility. Skin integrity is preserved by regular turning and careful positioning (Barbenel, 1990). Active and passive exercises, elevation of the affected limbs and the wearing of anti-embolus stockings by immobile patients can help in the prevention of deep vein thrombosis and maintain tone and a normal range of movement (McConnell, 1990). A sound nursing knowledge of the causative factors of constipation, namely dehydration, a low-fibre diet and reduced mobility as well as the effect of opioid and codeine-based analgesics, is essential in its prevention (see Chapter 8).

Cognitive changes

Cognitive changes following craniotomy are well documented and refer to higher functions such as memory, abstract reasoning, perception, orientation and thought (Hannegan, 1989). If surgery is in the frontal region of the brain or the patient experiences cerebral hypoxia or oedema, these changes can be permanent. A transient alteration in thought processes may also result from stress or anxiety and be a side-effect of medication, for example with dexamethasone. Nurses must be aware of this potential complication and report any changes in intellectual ability, memory, concentration and personality so that the cause may be investigated. Family members will almost certainly need much support and reassurance to cope with cognitive changes and may even benefit from more formal counselling (see Chapter 11). There is evidence that it may in some cases lead to depression and altered family dynamics, although these changes frequently resolve partially or even completely within 6 months of surgery (Hannegan, 1989).

Occupational therapists and clinical psychologists have an important part to play in the assessment and management of these problems.

Communication difficulties

With the location of two speech centres in the dominant parietal and frontal lobes, and hearing being in the temporal lobes, there is a significant possibility of some form of communication difficulty postoperatively, be it deafness or receptive or expressive dysphasia. This can be a major frustration for all concerned as it may prevent patients communicating their needs effectively. Nurses must take time to speak slowly and concisely and, where appropriate, be prepared to use other communication aids, for example picture boards or pen and paper. Speech therapy referrals are essential in the assessment of difficulties and the co-ordination of measures to aid the problem.

Psychological support

The psychological care given to patient and family prior to surgery must be actively continued into the postoperative phase. Once again, the emphasis is on individualised care meeting the specific needs of that patient and his or her family. They generally value opportunities to discuss the surgery with the medical staff concerned and appreciate regular progress updates and involvement in decision-making where appropriate. Nurses may need to make time to repeat and go over information that has been given by other staff members, ensuring that it has been fully understood and answering any questions patients may have. If the family feel supported and involved, they will be able to provide a higher level of support for the patient. However, in situations of severe distress, it may be appropriate to invite other professionals, for example the hospital chaplain or patient counsellor, to provide more formal support and counselling (see Chapter 11).

Ongoing care

The ongoing management of a patient, be it in another hospital setting or at home, should be carefully planned well in advance. This necessitates close liaison between patients, their carers and all multidisciplinary personnel to ensure that individuals' needs are met (see

Chapters 9 and 12). The specialist role of a neuro-oncology nurse specialist provides a smooth transition to adjuvant treatment.

Immediate post-surgical rehabilitation

Nursing care of patients has, over recent years, become holistic and patient focused. Rehabilitation is now part of that holistic nursing care, although it had previously been an aspect of nursing care that had been neglected. Rehabilitation should not be seen as an aspect of nursing that is left to tertiary centres but should be incorporated into the holistic care of the patient beginning at the time of admission (Davis, 1985).

Rehabilitation is described as being a process of relearning. It assists individuals to attain a meaningful life within their boundaries of an altered level of health by maximising their capabilities. The goals of rehabilitation (Davis, 1985; Sherburne, 1986) are:

- to improve the quality of life;
- to optimise physical abilities;
- to promote health preservation;
- to decrease health service costs.

In order to ensure that the goals of rehabilitation for a patient are met, a multidisciplinary approach is essential. Some of the professionals involved include medical staff, nursing staff, physiotherapists, speech and language therapists and occupational therapists (see Chapter 9). Some patients may require the support of social workers.

Patients undergoing neurosurgery are very susceptible to profound changes in their lifestyles. The location of the tumour and subsequent surgery may leave the patient with a permanent physical disability or transient cognitive changes that prevent the patient from returning to his or her normal life. This may have a significant impact upon the family, particularly if the patient is the main source of financial income. The most frequent concerns mentioned by patients prior to neurosurgery include loss of function, return of function and socioeconomic implications arising as a result of diagnosis and treatment (Markin, 1986). These concerns are not just restricted to the patients themselves but may be the source of a great deal of stress for the rest of the family. Fulfilling the goals of rehabilitation is therefore important for the whole family, including the patient, in order to reduce stress and enable the whole family unit to attain a meaningful life post-diagnosis and treatment.

In order to optimise patients' physical abilities post-surgery and ultimately improve their quality of life once treatment is completed, early rehabilitation is imperative. Physiotherapists and speech therapists working in conjunction with nursing staff can optimise physical abilities and speech impairments for patients following neurosurgery. However, as rehabilitation is a process of relearning, patients' emotional and cognitive state must also be considered in order to meet the objectives of rehabilitation.

Rehabilitation should also involve the family regardless of whether the patient returns home or remains in hospital. The family are often the main carers once the patient returns home, but they can also be involved in the nursing care of patients whose condition prevents them returning home. Involvement in the rehabilitation process can reduce the family's feelings of helplessness and stress and also provide them with some degree of control over a very stressful situation.

Conclusion

The role of the neurosurgical nurse is multifaceted, beginning at the patient's admission and ending on his or her transfer to other centres for adjuvant treatment or on discharge home. The range of professional skills and expertise needed is varied, from welcoming patients to the ward, attending to their physical and psychological requirements throughout all stages of care, to monitoring for any signs of neurological deterioration post-surgery. As such, nurses need substantial insight into not only the potential complications of the surgery, but also their role in recognising these problems and how best they are clinically managed. The nurses' skill in continuous neurological observation is crucial in the early identification of any deterioration, enabling problems to be dealt with without delay.

References

Arsenault L (1985) Selected postoperative complications of cranial surgery. Journal of Neurosurgical Nursing 17(3): 155–63.

Barbenel J (1990) Movement studies during sleep. Cited in Bader DL (Ed.) Pressure Sores – Clinical Practice and Scientific Approach. London: Macmillan, 249–60.

Braun V, Richter H (1995) Shaving the hair – is it always necessary for cranial neurosurgical procedures? Acta Neurochirurgica 135(1–2): 84–6.

Broderson J (1995) Surgical options for brain tumour treatment. Critical Care Nursing Clinics of North America 7(1): 91–102.

Carter L, Evans T (1996) Preoperative visiting: a role for theatre nurses. British Journal of Nursing 5(4): 204, 206–7.

Caunt H (1992) Preoperative nursing intervention to relieve stress. British Journal of Nursing 1(4): 171–2, 174.

Cochran R (1984) Psychological preparation of patients for surgical procedures. Patient Education and Counselling 5: 153–8.

Conie J (1991) Advances in Neurosurgery. British Journal of Theatre Nursing 1(3): 26–7.

Davis A (1985) Focus on rehabilitation in the acute care setting: the role of the neuro clinical nurse specialist. Journal of Neurosurgical Nursing 17(3): 244–6.

Depuis M, Barnier P, Givens H (1996) Brain surgery – a guide for patients and their families. Axon (September): 5–8.

Grossman R (1991) Principles of Neurosurgery. New York: Raven Press.

Gumnit R (1995) The Epilepsy Handbook: The Practical Management of Seizures. 2nd edn. New York: Raven Press.

Hannegan L (1989) Transient cognitive changes after craniotomy. Journal of Neuroscience Nursing 21(3): 165–70.

Hickey J (1986) Neuromedical and Neurosurgical Nursing. Philadelphia: JB Lippincott.

Hickey J (1996) The Clinical Practice of Neurological and Neurosurgical Nursing, 4th edn. Philadelphia: JB Lippincott.

Holloway K, Smith K, Wilberger J, Jensek J, Giguere G, Collins J (1996) Antibiotic prophylaxis during clean neurosurgery – a large multi-centre study using Cefuroxime. Clinical Therapeutics 18(1): 84–94.

Jacoby A (1993) Quality of life and care in epilepsy. In Chadwick D, Baker G, Jacoby A (Eds) Quality of life and quality of care in epilepsy: Update 1993. Royal Society of Medicine. pp 66–78.

Kane D (1991) Practical points in the postoperative management of a craniotomy patient. Journal of Post Anaesthesia Nursing 6(2): 121–4.

Kauffman H, Carmel P (1978) Aseptic meningitis and hydrocephalus after posterior fossa surgery. Acta Neurochirurgica 44: 179–96.

Kaye A (1997) Essential Neurosurgery, 2nd edn. New York: Churchill Livingstone.

Kondzidka D, Dade-Lunsford L (1993) Stereotactic radiosurgery for brain tumours. In Salcman M (Ed.) Current Techniques in Neurosurgery. Philadelphia: Current Practice.

League D (1995) Interactive, image-guided, stereotactic neurosurgery systems. AORN Journal 61(2): 360–70.

Lindsay K, Bone I, Callander R (1991) Neurology and Neurosurgery Illustrated, 2nd edn. Edinburgh: Churchill Livingstone.

McConnell E (1990) Clinical do's and don'ts: applying antiembolism stockings. Nursing 20(10): 92.

Markin D (1986) Preoperative concerns of the patient undergoing craniotomy. Journal of Neuroscience Nursing 18(5): 275–8.

Martin D (1996) Pre-operative visits to reduce patient anxiety: a study. Nursing Standard 10(23): 33–8.

Quiney N, Cooper R, Stoneham M, Walters F (1996) Pain after craniotomy. A time for reappraisal? British Journal of Neurosurgery 10(3): 295–9.

Radcliffe S (1993) Preoperative information: the role of the ward nurse. British Journal of Nursing 2(6): 305–9.

Raleigh E, Lepczyk M, Rowley C (1990) Significant others benefit from preoperative information. Journal of Advanced Nursing 15: 941–5.

Salmon P (1992) Anxiety and stress in surgical patients. British Journal of Hospital Medicine 48(9): 531–3.

Schofield P (1995) Using assessment tools to help patients in pain. Professional Nurse 10(11): 703–6.
Sherburne E (1986) A rehabilitation protocol for the neuroscience intensive care unit. Journal of Neuroscience Nursing 18(3): 140–5.
Stoneham M, Walters F (1995) Post operative analgesia for craniotomy patients: current attitudes among neuroanaesthetists. European Journal of Anaesthesiology 12: 571–5.
Syverud G (1991) Electrocardiographic changes and intracranial pathology. Journal of the American Association of Nurse Anaesthesia 59(3): 229–32.
Thomas D, Kitchen N (1994) Minimally invasive neurosurgery. British Medical Journal 308: 126–8.
Tortora G, Anagnostakos N (1987) Principles of Anatomy and Physiology, 5th edn, p 310.
Ward-Smith P (1997) Stereotactic radiosurgery for malignant brain tumours: the patient's perspective. Journal of Neuroscience Nursing 29(2): 117–22.
Waterlow J (1991) A policy that protects. Professional Nurse 6(5): 258–64.
Webb R (1995) Preoperative visiting from the perspective of the theatre nurse. British Journal of Nursing 4(16): 919–25.

Further reading

Black P, Rossitch E Jr (1995) Neurosurgery – an Introductory Text. Oxford: Oxford University Press, Chapters 7 and 11.
Kaye A (1997) Essential Neurosurgery, 2nd edition. London: Churchill Livingstone.

Chapter 6 Radiotherapy

Douglas Guerrero

Introduction

CNS tumours are generally infiltrative by nature, and some prove inaccessible to surgical intervention because of their position. Even with those CNS tumours which are amenable to surgery, complete excision may prove impossible. Tumours can recur even when apparently completely excised and may require further treatment with radiotherapy. The success of a radical course of radiotherapy depends on the tumour type, its extent and its sensitivity to radiation. The limitation to the successful use of radiotherapy is the radiation tolerance of surrounding normal brain structures (Brada and Robinson, 1991).

The aim of this chapter is to give nurses an understanding of CNS irradiation as well as to increase their knowledge of potential problems related to treatment and how best to support patients and families throughout radiotherapy.

Ionizing radiation

Cell sensitivity to irradiation varies with the stage of the cell cycle. Cells in mitosis (somatic cell division) and early synthesis are more vulnerable to ionising radiation damage than are those in late synthesis and early G2 (a second resting phase or premitotic phase).

Ionising (X-ray and gamma ray) radiation induces a variety of damage to intracellular Deoxyribonucleic acid (DNA). Cellular damage can manifest itself in a variety of forms, that is, by single- or double-stranded breaks of the double helix, by chemical alterations of the bases of DNA without necessarily causing any breakage of a strand, or by accelerating the process of apoptosis (programmed cell death). Single-stranded breaks are often completely repaired, but double-stranded breaks either may be repaired in a mutated form or are unrepairable, resulting in cellular death at the next mitotic phase. Mutated changes cause a permanent change in genotype that is transmitted to future generations of cells (Bomford et al, 1993).

Tumour radiosensitivity

The aim of any course of radiotherapy is to destroy tumour cells. Radiation cannot discriminate between normal and malignant cells, and potentially causes damage to all living cells. However, normal cells have a greater capacity for recovery than malignant cells. Radiotherapy is most effective in those cells which are well oxygenated. This is because, for radiotherapy to be more effective, it needs to convert oxygen into hydroxyl ions (highly reactive radicals). Body cells with a low oxygen concentration are said to be 'hypoxic'. Tumours may be hypoxic because they outgrow the local blood supply and/or because of their genetic make-up.

'Radiosensitive' is the term applied to cells that are injured or destroyed by ionising radiation. Intrinsic cellular radiosensitivity of tumours affects the patient's prognosis. Radiosensitivity of CNS tumours varies; for example, a single radiation dose of 2 Gy (Gray) will kill less than 50% of glioma cells compared with 70–80% of cells derived from lymphoma, germ cell tumours or embryonal tumours (Brada and Ross, 1996).

Normal brain tissue radiation tolerance is approximately 60 Gy at ≤2 Gy per fraction. The spinal cord level of tolerance is 2% risk of damage at 50 Gy. A Gy is the absorption of one joule (a unit of energy) per kilogram by material exposed to ionising radiation (Glance et al. 1986).

Fractionation

Conventional external beam radiotherapy is used either in the form of localised irradiation with two, three or four beams, or with extended field techniques treating the whole brain and the entire cranial axis (Brada and Thomas, 1995). Beams are directed towards the target volume (defined as the planning target volume, PTV), which normally exceeds the tumour volume (gross tumour volume, GTV). Radiation beams are aimed at the PTV from different directions in order to minimise the dose to normal CNS tissue (Figure 6.1).

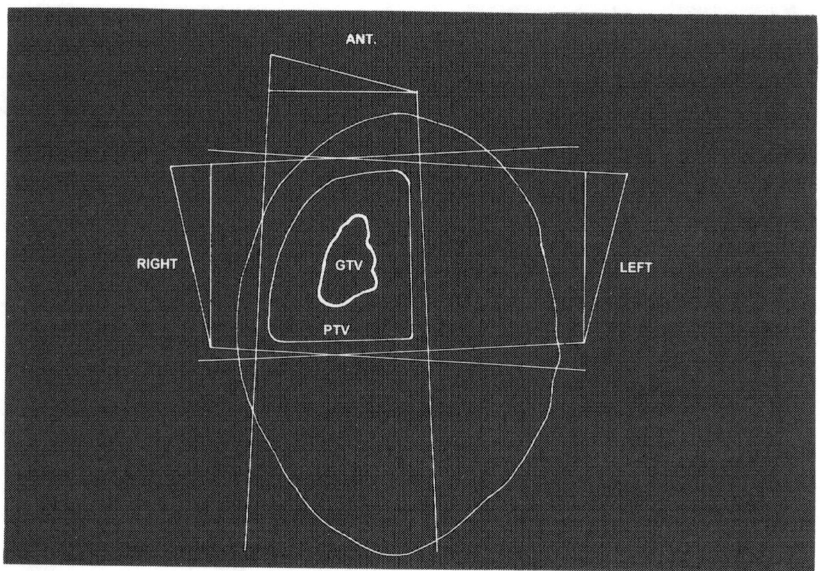

Figure 6.1 Direction of radiation beams.

In CNS tumours, the dose of radiation given is usually close to normal tissue tolerance. As such, radical irradiation is not generally repeated for fear of precipitating tissue breakdown (radionecrosis) (Bomford et al, 1993).

Radiotherapy technique

External beam technique

CNS tumours are generally irradiated by the external beam technique. External beam radiotherapy, also known as teletherapy, is given in the form of X-rays and electrons that are generated by linear accelerators (Linac) (Figure 6.2) and gamma rays emitted from a cobalt source.

External beam radiotherapy can comprise whole brain and spinal cord (craniospinal axis), whole brain or localised radiation. These can be given singly or in combination.

Craniospinal axis

Craniospinal axis irradiation is used to treat those brain tumours which have a high risk of spread via cerebrospinal pathways. While the rationale is currently under scrutiny in patients with cranial ependymoma, primary cerebral lymphoma and cranial germ cell

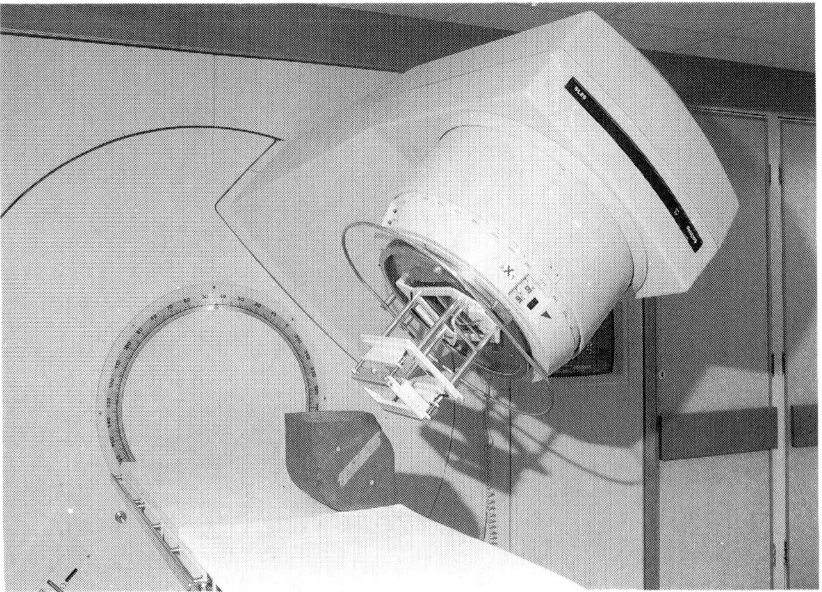

Figure 6.2 Linear accelerator (Linac).

tumours, it is of proven benefit in patients with medulloblastoma and other primitive neuroectodermal tumours (PNETs) (Jefferies et al, 1998). The 5 year survival rates with surgery alone for medullobiastoma were 10–20%, and this has increased with radiotherapy to 50–60% (Brada and Robinson, 1991). Oopheropexy (re-positioning of the ovaries) is sometimes undertaken prior to craniospinal axis irradiation. This is a surgical procedure and, although not standard practice, can prevent irradiation of the ovaries, which may result in sterility.

Whole brain and localised irradiation

The majority of studies utilising whole brain irradiation in malignant gliomas were performed prior to the availability of CT and MRI scanning (see Chapter 4). Modern-day CT and MRI provide much-improved information on the definition of the target volume (Leibel and Sheline, 1990). Thus most centres have adopted localised external beam treatment techniques with margins of 2–5 cm beyond the region of enhancement or low density on CT (Brada and Ross, 1996) (Figure 6.3).

Based on the presumed localised nature of glial tumours, attempts have been made to increase the dose to the tumour whilst minimising the dose to normal brain using the technique of intersti-

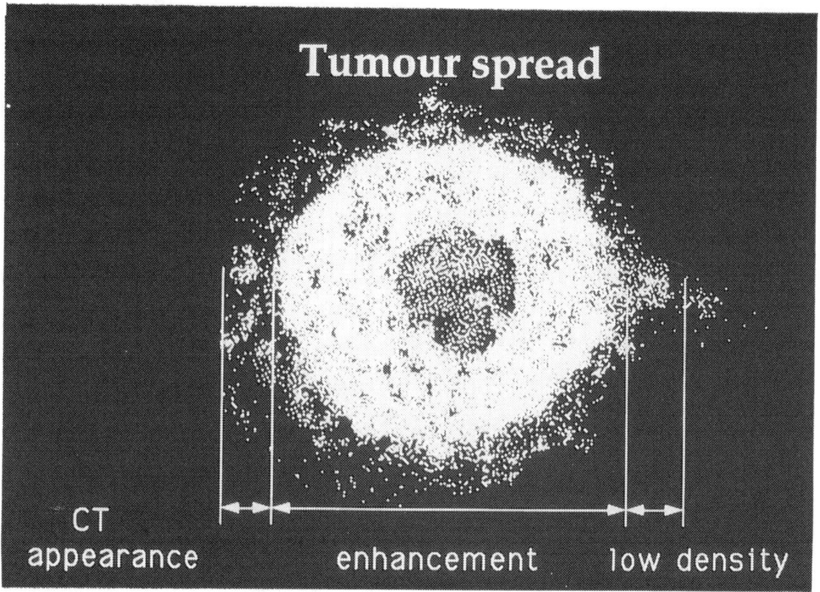

Figure 6.3 CT appearance of tumour spread.

tial radiotherapy or stereotactic external beam radiotherapy (Brada and Ross, 1996).

Interstitial radiotherapy

Interstitial radiotherapy (brachytherapy) involves the implanting of radioisotopes directly into the tumour bed. This form of treatment emits a continuous low-dose-rate radiation to the tumour and adjacent surrounding cells. Radioisotopes used in the therapeutic treatment of CNS tumours include ^{125}iodine and ^{192}iridium.

While the policy of interstitial irradiation may potentially prolong survival, it is a highly interventionist policy with a need for a number of operative procedures. In patients with high-grade glioma, where the treatment is not curative, it is questionable whether such a policy has a real benefit in terms of quality of life (Brada and Ross, 1996).

Fractionated stereotactic radiotherapy and single-fraction radiosurgery

Fractionated stereotactic radiotherapy and single-fraction radiosurgery increase the precision of tumour localisation and treatment (Brada and Graham, 1994). Fractionated stereotactic radiotherapy can be used for the treatment of recurrent gliomas and metastatic tumours. Single-fraction radiosurgery is used in the treatment of arteriovenous malformations (AVMs). Fractionated stereotactic radiotherapy is often used as an adjunct to other radiotherapy modalities, with the exception of AVM, for which single-fraction radiosurgery tends to be the treatment of choice. When given as a single-fraction radiosurgery for AVM, the dose given is much higher.

There is much controversy regarding the appropriate use of stereotactic radiotherapy. Therefore clinical studies comparing stereotactic with conventional methods of irradiation should be undertaken in order to identify its true role in the treatment of CNS tumours.

Radical radiotherapy

Treatment intended to cure the patient is known as radical radiotherapy. All CNS tumours, depending on their histology, can potentially be treated or cured with radical radiotherapy. In radical radiotherapy, the radiation dose given is up to tissue tolerance. As the radiation dose given is high, some side-effects are unavoidable, but these are accepted as an inevitable part of attempted cure (Griffiths and Short, 1994).

In the treatment of CNS tumours, radical radiotherapy includes daily or alternative fractionation schedules.

Daily

External beam radiotherapy is the most common method of radiotherapy treatment for CNS tumours. The patient is usually treated daily (Monday to Friday) over a period of 5–6 weeks to a total dose of 55–60 Gy.

Alternative fractionation schedules (hyperfractionation/accelerated radiotherapy)

Hyperfractionation refers to a fractionation schedule in which the number of fractions is increased to two or three daily treatments but the overall treatment period is maintained.

In accelerated radiotherapy, the fraction size and number remain the same but the treatment is given two or three times per day, thus reducing the overall treatment time. For example, in neuro-oncology, the patient receiving accelerated radiotherapy would, instead of having the treatment over 30 days and receiving 1.8 Gy per day, have the treatment twice a day for 17 days (34 fractions), receiving a total daily dose of 3.23 Gy.

Hyperfractionated schedules allow dose escalation, whereas accelerated radiotherapy aims to control the rapid repopulation of tumour cells. Accelerated radiotherapy in CNS tumours is usually confined to patients with high-grade gliomas, under 60 years of age and with a good performance status. This is because high-grade gliomas generally have a poor prognosis and the long-term risk of such treatment on potentially curable tumours is at present unknown.

Palliative radiotherapy (hypofractionated)

The aim of palliative radiotherapy is to improve symptoms and enhance the patient's overall quality of life. In treating CNS tumours with palliative radiotherapy, the actual treatment dose is lower in order to lessen side-effects (Thomas et al 1994).

Efficacy of treatment

Radiotherapy can effect a cure in the majority of patients with cranial germinoma and in a proportion of patients with medulloblastoma/PNETs, and produces excellent tumour control in patients with pituitary adenoma and craniopharyngioma. However, in patients with high-grade glioma, treatment is palliative in nature, although a radical dose may be used to maximise tumour control.

General treatment approaches

Glioma

In patients with a high-grade glioma, the treatment options are daily, twice daily (accelerated) or palliative (hypofractionated) radiotherapy given by the external beam method. As the prognosis for this group of patients is generally poor (median survival 40–50 weeks), treatment should be decided on the basis of disability as severe deficits are unlikely to improve. The expected benefits of treatment must be discussed carefully with the patient and family, and the patient's quality of life must not be compromised.

The role of radical radiotherapy in patients with asymptomatic low-grade glioma remains controversial. Whilst radiotherapy may be a useful treatment to inhibit tumour growth in progressive symptomatic disease, there is currently no clear survival benefit for immediate compared with delayed radiotherapy. Most centres would advise a 'watch' policy for asymptomatic patients. Patients on the 'watch' policy are monitored closely by regular imaging with CT or MRI scans. Therefore, the appropriate policy is not to offer radiotherapy treatment to patients with low-grade gliomas with asymptomatic static or indolent tumours, where there is no immediate threat to neurological dysfunction from progressive tumours. Radiotherapy is reserved for patients with progressive and/or symptomatic disease where surgery is not an option.

Radiotherapy treatment of other tumours

External beam radiotherapy is used as an adjuvant treatment in the management of other CNS tumours. Patients with medulloblastoma (PNETs) have craniospinal irradiation because of the tendency of the tumour to spread throughout the CNS. Primitive neuroectodermal tumours include medulloblastomas, ependymoblastomas and pineoblastomas, of which the medulloblastoma is the most common brain tumour in children.

Radiotherapy for pineal and germ cell tumours is either localised or by craniospinal radiation depending on whether the tumour has seeded to the rest of the CNS. In patients with CNS lymphoma, the whole brain is irradiated, a subsequent boost to the primary site with craniospinal irradiation being reserved for patients with positive CSF cytology (Brada, 1995a). For malignant meningiomas, patients are treated on a 'daily' basis as for gliomas. In adult patients with craniopharyngioma, radical local radiotherapy is given. The recommended radiotherapy treatment of non-secreting pituitary adenomas is 45–50 Gy in 25–30 fractions. In patients with optic nerve gliomas, intervention in the form of radiotherapy, surgery or chemotherapy should be reserved for progressive disease (Brada, 1995a) as such patients with optic nerve gliomas should be carefully monitored with ophthalmological examination and scanning. For spinal cord tumours (ependymomas, astrocytomas and metastatic tumours), local radiotherapy confined to the region of the tumour plus a margin is recommended.

Most tumours have surgical intervention prior to radiotherapy for debulking and biopsy in order to ascertain their true histology (see Chapter 5). Some tumours will require chemotherapy as part of a combined modality treatment or if the patient is involved in a research project (see Chapter 7).

Brain metastases

Common solid tumours such as lung and breast frequently metastasise to the brain. It is estimated that approximately 20–40% of patients with cancer develop brain secondaries. Patients may present with neurological problems resulting from a brain secondary as the first presentation of a silent primary tumour elsewhere in the body.

As clinicians are becoming more adept at treating systemic cancers, brain metastases may become a bigger concern as the brain may be the only organ where metastases can be relatively shielded from the effects of chemotherapy.

Various radiotherapy techniques, that is, whole brain, interstitial (brachytherapy) radiotherapy and stereotactic radiotherapy, have been employed usually to palliate with no known overall effect on survival. The prognosis for patients with brain secondaries remains poor, with a median survival of 4–6 months (Diener-West et al, 1989; Priestman et al, 1996).

Children and radiotherapy

Although the incidence of tumours of the CNS is numerically small in children, these are the most common solid childhood tumours. It is an overall principle, if possible, not to treat young children with radiotherapy. Thus radiotherapy is best avoided in any child, particularly in those children under the age of 3 years, because of the danger of the late effects of radiation on the developing CNS. Potential late effects of radiation include endocrine and fertility problems and growth disturbances as well as psychosocial problems and secondary tumours. However, radiotherapy is recommended in some paediatric CNS tumours, in particular medulloblastoma.

It is often difficult, because of fear or their young age, for children to remain still during radiotherapy. Play therapy to familiarise the child with the equipment and machinery is often employed in order to allow the child some degree of control.

Positioning of the child during treatment is of the utmost importance to ensure its constant reproducibility. It is occasionally necessary to sedate young children requiring radiotherapy, although general anaesthesia is preferred as it causes fewer problems with weight loss: sedated children are often too drowsy to eat properly. Older children are often intrigued by the technology involved during treatment so sedation is not usually required.

It is well accepted in paediatric oncology that long-term follow-up is a multidisciplinary concern that should involve the endocrinologist and neuropsychologist.

Practicalities of care

The majority of patients will undergo treatment on an outpatient basis and practical issues therefore need to be discussed before doctors prescribe a treatment schedule. Professionals often do not consider practical issues of care, and if they do, these are frequently deemed secondary in importance to treatment. To patients, 'doctor knows best' and they are understandably led by doctors when treatment options are being discussed.

It must be remembered that, if practical problems are experienced, it may be difficult to revert the patient to a different radiotherapy schedule once treatment has started. In such a situation, it may be necessary for the patient to be admitted to hospital to complete the prescribed treatment schedule.

For example, it may be reasonable and clinically indicated to prescribe accelerated radiotherapy for a young patient with a minimal disability as a consequence of a high-grade glioma. But the questions nurses need to ask are 'How easy will it be for the patient to attend the hospital twice a day for treatment?' and 'Who will be responsible for bringing the patient to the hospital for treatment?' Because of surgery and the risk of epilepsy, patients are not allowed to operate machinery or drive a car, regulations imposed by the Driving and Vehicle Licensing Authority (DVLA). Hospital transport cannot be relied on for patients undergoing accelerated radiotherapy as patients need to have their first treatment at around 9 am and their second at around 4 pm. This gap between treatments is crucial in order to allow normal cell recovery, so hospital transport cannot be depended on.

Patients are reliant on their families and friends for a variety of activities, of which chauffeuring and baby-sitting are just two examples. Patients who are mothers often need to make arrangements for their children to be taken to and collected from school so that they can attend for treatment. At times, carers themselves may be elderly or have health problems. It is a fact that caring for a sick partner or relative can be extremely exhausting as well as time-consuming. Professionals must recognise and acknowledge this and make appropriate supportive arrangements for patients and their families (see Chapter 12).

Once the treatment schedule has been decided, the importance of prompt attendance at the radiotherapy department should be emphasised to the patient. Delays in attending for treatment can give rise to an increase in waiting times for other patients. Treatment omissions, unless medically indicated, should be avoided as this may prolong treatment, which may require adjustment to the treatment dosage.

Patients often believe that treatment will commence at the time of their first appointment at the neuro-oncology clinic. However, the

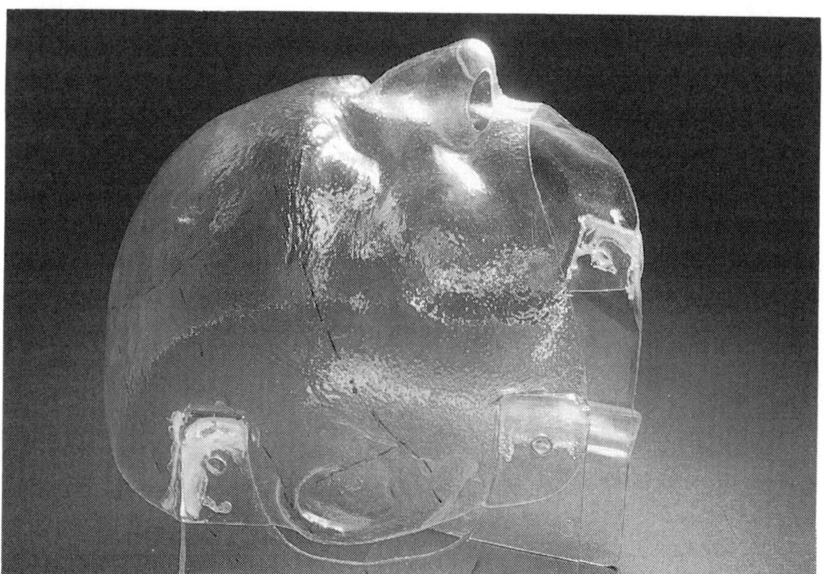

Figure 6.4 Face mould (supine).

preparation for treatment usually takes at least a couple of weeks. This is because the majority of patients will require a face mask (mould) as well as attending various planning visits to the simulator. For many patients, the thought of having to wait a few weeks to commence treatment can prove disturbing as they fear tumour recurrence. The nurse needs to understand such fears and must reassure patients that treatment preparation is vital in order to guarantee its accuracy and minimise normal tissue sequelae. However, it is important for professionals also to consider long waiting times prior to the initial commencement of treatment as being unacceptable.

Before the start of any treatment, professionals must discuss with patients and families the expected benefits as well as the side-effects of radiotherapy. It is unacceptable to submit patients with major disabilities and poor prognoses to a course of radical treatment. In such instances, 'care' is even more crucial and it may therefore be more appropriate to discuss palliative care issues (Brada and Guerrero, 1997).

Face masks

The first visit during the preparation for radiotherapy is to the mould room department. A face mask is necessary for accurate planning and reproducible delivery of treatment as well as sparing the patient the necessity of skin marks on his or her head (Figure 6.4).

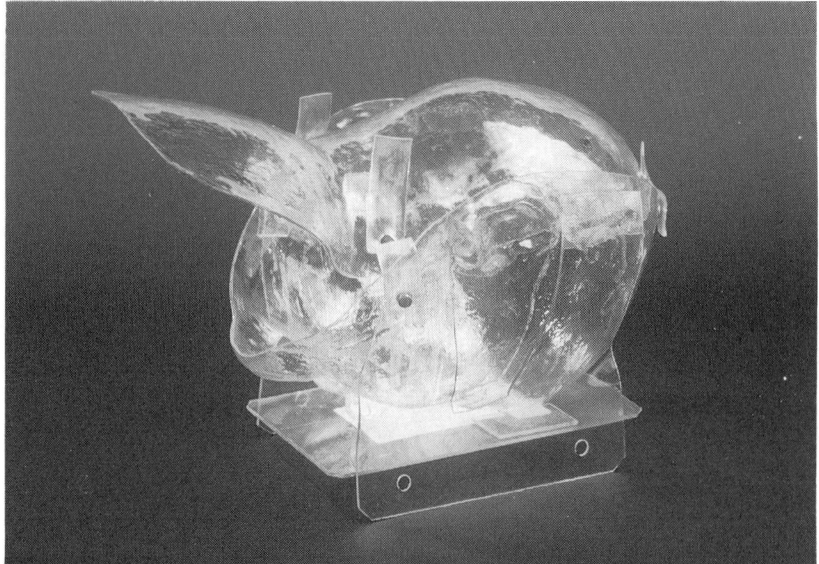

Figure 6.5 Mould: craniospinal axis irradiation (prone).

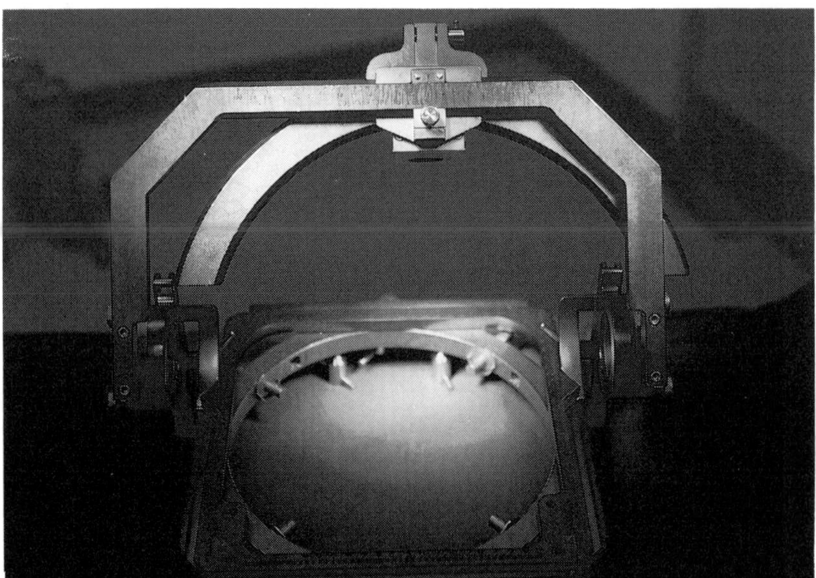

Figure 6.6 Fixed stereotactic frame.

The design of the mask and its method of attachment to the headrest system influences its effectiveness (Griffiths and Short, 1994). Many patients suffer claustrophobia and find the idea of having to wear a face mask frightening. Vision through the mask is distorted, which

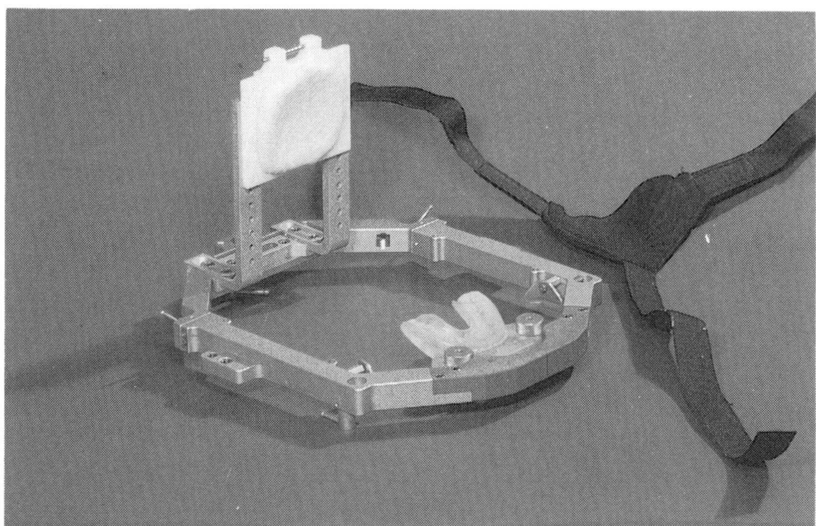

Figure 6.7 Relocatable stereotactic frame.

adds to anxiety. In such a situation if treatment permits, it may help to remove the perspex around the orbital areas to allow patients to see more clearly. Some patients, especially those with medulloblastoma and other posterior fossa tumours, will be treated in the prone position, this can cause even further anxiety (Figure 6.5).

For those patients undergoing stereotactic radiotherapy, the form of immobilisation is by means of either a fixed or a relocatable frame. If the treatment is to be given in one fraction, the immobilisation used may be in the form of an invasive frame indented into the skull with steel-tipped screws, which stays on the patient from imaging to treatment (Griffiths and Short, 1994) (Figure 6.6). For fractionated stereotactic treatment, immobilisation with a relocatable frame held in position by an occipital head support, and a dentition mould used as a mouthbite, is preferable as the patient will require daily treatment (Figure 6.7). With the relocatable frame, problems can be experienced in those patients with no dentition as it is difficult to rely on gums or dentures for treatment accuracy.

Simulation

Simulation is the next stage in the treatment planning process. Patients usually need to attend an X-ray machine known as a simulator two or three times, this figure varying between treatment centres and each visit lasting between 15 and 40 minutes. During the planning process, the proposed treatment target area in relation to the location of the tumour is decided on, and X-rays are taken to assist the radiologist and physicist. It may also be necessary at this stage to have further CT planning imaging, but conventional planning using preoperative scans is generally used. The treatment simulator is for the localisation of the target tissues and the verification of the treatment plan. It is general practice for the treatment volume to include the radiological abnormality with margins of 2–3 cm (see Figure 6.3).

The visits to the simulator give patients an understanding of what will be expected of them once treatment starts.

Nursing care

It is important for nurses to understand what the treatment experience is like for patients. Nurses should observe patients during all the stages of the planning and treatment process so that they can support patients during treatment. Such first-hand experience will place nurses in a better position when discussing treatment and answering patients' questions. Patients are generally frightened and feeling vulnerable, and nurses have a major responsibility to discuss practical issues with patients in order to avoid unnecessary anxiety and any future crises.

Simple things like showing patients a face mask and reassuring them that the treatment is painless can often help to alleviate anxiety. Patients should be told that the actual treatment time takes just a few minutes but that the process of positioning them on the treatment table to ensure treatment accuracy will take longer. Patients should also be told that the treatment machine, while operational, may rotate as well as make different noises. Such information may appear trivial but is in fact very important as any alteration in the level and type of sound can cause major anxiety to patients undergoing radiotherapy treatment. Recall how your heart misses a beat when you are in an aeroplane and it suddenly makes a new noise. The air crew are familiar with such a diversity of noises, but to you, the passenger, this new noise can be fear-provoking; the situation is no different for patients.

Patients should be reassured that they will be continuously monitored during treatment by means of a video and sound system. Many patients enjoy having their favourite music played during radiotherapy as they find this relaxing and it helps to make the treatment experience more bearable. Such diversion can easily be arranged following discussion with the radiographers.

As an *aide-mémoire*, it may help to encourage patients and families to write down those pertinent questions that they may wish to ask when phoning and/or attending a treatment or clinic. Patient information booklets should also be made available for them to read at their leisure.

Monitoring of patients during radiotherapy

During radiotherapy treatment, patients should be monitored regularly, usually on a weekly basis, to provide continuous information and support, and to familiarise them with what to expect during treatment. Information and education are vital as they allow patients to have a better sense of control during the treatment experience. Patients who are uninformed could misconstrue side-effects of treatment as being those of tumour recurrence. Research indicates that the provision of information, education and treatment monitoring can be carried out effectively by trained nurse specialists within an outpatient and telephone setting (Guerrero, 1994; James et al, 1994).

Treatment-related problems

There are various side-effects that are associated with CNS irradiation. These are classified as acute reactions, early delayed reactions and late delayed reactions.

Acute reactions occur within 24–48 hours of the commencement of treatment. Early delayed reactions occur during the course of radiotherapy and can last for a few months after treatment, and late delayed reactions can occur months to years after the completion of radiotherapy.

There are various factors that can contribute to the degree of neurotoxicity that patients can experience, including the dose per fraction, the total dose of radiation given, the volume of CNS irradiated and any other pre-existing medical problems.

Acute reactions

The aetiology of the acute reactions is not clear but may be tumour or brain oedema causing elevation of the intracranial pressure (Posner, 1995). Acute reactions are transient and tend to resolve after a few days and occasionally after a short course of corticosteroids.

The acute reactions are often very frightening for patients. What usually happens is that the patient experiences an exacerbation of the presenting symptoms. For example, those patients presenting with an expressive dysphasia that may have resolved or improved after surgery and/or steroid therapy may find that their speech deteriorates on commencement of radiotherapy. Other patients may experience severe headaches, whilst those patients who presented with epilepsy may experience an initial increase in the number of seizures.

Headaches and other focal symptoms can occasionally be attributed to a rapid decrease of steroids at the commencement of radiotherapy. Nurses have a responsibility to monitor steroid therapy and corticosteroids must be decreased gradually in order to minimise the potential of an Addisonian crisis. Corticosteroid in the form of dexamethasone is used. Dexamethasone, a synthetic glucocorticoid, has a potent anti-inflammatory action that reduces the amount of oedema around the tumour (see Chapter 8).

It is a wise practice to ensure that patients on corticosteroids are taking either prophylactic H_2 antagonist or appropriate symptomatic treatment for dyspepsia (see Chapter 8). Patients on corticosteroids are more prone to oral candidiasis and steroid-induced diabetes. Nurses should therefore check the patient's mouth weekly as well as testing their urine for sugar, particularly if the steroid dose is increased. Steroid-induced psychosis may occasionally be observed; although rare, it is nevertheless very distressing for both patients and families when it occurs.

To reduce the anxiety that patients and families may experience, it should be standard practice for nurses to arrange appropriate community and/or hospital support (see Chapters 9 and 12). There should also be a designated key person in the form of a clinical nurse specialist whom patients and families can contact.

Early delayed reactions

Alopecia

Hair loss is an inevitable consequence of cranial irradiation and generally causes the greatest distress to patients. Alopecia usually commences within 10–14 days of commencing treatment. Following radical treatment, alopecia can be permanent.

Scalp shielding is a technique employed by some radiotherapy centres. This involves the use of lead blocks to protect parts of the scalp receiving the highest dose during irradiation in order to prevent permanent hair loss. With scalp shielding, initial hair loss occurs during treatment, but the hair may eventually grow back after a period of a few months. Scalp shielding is a time- and manpower-consuming process that requires extra time in preparing the radiotherapy machine and the patient. It tends to be used in younger patients with good prognostic tumours and only if the treatment to the tumour is not compromised.

Hair and scalp care

Historically, patients were advised not to wash their hair during treatment, and such advice often caused much distress. However, most centres will now allow patients to wash their hair as long as they do not use dyes or perms during treatment. To minimise scalp irritation, patients should use tepid water and a mild shampoo and not rub but pat their hair and scalp dry with a soft towel. They should be discouraged from using hair dryers as even a low setting on the dryer can irritate the scalp.

Many patients opt to have their hair cut before the commencement of radiotherapy. Simple measures such as wearing a hair net at night to catch falling hairs often help the distress of waking up in the morning and finding hairs all over the pillow.

The scalp will be more sensitive to the effects of ultraviolet rays as a result of irradiation. Patients should always be advised to protect the treatment area from the sun during and for up to a year following radiotherapy. Such advice often gives patients positive hope that things will generally improve after treatment.

As a means of scalp protection, ladies generally tend to be extremely adventurous, and often it is a good excuse for them to go shopping for hats, turbans and scarves. Wigs tend not to be very comfortable to wear during treatment because of the inevitable skin reaction resulting from radiotherapy. Some patients report that wigs, if used during treatment, can cause worsening of scalp irritation as well as constriction and tightness around hypersensitive skin. However, it may still be sensible to encourage females to purchase a wig as this may be more useful when dining out or on social occasions.

Although baldness is more acceptable in men, some still find treatment-induced alopecia very distressing and they should therefore also be given the opportunity of ordering a wig. However, most men tend to wear hats as a means of scalp protection from the sun. Occasionally, some men worry about undertaking facial wet shaves during treatment as they are not clear where the radiation beams are being aimed. They should be reassured and advised that facial wet shaves are safe. The importance of scalp and skin care should be emphasised and patients given the opportunity to meet with the appliance officer to discuss the use of wigs.

Psychological impact of hair loss

Professionals should never underestimate the impact of treatment-induced alopecia. For many people hair is associated with body image and sexuality (see Chapter 10), and its loss can severely affect self-esteem (Guerrero, 1996).

Patients are occasionally so anxious to commence treatment that they tend to say that hair loss is the least of their worries, and some may believe that it will not happen to them. However, once their general condition starts to improve and alopecia commences, hair loss can become a major cause of anxiety. This is because the impact of hair loss is not just restricted to the patient but is a family concern, children often becoming very distressed when daddy or (especially) mummy is losing his or her hair.

One child refused to allow his mother to fetch him from school as other children had noticed that she was going bald and had been making fun of her. Another child was so upset over his mother's hair loss that he had screaming fits every time she tried to remove her turban when at home.

It may thus at times be necessary to refer patients and families for psychological support as hair loss can give rise to major altered body image effects (see Chapters 10 and 11).

Skin reactions

There are three distinct stages of skin reaction during and after radiotherapy: erythema, dry desquamation and moist desquamation. The majority of patients undergoing cranial irradiation will not experience moist desquamation. Patients should be made familiar with the first two stages in order to avoid unnecessary anxiety.

Erythema

Scalp erythema is the first stage of skin reaction and usually precedes alopecia. Erythema occurs at the site of entry and exit of the radiation beams. At this stage, the skin becomes red and inflamed, and patients will complain of a hot, burning sensation as well as tightness of the skin. Erythema may make the patient scratch the affected area, which can cause excoriation and may become a focus for infection.

It is treated with topical hydrocortisone cream 1%, spread thinly over the affected area two or three times a day. Hydrocortisone cream reduces the discomfort associated with the skin radiation reaction. Patients should be advised not to scratch the affected skin, and it is often advisable to instruct patients to apply the hydrocortisone cream at bedtime as this may prevent patients scratching while asleep.

Hydrocortisone cream is often more effective once alopecia commences as the cream is otherwise smeared onto the hair, thus avoiding the scalp.

Some patients worry about the use of topical steroids. Applying hydrocortisone cream is only necessary for a short while during the stage of scalp erythema (usually 2–3 weeks), and side-effects are related to long-term use. However, treatment should be monitored regularly for, in this instance, the presence of other potential skin complications.

Dry desquamation

Dry desquamation is the second stage of skin reaction. This stage usually occurs 2–4 weeks after the completion of radiotherapy. The skin becomes dry and flaky, and may appear unsightly. If there is no redness of the scalp and the skin is intact, patients should be advised to apply a good-quality, unperfumed moisturising cream and to spread this liberally over the treatment area. This should help to keep the scalp supple.

Moist desquamation

Moist desquamation is rarely a problem associated with cranial irradiation. With moist desquamation, patients develop skin blisters and ulceration within the irradiated areas.

In those patients who wear spectacles and are receiving temporal lobe irradiation, blistering behind the ears can occasionally be observed. This results from patients sliding their spectacles rather than lifting them on and off their ears. The motion of sliding spectacles on and off gives rise to friction; this can in turn cause blistering and breakage of the skin, which can become a focus for infection. In this instance, Proflavine lotion applied to the affected skin is usually very effective.

Somnolence

Somnolence syndrome is described as excessive sleep, drowsiness, lethargy and anorexia (Faithfull, 1991). Although not well documented, this phenomenon is believed to be a consequence of transient damage to the oligodendroglial cells. One of the major roles of oligodendroglial cells is the production of myelin for neuronal conduction. Radiation may therefore lead to transient demyelination affecting the complex neuronal communication pathways, giving rise to transient fatigue and exhaustion.

Somnolence is the most debilitating condition that patients undergoing cranial irradiation will experience. It often commences halfway during the course of radiotherapy, occasionally improving towards the end of irradiation, only to peak again after completion of treatment. The effects of somnolence can last for 6–8 weeks after the completion of cranial irradiation.

The severity of somnolence can vary from patient to patient. This could be due to radiation sensitivity of specific critical brain structures within the treatment areas.

Somnolence can lead to fear and anxiety as patients often believe that there is tumour progression as a result of treatment failure. Somnolence needs to be discussed often and in detail with patients and families before, during and after radiotherapy treatment.

It is often difficult to describe the somnolence experience to patients as, for those severely affected, such intensive fatigue and exhaustion have often never been experienced before and even minor daily tasks can pose a major struggle. As such, patients should be told that there are degrees of fatigue and tiredness (and occasionally other symptoms) that can vary in intensity in different individuals. Thus professionals cannot predict how severely somnolence can affect an individual patient, and patients must be reassured that this is a normal and expected reaction to treatment. Even well-prepared patients can, when severely affected, find the experience of somnolence catastrophic. One patient reported somnolence as 'being a constant hang-over without the benefits of having enjoyed the night before'.

Many patients feel very vulnerable as well as tearful during somnolence, and they often report not feeling in control of their lives.

Corticosteroids (dexamethasone) are occasionally prescribed or increased in those patients with evidence of increased focal signs to reverse the possible side-effects of intracranial pressure (see Chapter 8). Many patients are on varied assortment of medications that may include anxiolytics as well as hypnotics; these may well exacerbate somnolence.

The effects of somnolence must be carefully considered and the the patient's condition regularly evaluated. There should also be a means of post-radiotherapy contact with the patient especially during the acute phase of somnolence and prior to the first post-treatment clinic evaluation. This contact should preferably be by means of a telephone consultation in order to support and reassure patients during the somnolence experience and to avoid unnecessary visits to the hospital (James et al, 1994; Brada, 1995b).

Other treatment-related issues

Apart from those side-effects expected, patients may report other radiation problems that are often related to the specific area of the CNS that is being treated. At times, some problems may be exacerbated by anxiety and fear, but this should not make them less important. Continuous patient monitoring and education are therefore of paramount importance and must be viewed by nurses as a major ongoing process of care. Such monitoring and education may reduce stress-related problems as well as helping patients to maintain some degree of control throughout the illness experience.

Otitis externa and media

Although not well documented, otitis externa and/or media can be experienced by some patients during treatment. Such problems often cause much anxiety, particularly to those patients with failing hearing or a previous history of deafness.

Otitis externa is caused by radiation-induced erythema, giving rise to swelling and narrowing of the external auditory meatus. There is often wax retention within the ear, which may cause abrasion of the skin, particularly in those patients who tend to insert objects such as cotton buds in their ears. If, on examination, there is no evidence of tympanic membrane perforation, sodium bicarbonate or olive oil ear drops can be given to loosen the ear wax. Ear syringing should be avoided during radiotherapy and most definitely in those patients with a history of tympanic membrane perforation. If there is evidence of ear infection, a swab should be taken for culture and sensitivity and the patient commenced on a combination of anti-infective and corticosteroid ear drops. Patients requiring ear drops should be instructed to lie with the affected ear uppermost for a few minutes after the administration of the drops in order to allow complete distribution of the drops throughout the external auditory meatus.

Patients with secretory otitis media present with deafness due to radiation-induced oedema causing obstruction of the eustachian tube. The condition is often unilateral and tends to clear itself 4–6 weeks post-radiotherapy when the eustachian tube opens and allows the fluid to drain. If the condition persists, the patient should be referred to an ear, nose and throat department as it may be necessary to undertake myringotomy and the insertion of grommets.

Irregularities in menstrual cycle

Premenopausal women will occasionally report cessation of their menstrual cycle. In the first instance, pregnancy should be excluded with a pregnancy test. This can easily be undertaken with a pregnancy kit. If the test proves negative, the patient should be reassured that the irregularity of the menstrual cycle usually corrects itself after the completion of radiotherapy. Although not well documented, menstrual cycle cessation may well depend on radiation sensitivity of the pituitary/hypothalamic region. Menstrual irregularities can also be experienced during glucocorticoid therapy.

Headaches

Headaches are common in patients with brain tumours. First, they require assessment and evaluation to ascertain the cause. The most frequent cause is raised intracranial pressure as a direct effect of the tumour or treatment (see Figure 6.8). Corticosteroids are usually the

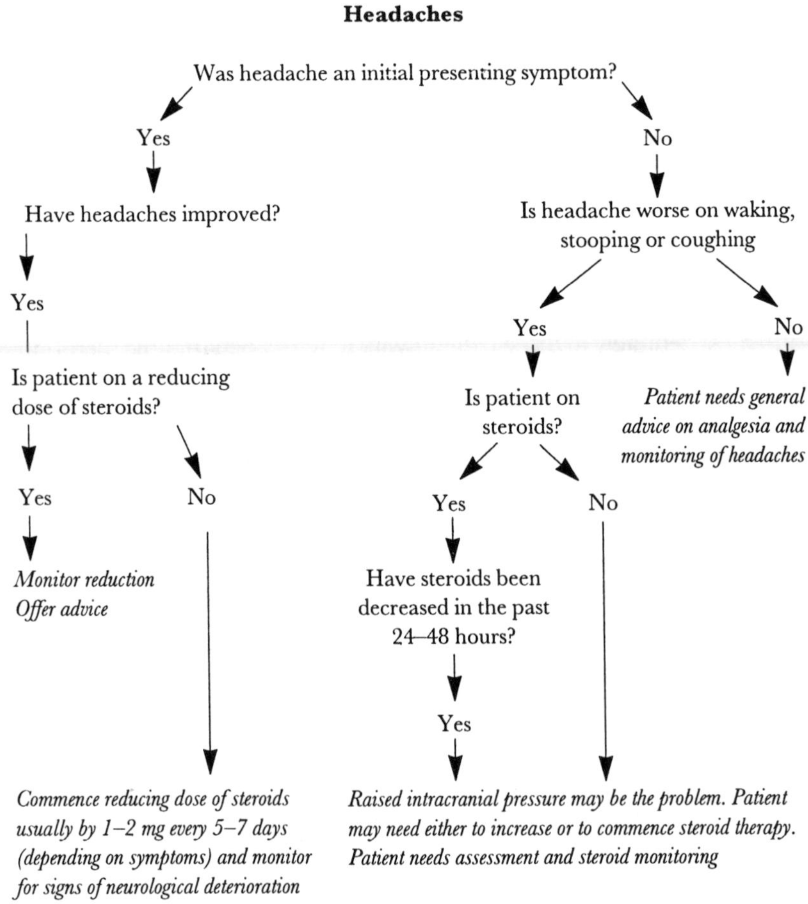

Headaches

Was headache an initial presenting symptom?

- Yes → Have headaches improved?
  - Yes → Is patient on a reducing dose of steroids?
    - Yes → *Monitor reduction* / *Offer advice*
    - No → *Commence reducing dose of steroids usually by 1–2 mg every 5–7 days (depending on symptoms) and monitor for signs of neurological deterioration*
- No → Is headache worse on waking, stooping or coughing
  - Yes → Is patient on steroids?
    - Yes → Have steroids been decreased in the past 24–48 hours?
      - Yes → *Raised intracranial pressure may be the problem. Patient may need either to increase or to commence steroid therapy. Patient needs assessment and steroid monitoring*
    - No → *Raised intracranial pressure may be the problem. Patient may need either to increase or to commence steroid therapy. Patient needs assessment and steroid monitoring*
  - No → *Patient needs general advice on analgesia and monitoring of headaches*

Figure 6.8 Headaches.

initial treatment of choice (see Chapter 8). However, in the absence of neurological deterioration, headaches are best treated with reassurance and simple analgesia. Therapeutic massage and/or aromatherapy are often of benefit.

Change in the severity of headaches and/or development of a neurological deficit and a change in the level of consciousness should be discussed with the medical staff and acted on immediately.

Questions to ask

- Is there a pattern to the headaches?
- Where is the pain in the head?
- How long does the headache last?
- How often do the headaches occur?
- Is there a warning of their onset?
- Does simple analgesia resolve the headache?

Points to note

- It is always sensible to keep those patients taking steroids on a prophylactic H_2 antagonist.
- Steroids should not be taken late in the day (last dose 5–6 pm) as they often keep patients awake.
- Test the patient's urine for sugar, particularly if the dose of steroid is increased.
- Check the patient's oral cavity weekly for any signs of candidiasis.
- All patients on steroids should have a medication chart indicating the dosage, frequency and contact telephone numbers.

Taste alterations

Taste alterations or ageusia (loss of taste) is often reported by patients during cranial irradiation. Alterations in taste can range from increased sensitivity to taste, to foods having a bland or metallic taste. Patients with taste alterations or taste loss are more prone to anorexia, which can lead to weight loss. Patients should be reassured that taste changes are a normal feature of treatment and often persist for a period of time after the completion of cranial irradiation.

Candidiasis can at times be a contributing factor to taste changes. The patient's oral cavity should be inspected regularly, especially in those patients taking corticosteroids. If a patient's condition necessitates antifungal preparations, education and advice to both patient and family on the proper usage of the medication, including the treatment of dentures, should be undertaken (see Chapter 8). Patients should if necessary be referred to a dietitian for dietary advice.

Smell

Loss of smell (anosmia) or hypersensitivity to smell is a commonly reported problem. Patients often report smelling 'ozone' during radiotherapy treatment. Hypersensitivity to smell is probably caused by stimulation of olfactory nerve (cranial nerve I) endings by the radiation (Posner, 1995).

Loss of smell can be particularly distressing, and professionals often trivialise its impact on patients. One young mother derived great pleasure from the smell of her baby after being bathed and was distraught at the occurrence of anosmia.

Nausea

Nausea is not often associated with CNS irradiation, although it may accompany raised intracranial pressure. Nausea can be aggravated by anxiety at the thought of having to attend hospital for treatment. However, if reported it must be investigated to rule out a specific aetiology. Taste and smell alterations as well as candidiasis can at times contribute towards the feeling of nausea. Referral to a dietitian and/or anti-emetic therapy, as well as reassurance, is often helpful.

Bone marrow suppression

Bone marrow suppression is a complication of craniospinal axis irradiation because of the large volume of bone marrow within the radiation area. Of 210 patients undergoing craniospinal axis irradiation studied at the Royal Marsden NHS Trust between 1965 and 1994, 66 patients developed grades 3 and 4 haematological toxicity (Jefferies et al, 1998). These authors reported the risk being higher in children and those patients who received chemotherapy prior to radiation.

Patients undergoing craniospinal axis irradiation should have full blood count values checked weekly to detect suppression of white blood cells and/or platelets. If the full blood count values are below accepted levels, the patient should be rested for a few days from treatment to allow the blood count to recover.

Difficulty in swallowing.

Difficulty in swallowing (dysphagia) and oesophagitis during craniospinal irradiation result from the exit dose of radiation passing through the pharynx and oesophagus. Simple measures such as mucaine suspension often alleviate this condition.

Lhermitte's phenomenon

Lhermitte's sign is characterised by transient, electric-like shocks that spread down the body when the head is flexed forward. Lhermitte's sign is usually a feature of multiple sclerosis but is reported following spinal irradiation. Although there is no research evidence to support a demyelination hypothesis, it is generally believed that Lhermitte's sign probably results from demyelination of the spinal posterior columns leading to the spontaneous discharge of sensory axons when the spinal cord is stretched by neck flexion (Posner, 1995).

Lhermitte's sign occurs 12–20 weeks after spinal irradiation in up to 25–40% of patients receiving over 35–40 Gy to significant lengths of the cord (Kun, 1994). Although unpleasant, Lhermitte's phenomenon is not painful and usually resolves after a few months to a year, although in some patients it may persist for longer.

Late delayed reactions

The late effects of radiation are multiple and may occur months to years after irradiation. Late delayed reactions often depend on the site, total dose and volume of CNS irradiated.

In the brain, necrosis is of particular concern as it can sometimes be mistaken for tumour recurrence. Surgery and/or steroid therapy is occasionally an option for patients presenting with necrosis. Radionecrosis cannot be accurately distinguished from recurrent tumour by CT or MRI. However, positron emission tomography (PET) can help to make the distinction between radionecrosis and recurrent tumour (see Chapter 4).

Leucomalacia (white matter changes) causes dementia. Dementia is often extremely distressing for partners and families and can lead to family breakdown as families cannot cope with the constant demands now posed by patients. This understandably causes much grief and pain in already shattered lives (Guerrero, 1996).

Other late delayed reactions includes motor and sensory changes as well as problems with neuropsychological development; this is often a major concern when treating children. Patients whose visual pathways are within the treatment area should have baseline ophthalmological assessment as damage to the optic nerves (cranial nerve II) is possible if they are irradiated above tolerance level.

Endocrine dysfunction as a consequence of hypothalamic radiation can be treated with hormone replacement therapy and, as such, an initial baseline endocrinological assessment and monitoring of patients for their entire life span by an endocrinologist are of vital importance.

When the spinal cord is within the treatment area, radiation myelopathy, necrosis and paralysis are of major concern. Also of particular concern is the long-term development of secondary tumours as a consequence of CNS irradiation.

Professionals have a major responsibility to discuss long-term effects with patients prior to the commencement of CNS irradiation. For those patients with extremely aggressive tumours such as high-grade gliomas, late delayed reactions do not often pose a major problem as the prognosis for this group of patients is unfortunately often poor. However, for those patients with low-grade gliomas as well as potentially curable tumours such as medulloblastomas and pineal tumours, the potential late delayed reactions of treatment are a major issue and have to be carefully addressed.

Conclusion

Nurses should not underestimate their role during the patient's radiotherapy. The major issues during treatment are often those of proper nursing assessment, good-quality patient care, education and treatment preparation. The needs of carers must also be taken very seriously as long-term care may depend on a well-prepared family (Guerrero, 1996).

Patients will often feel vunerable, frightened and not in control of their lives. Nurses therefore have an ongoing responsibility to identify those issues of concern and to support and refer patients and families as appropriate to other team members in order to avoid the occurrence of a crisis.

Doctors are predominantly concerned at developing radiotherapy treatments that aim to minimise the amount of normal tissue in the target volume as well as exploring better ways of fractionated therapy. Nurses have a responsibility to work closely with doctors by undertaking and/or collaborating in research studies. Such research could include new ways of reducing treatment-related problems experienced by patients as well as better ways of supporting patients and families through the treatment experience.

It is only by professionals working together that we can provide the best and most cost-effective care to our patients.

References

Bomford CK, Kunkler IH, Sherriff SB (1993) Walter and Miller's Textbook of Radiotherapy, Radiation Physics, Therapy and Oncology. London: Churchill Livingstone.

Brada M (1995a) Central nervous system tumours.In Horwich A (Ed.) Oncology, a Multi-disciplinary Textbook. Oxford: Chapman & Hall, Chapter 29.

Brada M (1995b) Is there a need to follow up cancer patients? European Journal of Cancer 31A(5): 655–7.

Brada M, Graham JD (1994) Stereotactic external beam radiotherapy in the treatment of glioma and other intracranial lesions. In Tobias JS, Thomas PRM (Eds) Current Radiation Oncology, Volume 1. London: Edward Arnold, pp 86–100.

Brada M, Guerrero D (1997) One model of follow-up care. In Davies E, Hopkins A (Eds) Improving care for Patients with Malignant Cerebral Glioma. London: Royal College of Physicians of London, pp 93–8.

Brada M, Robinson MH (1991) Radiotherapy. Medicine International 94: 3834–9.

Brada M, Ross G (1996) Radiation therapy in the management of malignant gliomas. Baillière's Clinical Neurology. 5(2): 319–43.

Brada M, Thomas DGT (1995) Tumours of the brain and spinal cord in adults. In Peckham M, Pinedd B, Veronesi U (Eds) Oxford Textbook of Oncology, Vol. 2. Oxford: Oxford University Press, pp 2063–94.

Brada M, Thomas D, Bleehan N (1998) Medical Research Council (MRC) randomised trial of adjuvant chemotherapy in high grade glioma. BRO5, ASCO 1998. Los Angeles California. 400a.

Diener-West M, Dobbins TW, Phillips TL, Nelson DF (1989) Identification of an optional subgroup for treatment evaluation of patients with brain metastases using RTOG study 7916. International Journal of Radiation Oncology, Biology, Physics 16: 669–73.

Faithfull S (1991) Patients' experiences following cranial radiotherapy: a study of the somnolence syndrome. Journal of Advanced Nursing: 939–46.

Glance WD, Anderson KN, Anderson LE, Urdang L, Harding, Swallow H (Eds) (1986) Mosby's Medical and Nursing Dictionary, 2nd edn. St Louis: CV Mosby.

Griffiths S, Short C (1994) Radiotherapy: Principles to Practice. Edinburgh: Churchill Livingstone.

Guerrero D (1994) A nurse led service. Nursing Standard 9(6): 21–3.

Guerrero D (1996) Brain tumours. In Tschudin V (Ed.) Nursing the Patient with Cancer, 2nd edn. London: Prentice Hall, pp 146–61.

James ND, Guerrero D, Brada M (1994) Who should follow up cancer patients? Nurse specialist based out-patient care and the introduction of a phone clinic system. Clinical Oncology 6: 283–7.

Jefferies S, Rajan B, Ashley S, Traish D, Brada M (1998) Haematological toxicity of cranio-spinal irradiation. Radiotherapy and Oncology 48. pp23–27.

Kun LE (1994) Principles of radiation therapy. In Cohen ME, Duffner PK (Eds) Brain Tumors in Children, Principles, Diagnosis and Treatment, 2nd edn. New York: Raven Press, pp 95–115.

Leibel SA, Sheline GE (1990) Radiotherapy in the treatment of cerebral astrocytomas. In Thomas DGT (Ed.) Neuro-oncology. Primary Malignant Brain Tumours. London: Edward Arnold, Chapter 12.

Posner J (1995) Neurologic Complications of Cancer. Philadelphia: FA Davis.

Priestman TJ, Dunn J, Brada M, Rampling R, Baker PG (1996) Final results of the Royal College of Radiologists' trial comparing two different radiotherapy schedules in the treatment of cerebral metastases. Clinical Oncology 8: 308–15.

Thomas R, James ND, Guerrero D, Ashley S, Gregor A, Brada M (1994) Hypofractionated radiotherapy as a palliative treatment in poor prognosis patients with high grade glioma. Radiotherapy and Oncology 33: 113–16.

Chapter 7
Chemotherapy

Douglas Guerrero, Sue Sardell and Frances Hines

Introduction

CNS tumours range from the relatively chemosensitive tumours such as germinomas, primary CNS lymphomas and primitive neuro-ectodermal tumours (PNETs) to the relatively chemoresistant gliomas (see Chapters 3 and 4). Even in those tumours which are relatively chemosensitive, the current chemotherapeutic treatments available are not very effective. Thus, for the majority of patients with CNS tumours, current chemotherapy treatments are not curative in intent.

This chapter aims to provide nurses with a wider understanding of the chemotherapeutic treatment of CNS malignancies. It will also explore the value of such treatment, the expected side-effects and the nurse's role in the maintenance of patients' quality of life.

Mechanism of action of chemotherapeutic agents

All proliferating cells go through a series of events that comprise the cell cycle (Steward et al, 1995). Following mitosis (M), the cell enters the G_1 phase (resting period) during which ribonucleic acid (RNA) and proteins are made. On entering the synthesis (S) phase, deoxyribonucleic acid (DNA) and RNA synthesis occurs. This is followed by the G_2 phase during which the cell ceases DNA synthesis and undertakes final checks and repair of the DNA prior to mitosis. Cells in G_0 are in a resting phase out of the cycle. However, these cells can actively synthesise RNA and proteins, can differentiate and are typically resistant to the cytotoxic effects of chemotherapy (Tortorice, 1997).

Chemotherapy acts at the level of the DNA by damaging cellular DNA or preventing its repair. Therefore, when the damaged cell attempts to undergo mitosis, drug-induced apoptosis (cell death) occurs.

Classification of cytotoxic drugs

Cytotoxic drugs are divided into certain groups depending on their mechanism of action.

Alkylating agents

Alkylating agents act by transferring alkyl groups onto amino acid residues of cellular proteins, resulting in covalent bond formation with cellular molecules. It is the reaction of the drug with the DNA that determines the cytotoxic effect. Alkylating agents form cross-links with DNA, preventing transcription and mitosis. They are therefore most effective in cycling cells.

There are a number of different types of alkylating agent, which differ in their pharmacokinetics and toxicity profile. They include the nitrogen mustards, cyclophosphamide, ifosfamide, melphalan, chlorambucil and the nitrosoureas BCNU (carmustine) and CCNU (lomustine), and other such drugs as dacarbazine, mitomycin C and busulphan.

Mesna (mercaptoethane sulphonic acid) rescue is administered parenterally to reduce the risk of haemorrhagic cystitis associated with cyclophosphamide.

In neuro-oncology, the nitrosoureas are of specific interest because they are highly lipid soluble and therefore able to cross the blood–brain barrier easily.

Antimetabolites

Antimetabolites interfere with the normal metabolism of RNA and DNA precursors because of their structural similarity to intermediates in the synthetic pathway (Peters, 1995). These structural analogues interfere with the action of a key enzyme in the synthetic process. Because of the differences in metabolism between normal cells and cancer cells, several antimetabolites have the ability to act with a certain degree of specificity on cancer cells (Peters, 1995).

Antimetabolites include methotrexate, fluoropyrimidines (5-fluorouracil), cytidine analogues (cytarabine) and thiopurines (6-mercaptopurine and 6-thioguanine).

The antifolate agent methotrexate is the most commonly used antimetabolite in neuro-oncology as it may be delivered intrathecally or intravenously and in high dose may effectively cross the blood–brain barrier. Folinic acid rescue is given to prevent life-threatening toxicity and acts by bypassing the blocking activity of methotrexate (Steward et al, 1995). Folinic acid rescue is continued if methotrexate levels fail to fall by 48 hours post-infusion.

Antitumour antibiotics

The antitumour antibiotics are considered to produce their effect by binding components of the DNA (intercalating), by generating intracellular free radicals or by interacting with the DNA repair enzyme topoisomerase II.

The antitumour antibiotics include the anthracycline antibiotics (epirubicin, doxorubicin and idarubicin), the n-anthracycline antibiotics (bleomycin) and the anthracenediones (mitozantrone).

Vinca alkaloids

The vinca alkaloids bind to tubulin, which is an intracellular protein that polymerises (linking intracellular molecules) to form microtubules (Priestman, 1989). Microtubules are involved in a number of cellular functions including mitosis, and the inhibition of tubulin function by vinca alkaloid binding prevents successful mitosis.

The vinca alkaloids include vincristine, vinblastine and vindesine.

Podophyllotoxins

Podophyllotoxins interact with the DNA repair enzyme topoisomerase II and produce single- and double-strand breaks in the DNA (Steward et al, 1995). Podophyllotoxins include VP16 (etoposide) and VM26 (teniposide).

Miscellaneous agents.

Miscellaneous compounds include procarbazine, a methylating agent (alkylating-like drug) that is a weak monoamine oxidase inhibitor (MAOI) and acts by inhibiting the action of both RNA and DNA, and by depressing protein synthesis. As procarbazine is a weak MAOI, patients will require advice on dietary restrictions.

The mode of action of both cisplatin and carboplatin is unknown, but they are considered to act on DNA cross-links in a manner similar to that of the alkylating agents. Patients treated with cisplatin or carboplatin will require adequate hydration and osmotic diuresis to prevent renal toxicity.

Combination chemotherapy

Effective cancer chemotherapy often consists of employing more than one drug. Combination chemotherapy has been developed empirically during controlled clinical trials (see chapter appendix). The aim of combination chemotherapy is to deliver a cocktail of cytotoxic drugs that can interfere at different stages of the cell cycle. As such, three general principles govern the use of combination chemotherapy. The drugs included should be active against the tumour when used alone, have different mechanisms of action and have minimally overlapping toxicities (Steward et al, 1995).

Mechanism of cytotoxic drug resistance

There are various reasons why cytotoxic chemotherapy is limited in its effectiveness. Such limitations result from the tolerance of normal tissue, the intrinsic sensitivity of the tumour cells, acquired resistance to cytotoxic chemotherapy and the accelerated growth of the tumour cells after treatment with cytotoxic drugs (Cleton, 1995). The dose, dose rate, schedule of administration and duration of treatment may all have a profound effect on the success of chemotherapy (Cleton, 1995).

The nervous system consists of cells that either do not divide, such as most neurones (although olfactory neurones undertake mitosis), or divide slowly, such as neuroglia (Posner, 1995). Cytotoxic agents are much more effective in dividing cells. As such, cytotoxic chemotherapy at present offers little survival benefit for most CNS tumours.

Limitations in the treatment of CNS tumours include the blood–brain and blood–tumour barriers.

Blood–brain barrier

The blood–brain barrier is formed by tight junction between endothelial cells. Its purpose is to maintain a constant chemical environment in the brain by forming a barrier between the blood and brain. Without the blood–brain barrier, nerve cells would be subjected to fluctuations in concentrations of glucose, amino acids and hormones as well as other compounds, leading to uncontrolled nervous activity and even fits (Ramlakhan and Altman, 1990). In the treatment of CNS tumours, the blood–brain barrier excludes the delivery of most drugs to the brain.

Most cancer drugs are hydrophilic (water soluble), and cell membrane is composed of fatty substances. Drugs therefore need to be lipophilic (fat soluble) to penetrate the blood–brain barrier. Alteration of the blood–brain barrier permeability is achievable, for example by the use of high doses of mannitol. However, alterations to the blood–brain barrier can lead to toxic drug concentrations in normal brain tissue as drugs cannot be targeted at the tumour cells alone.

Blood–tumour barrier

The permeability of brain vasculature varies in different regions of a tumour as well as between tumours. It is the transfer of drugs across the endothelial membrane which is of most relevance to drug delivery, and the precise role of the blood–tumour barrier in determining chemoresponsiveness is not known (Brada and Thomas, 1995). The slower blood flow in tumours reduces the delivery of lipid-soluble drugs, whereas the variable permeability of the blood–tumour barrier restricts the entry of water-soluble drugs (Shapiro et al, 1995).

Novel drug strategies

New agents are continually being developed for clinical trials (see chapter appendix). These agents have been derived from molecular biology studies and are designed either to interrupt the aberrant cellular activity or to restore normal cellular function by either stimulating an activity or replacing it (Shapiro et al, 1995). These include immunotherapy, tumour necrosis factor (TNF), monoclonal antibodies and antisense and gene therapy. The development of stereotactic localisation procedures that can precisely define tumour position and size, and the feasibility of siting intratumoral catheters using this technology, have opened the possibility of administering antibodies and a range of antisense and gene therapies (Brada and Ross, 1996). Such developments are important as it is unlikely that a breakthrough in cancer chemotherapy will be achieved with the use of existing drugs or their analogues (Cleton, 1995). For specialist nurses, these developments will give rise to new demands in the areas of knowledge and education (Guerrero, 1996).

Route of administration

The route of administration of cytotoxic chemotherapy depends on various factors, including the stability, size, molecular charge and sclerosant characteristic of the drug (Steward et al, 1995). In neuro-oncology, most routes have been explored in an attempt to deliver a higher concentration of drugs to the tumour as well as to bypass and/or modify the blood–brain barrier. Routes of administration have included oral, intra-arterial, intravenous, intrathecal and intra-tumoral.

Although the oral route (in some cancers) is often used infrequently because of the fear of poor patient compliance and uncertain absorption, it is nevertheless often used in neuro-oncology, particularly in the treatment of patients with a high-grade glioma. This is because the prognosis is generally poor for most patients with a high-grade glioma and the emphasis is on care and support, whenever possible maintaining patients at home whilst reducing the number of hospital admissions (Brada and Guerrero, 1997). However, good-quality education for both patients and carers is paramount in order to decrease the risk of non-compliance with medication and also to ensure the administration of a correct drug dosage.

The route and schedule of cytotoxic drug administration can be crucial and dependent on tumour chemosensitivity as dose, drug absorption and time interval may be critical when attempting to improve disease survival.

Extravasation

Care must always be taken when drugs are given by any route. However, when drugs are given intravenously, added precautions must be observed as any leakage of a vesicant drug into the tissues can cause severe ulceration and necrosis. As such, the nurse should, before the administration of cytotoxic drugs, know which agents are capable of producing tissue necrosis (Dougherty, 1996) (Table 7.1). Intravenous cytotoxic chemotherapy should be administered by trained personnel as the prevention of extravasation is of major importance. Ulceration caused by drug extravasation may cause severe necrosis and long-term pain, and may take months to heal. Thus most hospitals engaged in cancer treatment will have specialist nurses with expert knowledge in the management of cytotoxic drugs. Cancer patients may be more prone to drug extravasation because of multiple venepunctures, phlebitis limiting future sites of venous access, lymphoedema from prior surgery and generalised debility (Clamon, 1996).

Extravasation should be suspected if the patient complains of a burning or stinging sensation around the needle or cannula site. However, the time course of the injury after drug extravasation varies; injury may not be immediate but may come on gradually depending on the chemotherapy employed (Clamon, 1996). Other signs to observe for are swelling or leakage around the administration site, resistance during bolus administration, stopped infusion and no flashback of blood with a pull back on the syringe.

The management of extravasation is controversial and its treatment may vary according to different hospital policies.

Investigations

Patients will require investigations prior to the commencement of any chemotherapy treatment. A full blood count and full blood chemistry are standard and are routinely conducted. A height and baseline weight should be recorded, not only for body surface area calculation for drug dosage, but also because many patients are receiving corticosteroids (see Chapter 8). Fluctuations of body weight during courses of treatment may necessitate further drug dosage calculations. Certain regimens will require a nadir count.

Individual drugs may require specific investigations prior to treatment. For example, patients receiving platinum-based chemotherapy should have baseline ethylene diamene tetra-acetic acid (EDTA) test to assess renal function. Baseline audiogram tests are also conducted to determine the patient's hearing level and are repeated at intervals during treatment. Such investigations are important as platinum-based drugs can cause nephrotoxicity and ototoxicity.

Imaging, CT or MRI (see Chapter 4) will be required in the majority of patients prior to the commencement of cytotoxic chemotherapy. This acts as a baseline for the future assessment of the radiological response to treatment. CSF cytology is required whenever possible from those patients with CNS lymphoma and germ cell tumours. The latter will also require blood and CSF tumour markers alphafetoprotein (AFP) and human chorionic gonadotrophin (β-HCG) to be ascertained. For those patients entering clinical trials (see chapter appendix), baseline investigations can be more extensive, often including an ECG and chest X-ray.

Provision of information

Patients and families should always be provided with clear verbal and written information, and be given the opportunity to return to the clinic to discuss proposed treatment further. If possible, a contact telephone number should be provided so that they can phone to

Table 7.1 Most common cytotoxic drugs used in neuro-oncology

Generic name	Route of administration	Emetic potential	Side-effects	Special considerations
Lomustine	Oral	High	Moderate to severe myelosuppression. Permanent bone marrow depression with long-term use Delayed renal and pulmonary toxicity	Requires nadir count
Carmustine	Intravenous	High	Cumulative myelosuppression Pulmonary toxicity leading to fibrosis Renal toxicity	Irritant, avoid extravasation Requires nadir count Can cause burning and hyperpigmentation of exposed skin
Methotrexate	Oral Intravenous Intrathecal Intra-arterial	Moderate	Neutropenia, thrombocytopenia, anaemia Mucositis Diarrhoea Renal toxicity with high-dose regimen Common side-effects for intrathecal administration include headache and fever. More serious side-effects include paralysis, cranial nerve palsies, epilepsy and coma.	Requires nadir count With high-dose Methotrexate, folinic acid rescue is given to diminish myelotoxicity Hydration and urine alkalinisation are undertaken to diminish renal toxicity Irradiation followed by Methotrexate can increase the incidence of leucoencephalopathy
Vincristine	Intravenous	Low	Peripheral neurotoxicity Hoarseness, diplopia, deafness, jaw pain, pharyngeal pain, parotid pain and facial palsies Constipation Bone, back, limb and abdominal pain Myelosuppression, leucopenia and thrombocytopenia. Polyuria, dysuria, incontinence and acute urinary retention Hypertension and hypotension	Vesicant, avoid extravasation Although rare, confusion, depression, agitation, epilepsy and coma have also been reported

Etoposide	Oral Intravenously	Moderate	Hypersensitivity Myelosuppresion Granulocytopenia anorexia, diarrhoea, stomatitis, abdominal pain, dysphagia and constipation Mucositis in high doses Reversible alopecia Pruritus Reversible hepatotoxicity	Requires nadir count Irritant, avoid extravasation Renal excretion is major route: approximately 40–60% of the drug excreted is unchanged in urine Administer over 30–60 minutes to avoid hypotension. Use gloves and avoid skin or mucosal contact. May cause rash
Procarbazine	Oral	Low	Myelosuppression Flu-like symptoms Peripheral neuropathy Psychotic reaction Hyperpyrexia	Mild MAOIs will require dietary advice Azoospermia and infertility
Doxorubicin	Intravenous	Moderate	Bone marrow suppression mucositis, stomatitis, alopecia and anorexia Flushing of face and torso. Vein itching (acute reactions) Cardiotoxicity	Vesicant, avoid extravasation Radiation recall reaction, i.e. pain at the previously irradiated area
Cisplatin	Intravenous	High	Nephrotoxicity Irreversible ototoxicity Raynaud's syndrome Urticaria Anaphylaxis	Renal excretion is primary route of elimination. Dose reduction in patients with compromised renal function Adequate patient hydration with diuretics, i.e. mannitol Azoospermia
Carboplatin	Intravenous	High	Thrombocytopenia, Neutropenia	Renal excretion primary route of elimination. Dose reduction in patients with compromised renal function. Adequate patient hydration with diuretics i.e. mannitol.

clarify any issues of concern. The staff should be skilled in dealing with patients with CNS tumours and have knowledge of the problems that relate to the disease and its treatment (Brada and Guerrero, 1997). If the patient is to be entered into a clinical trial, detailed information regarding the trial should also be made available. The description of any proposed drugs and route of administration should be given, along with appropriate advice regarding side-effects, mode of action, dietary restrictions, drug interactions and so on. What may appear basic information, such as what time of day it is best to take the drug, how long before taking the drug it is best to take anti-emetics, when the nausea and vomiting will commence, how long the nausea and vomiting will last and how the patient should discuss treatment issues with family and friends, are all important areas of concern and should be dealt with understanding and sensitivity without giving the impression that the nurse is pressed for time.

It is often very reassuring for patients to receive a telephone call prior to or during their treatment. Such contact will enable the nurse to monitor the patient's progress and allow the patient time to discuss any problems. Such calls often help to reassure patients that all is well and make them feel that someone cares (Brada and Guerrero, 1997).

Informed consent

It is the responsibility of professionals to provide patients with the necessary information prior to the commencement of any treatment. This includes standard approved treatment as well as new cancer treatments undergoing clinical trials (see chapter appendix). This information should, as far as possible, be provided in layman's terms without the use of medical jargon that may confuse patients. In neuro-oncology, the patient's partner and family should be included in the process of informed consent as patients may have subtle cognitive and/or personality changes and may not truly comprehend the implications of the proposed treatment.

Patients and families should not be expected to agree to enter a clinical trial or necessarily undertake treatment during this visit. However, written as well as verbal information should be provided and a further appointment arranged in order to allow them time to consider the implications of the treatment discussed. At all times, particularly when discussing a clinical trial, patients should be reassured that refusal to enter a trial does not mean exemption from further treatment or substandard care and therapy in the future. Nurses play an important role in patient advocacy, often explaining and clarifying the treatment being offered; as such, nurses should always be present when treatment discussions are undertaken.

Quality of life

Failing survival, the major aim of any treatment should be care and quality of life. As cure is not often achievable for many CNS tumours, quality of life issues for this group of patients remain even more crucial. Quality of life must be viewed from a holistic perspective rather than solely from a medical viewpoint. Professionals should not just concentrate their efforts on the impact of cancer treatment on the disease but must, very importantly, also be attending to the broader issues of care. When viewing quality of life, the needs of not only the patient, but also the family need to be considered, and appropriate psychosocial support and care must always be made available (see Chapter 11).

Children and chemotherapy

Paediatric brain tumours are generally managed on the same lines as adult brain tumours of a similar histology. The principal exception to this is tumours arising in children under 3 years of age for whom the treatment is with primary chemotherapy.

Ideally, all children with CNS tumours should be treated in dedicated specialist units and entered, when eligible, into national and international trials in order to determine whether chemotherapy improves prognosis and quality of life. Despite the intensity of many childhood chemotherapy regimens, most children are treated as outpatients, with dedicated nurse specialists visiting and supporting the child and family through treatment.

The child will almost always have a central venous catheter or skin tunnelled catheter inserted in order to avoid the trauma of frequent cannulation and for ease of drug administration. The play therapist is an important member of the multidisciplinary team, devising various distractions in order to make the treatment experience more tolerable. If the child needs inpatient care, every effort should be made to accommodate parents and other siblings and thus reduce the trauma of admission. Whenever possible, chemotherapy is administered overnight so that the child can have the day free for play activities.

CNS tumours

Gliomas

High-grade gliomas

The optimum role of cytotoxic chemotherapy in the management of high-grade gliomas is still to be determined. Chemotherapy is not curative, but its role has been investigated widely in both adjuvant and palliative settings.

There is at present no proven role for adjuvant chemotherapy following surgery and radiotherapy for high-grade gliomas. The Medical Research Council (MRC) trial of randomised adjuvant chemotherapy in high-grade glioma closed in 1997 (Brada et al. 1998). Over 670 patients with high-grade gliomas were recruited into this multicentre trial over a period of 9 years, of whom 335 were randomised for adjuvant chemotherapy commencing 4 weeks after the completion of radiotherapy, and 339 patients were allocated to the no-chemotherapy arm. The chemotherapy group were treated with a combination of procarbazine, CCNU (lomustine) and vincristine (PCV). There was no statistically significant difference in survival between the two treatment arms, suggesting no benefit for adjuvant chemotherapy. The current policy is not to offer chemotherapy as part of the initial treatment of high-grade gliomas.

Palliative chemotherapy remains a conventional treatment for patients with recurrent high-grade gliomas because recurrent tumours are usually large and re-excision is rarely indicated.

At present, the only proven effective agents against high-grade gliomas in phase III studies have been the nitrosoureas. Although chemotherapy does not have a curative role, patients may have a 20–40% probability of a short-term response, with oligodendrogliomas responding more favourably (Brada and Thomas, 1995). Combination chemotherapy is not clearly superior to that with single agents (Brada and Thomas, 1995).

As oligodendrogliomas appear to respond more favourably to chemotherapy, a new randomised study of adjuvant PCV is currently being undertaken under the auspices of the European Organisation for Research and Treatment of Cancer (EORTC). The major aim of this study is to determine whether adjuvant PCV chemotherapy prolongs overall survival time and time to first progression in patients with anaplastic oligodendroglioma following surgery and radiation therapy. The study will also determine the toxicity of adjuvant PCV chemotherapy and investigate the effect on quality of life and neurological function.

Low-grade gliomas

Following surgery, the role of adjuvant treatment for low-grade gliomas remains controversial. Most centres will adopt a 'watch' policy (see Chapter 6) prior to undertaking further treatment. There is at present little objective information regarding the benefits of cytotoxic chemotherapy in terms of survival or quality of life for this group of patients.

Primitive neuroectodermal tumours

The standard treatment for most PNETs is craniospinal axis irradiation, but the additional role of chemotherapy is under investigation, particularly in the treatment of poor-prognosis PNET, which includes supratentorial PNET and extensive medulloblastoma (see Chapters 3, 4 and 6). Chemotherapy offers excellent palliation for recurrent disease as these tumours are chemosensitive. However, there is much debate about the value of chemotherapy as an adjuvant treatment. There are at present no good randomised data that prove efficacy (Evans et al, 1990; Tait et al, 1990), but phase II results (Packer et al, 1991) have led to the routine use of cytotoxic chemotherapy in some countries.

Current chemotherapy for medulloblastoma includes a combination of carboplatin, etoposide, cyclophosphamide and vincristine, and scheduling with radiotherapy needs to be determined.

Primary CNS lymphoma

These tumours are highly sensitive to corticosteroids and radiotherapy, although the prognosis unfortunately remains poor. Combination chemotherapy may be employed and followed by consolidation radiotherapy in the hope of improving the patient's quality of life and survival (see Chapter 6). However, many patients with primary CNS lymphomas are elderly and unfortunately tolerate chemotherapy poorly, so they may thus not be suitable for such aggressive treatment.

Current chemotherapy for primary CNS lymphoma includes a combination of doxorubicin, cyclophosphamide, high-dose methotrexate, vincristine and prednisolone.

Germ cell tumours

Germ cell tumours are extremely sensitive to radiotherapy and chemotherapy, with germinomas generally having a more favourable prognosis than non-germinomas.

Current chemotherapy for germ cell tumours includes a combination of carboplatin, vincristine, bleomycin and hydrocortisone.

Brain metastases

Surgery and radiotherapy are often the treatment of choice for brain metastases (see Chapters 5 and 6). However, for patients with chemoresponsive tumours, such as small cell lung cancer, treatment with the cytotoxic drug appropriate for the tumour may be considered.

Practicalities of care

The decision for patients to be given cytotoxic chemotherapy and/or entered into clinical trials should not be taken lightly. In particular, as is often the case for most of these patients, treatment is palliative in nature. As such, issues of care and support are paramount, and a holistic approach to patient management, requiring the skills of different members of the multidisciplinary and primary health care team, is vital (see Chapter 9). Other practical issues that may contribute towards quality of life can then be further addressed. The emphasis should be on minimising inconvenience and unnecessary visits to the hospital (Brada and Guerrero, 1997). For example, the patient's nadir full blood count and chemistry could be done by the general practitioner or district nurse and the results faxed or telephoned to the hospital. This would avoid unnecessary hospital visits for the patient, especially if haemoglobin, white cell and platelet levels are at a low range for treatment. It is therefore important to alert local community services and voluntary organisations at an early stage to provide appropriate care and support (Brada and Guerrero, 1997).

Nurses therefore play a complex and demanding role during chemotherapy, balancing the care and support of the patient and family with the educational preparation required to assist the patient through the various treatment experiences. Nurses' knowledge must therefore be 'expert' and their judgement backed by research-based practice.

Treatment-related problems

Nurses, whether working in hospital, community or hospice, are in a pivotal position to monitor and observe patients for potential treatment-related side-effects. Patients, unless told, will often not know or may have forgotten what is significant and what they need to report. Side-effects can be unpleasant as well as frightening for those patients with little information. Patients need to be reassured that such side-effects are often transient and that they can be prevented or alleviated by appropriate intervention.

Gastrointestinal

Nausea and vomiting

Apart from being the most common side-effects of chemotherapy, nausea and vomiting are also often the most distressing side-effects of treatment for many patients. In neuro-oncology, some patients will have speech and/or swallowing difficulties; as such, nausea and vomiting are of particular concern because of the danger of aspiration. The incidence and severity of nausea and vomiting vary between different cytotoxic drugs (see Table 7.1) and can be dose related and dependent on the drug schedule. It is always advisable to provide patients with adequate anti-emetic medication to prevent and/or control any acute or delayed nausea and vomiting that may be experienced during treatment (see Chapter 8).

Support, advice and reassurance are paramount as many patients neglect their diet and fluids, which can contribute towards weight loss and dehydration. Carbonated drinks can at times help, and advice should be provided regarding a light diet with an emphasis on small, frequent, appetising meals. The dietitian should be involved as nausea and vomiting can often exacerbate anorexia.

Other non-pharmacological interventions, such as relaxation therapy, massage and diversional therapy, can at times prove helpful: patients should be referred for alternative therapy as necessary.

Mucositis

Oral hygiene is of paramount importance as some chemotherapeutic agents, in particular methotrexate, will give rise to mucositis. As well as being a distressing side-effect of therapy, oral infection may provide a route of spread for severe systemic sepsis and may also lead to functional problems including dysphagia. Mouth hygiene should be encouraged and the patient's oral cavity regularly inspected for the presence of fungal, viral and bacterial infections. The use of appropriate oral care agents and topical nystatin will help to minimise superimposed infection (Porter 1996).

Mucositis can be very distressing and painful as well as exacerbating anorexia. It may at times be necessary to provide analgesia to alleviate the pain associated with mucositis; in severe cases, the temporary use of opiates may improve the discomfort experienced.

Bowel

It should be routine practice for nurses to ascertain a patient's normal bowel habit. Many patients with CNS tumours are, because of mobility problems, prone to constipation. The use of pharmacological agents often predisposes to constipation, and for those patients undergoing chemotherapy, especially with vinca alkaloids, this problem can be exacerbated. Advice on diet and the use of laxatives such as co-danthramer elixir or capsules often improves the situation (see Chapter 8).

Diarrhoea is not common, but if it is experienced as a consequence of cytotoxic chemotherapy, patients may require treatment with codeine phosphate tablets and be encouraged to drink fluids in order to avoid dehydration. If the diarrhoea persists, a stool sample should be obtained to exclude infection.

Haematological

For the majority of cases of cytotoxic chemotherapy, bone marrow suppression is the most important dose-limiting toxicity (Steward et al, 1995). It is therefore important that patients have a full blood count taken prior to the commencement of chemotherapy. It is often also important that the appropriate nadir count is undertaken, as certain drugs, such as nitrosoureas, may have a delayed nadir, whereas alkylating agents have a cumulative effect on the bone marrow stem cells (Steward et al, 1995).

The blood count will often recover of its own accord given time, the only action necessary being to delay chemotherapy treatment for a week and then repeat the blood count. It may occasionally be necessary, because of the risk of acute toxicity, to reduce the chemotherapy dose. However, such action may be detrimental to patients' outcomes, especially in those with potentially curable tumours. Although it is not at present standard practice in neuro-oncology, haemopoietic growth factors can be used with chemotherapy to maximise the appropriate treatment delivery. Patients at risk of thrombocytopenia (a low platelet count) should be asked to report any signs of bruising, petechiae, nose bleeds, bleeding gums and haematuria. Those at risk of neutropenia (a low neutrophil count) should be asked to report any signs of fever, sore throat and 'flu-like symptoms. It should be noted that, although they are not necessarily neutropenic, patients on steroid therapy because of the risk of immunosuppression are also vulnerable to infection.

Alopecia

Chemotherapy-induced alopecia is a well-recognised problem. Treatment-induced alopecia can be very distressing, and the patient should be given the opportunity to discuss the practical issues and psychosocial effects of hair loss (see Chapters 6, 10 and 11). Unlike the case in radiotherapy, it is possible to reassure patients that their hair will grow back. However, the majority of patients with CNS tumours will have undergone radiotherapy prior to chemotherapy and may as such have already experienced some degree of permanent hair loss (see Chapter 6). Cytotoxic drugs such as etoposide (VP16), epirubicin, cyclophosphamide, doxorubicin and vincristine are commonly associated with alopecia.

Pulmonary toxicity

Cytotoxic drugs such as bleomycin, busulphan, cyclophosphamide and methotrexate may all cause pulmonary changes, which may be transient or may progress to pulmonary fibrosis (Steward et al, 1995). Pulmonary toxicity is related to drug dosage with an increased risk when combination chemotherapy is being used. Those patients at risk of pulmonary toxicity should have baseline chest X-ray and pulmonary function tests, which may need to be repeated prior to each chemotherapy treatment. Nurses must be vigilant and observe patients as well as asking them to report any symptoms, for example shortness of breath and wheezing. It must be remembered that shortness of breath can also be a side-effect of corticosteroid therapy or infection (see Chapter 8).

Cardiac toxicity

Cardiomyopathy may be seen with the anthracyclines, that is, doxorubicin, daunorubicin and epirubicin (Steward et al, 1995). Cardiomyopathy is often associated with accumulating doses of the drug. Those patients at risk of cardiac toxicity should have a baseline ECG and Muga (multigated acquisition) scan before commencing treatment.

Renal and bladder toxicity

Chemotherapeutic drugs associated with renal and bladder toxicity include cisplatin, high-dose methotrexate, ifosfamide and cyclophosphamide. Cisplatin may cause a fall in glomerular filtration rate and tubular dysfunction, leading to hypokalaemia and hypomagnesaemia (Steward et al, 1995). Methotrexate can cause renal damage as a result of the deposition of methotrexate metabolites in the collecting tubules. Ifosfamide and cyclophosphamide may cause chemical cystitis (Steward et al, 1995).

Those patients at risk of renal and bladder toxicity should have a baseline renal function test (EDTA) prior to chemotherapy. With some regimens, adequate hydration with forced diuresis using a diuretic such as mannitol (see Chapter 8) is undertaken. It is important to maintain a record of the patient's fluid intake and output during treatment. The patient's urine should also be tested for pH as alkalinisation using sodium bicarbonate may be required during treatment. Sodium bicarbonate increases methotrexate excretion. The use of Mesna rescue by ensuring adequate diuresis may alleviate or prevent any chemical cystitis associated with chemotherapy since it prevents the acrolein metabolite of ifosfamide from damaging the bladder mucosa (Yarbro, 1996).

Neurological toxicity

Added neurotoxicity can be devastating for patients with existing CNS deficits. Because regeneration of nervous system structure is poor, recovery is unlikely once an agent has caused severe damage to the nerve cells or supporting structures (Posner, 1995). The vinca alkaloids, especially vincristine, can cause peripheral neuropathy. Loss of tendon reflexes, paraesthesia and numbness in the fingers and toes are signs of peripheral neuropathy and are an indication to reduce the drug dose (Steward et al, 1995).

Other complications include drowsiness, confusion and encephalopathy, which usually revert once the treatment is discontinued. The patient should be given the opportunity to talk, and referral for psychological counselling may need to be considered if appropriate as mood swings and depression can nearly always be observed (see Chapter 11).

The combination of intrathecal or high-dose systemic methotrexate with radiotherapy may cause arachnoiditis, cerebral atrophy and necrosing encephalopathy (Steward et al, 1995).

Long-term side-effects

Long-term side-effects of treatment must also be discussed with patients prior to the commencement of cytotoxic chemotherapy.

Although treatment for many CNS tumours is palliative in nature, this is no excuse to avoid discussing long-term issues.

It must not be assumed that this group of patients has no interest in or desire to discuss fertility issues. Issues such as pregnancy and sperm banking must be discussed and appropriate personnel, such as the tissue collector, involved in care. Female patients of childbearing age may require a pregnancy test prior to the commencent of treatment. Advice on appropriate contraceptive measures should be provided. Females should also be informed that chemotherapy may well cause disruption to their menstrual cycles.

In men, the alkylating drugs have been widely recognised as producing some damage to seminiferous epithelium. The duration and extent of the damage appear to be related to the age of the patient and the amount of drug received (Klein, 1996). Cyclophosphamide and chlorambucil have been associated with azoospermia, whereas procarbazine appears to be the single most toxic chemotherapeutic agent to the adult male gonad (Klein, 1996).

In women, as in adult men, alkylating agents are the most gonadotoxic of cytotoxic drugs as well as being associated with mutagenesis and teratogenesis (Klein, 1996).

The increased risk of secondary malignancies as a long-term side-effect of cytotoxic chemotherapy cannot be ignored in those patients with potentially curable tumours and, as such, this needs to be discussed. By far the most frequently reported cancers following chemotherapy are leukaemia and the associated myelodysplastic syndromes (Boice and Shriner, 1996).

Conclusion

Nurses play a valuable role when caring for patients undergoing cytotoxic chemotherapy treatment. They, as the patient's advocate, can listen, explain, clarify, support, express the patient's and family's concern, and, very importantly, clearly document those side-effects reported by patients during conventional chemotherapy treatment and clinical trials. Nurses, as expert practitioners, also have a responsibility to conduct their own research and/or clinical audits. The information gained will help to improve the quality of life of existing patients as well as explore new strategies for future intervention.

Appendix: clinical trials

There is a standardised sequence for evaluating new cytotoxic drugs, which allows the progressive and continuous assessment of toxicity and efficacy. These stages are referred to as phases I, II and III (Schold, 1994).

Phase I studies

The major aim of phase I studies is to determine the maximum safe dose of the drug that can be given before toxicity is encountered. As such, a significant number of patients receive an ineffective dose (Workman et al, 1995). Those patients entered into phase I studies usually have advanced disease and have failed conventional therapy.

Phase II studies

Before a new drug is added to and evaluated in a drug combination, it should be proved in single agent (phase II) studies that it has some intrinsic activity in a given tumour type (Winograd, 1995). In phase II studies, the actual dose of the drug is determined from the phase I trial. Patients being treated are selected to be as homogeneous as possible, thus avoiding an element of bias; this should ensure that results do not just overemphasise benefit. However, some patients may have failed previous treatment, and the response rate to second-line cytotoxic chemotherapy is usually less than that to the first; this could minimise potential results. The end-point used in phase II studies is a measurable and reproducible decrease in tumour size (Workman et al, 1995).

Phase III studies

Phase III studies are the definitive tests of a drug's efficacy (Schold, 1994). Phase III studies are controlled randomised studies involving the comparison of results between the new experimental agent and a control therapy that is known to have some tumour effect.

Determining the response in the treatment of CNS tumours is difficult. Response evaluation is often based on a combination of CT or MRI and the patient's clinical assessment (see Chapter 4). Of importance in phase III studies, in order to demonstrate drug effectiveness, are survival, time to treatment failure and disease-free survival, complete response rate, response rate and beneficial effects on disease-related symptoms or quality of life (O'Shaughnessy, 1991).

References

Boice JD Jnr, Shriner DA (1996) Second malignancies after chemotherapy. In Perry MC (Ed.) The Chemotherapy Source Book, 2nd edn. Baltimore: Williams & Wilkins, pp 785–802.

Brada M, Guerrero D (1997) One model of follow-up care. In Davies E, Hopkins A (Eds) Improving Care for Patients with Malignant Cerebral Glioma. London: Royal College of Physicians of London, pp 93–8.

Brada M et al. (1998) Medical Research Council Randomised Trial of Adjuvant Chemotherapy in High Grade Glioma (HGG) Proceedings of ASCO 17.

Brada M, Ross G (1996) Radiation therapy and the management of malignant gliomas. Baillière's Clinical Neurology 5(2): 319–43.

Brada M, Thomas DGT (1995) Tumours of the Brain and Spinal Cord in Adults. Oxford Textbook of Oncology. Oxford: Oxford University Press.

Clamon GH (1996) Extravasation. In Perry MC (Ed.) The Chemotherapy Source Book, 2nd edn. Baltimore: Williams & Wilkins, pp 607–11.

Cleton FJ (1995) Chemotherapy: general aspects. In Peckham M, Pinedo H, Veronesi U (Eds) Oxford Textbook of Oncology. Volume 1. Oxford: Oxford University Press, pp 445-53.

Dougherty L (1996) Cytotoxic drugs. In Mallet J, Bailey C (Eds) Manual of Clinical Nursing Procedures. The Royal Marsden NHS Trust, 4th edn. Oxford: Blackwell Science.

Evans AE, Jenkin DT, Sposto R et al (1990) The Treatment of Medulloblastoma. Results of a prospective randomized trial of radiation therapy with and without CCNU, vincristine and prednisone. Journal of Neurosurgery 72: 572–82.

Guerrero D (1996) Brain tumours. In Tschudin V (Ed.) Nursing the Patient with Cancer. London: Prentice Hall.

Klein C (1996) Gonadal complications and teratogenicity of cancer therapy. In Perry MC (Ed.) The Chemotherapy Source Book, 2nd edn, pp 813–32. Baltimore: Williams & Wilkins.

O'Shaughnessy JA (1991) Journal of Clinical Oncology 9: 2225–32. Cited in Peckham M, Pinedo H, Veronesi U (Eds) Oxford Textbook of Oncology, Volume 1. Oxford: Oxford University Press.

Packer RJ, Sutton LN, Goldwein JW et al (1991) Improved survival with the use of adjuvant chemotherapy in the treatment of medulloblastoma. Journal of Neurosurgery 74: 433–40.

Peters GJ (1995) Antimetabolites. In Peckham M, Pinedo H, Veronesi U (Eds) Oxford Textbook of Oncology, Volume 1. Oxford: Oxford University Press, pp 524–53.

Porter H (1996) Mouth care. In Mallet J, Bailey C (Eds) Manual of Clinical Nursing Procedures. The Royal Marsden NHS Trust, 4th edn. Oxford: Blackwell Science.

Posner J (1995) Side effects of chemotherapy. In Posner J, Neurologic Complications of Cancer. Philadelphia: FA Davis, pp 282–310.

Priestman TJ (1989) Cancer Chemotherapy: an introduction, 3rd edn. London: Springer-Verlag.

Ramlakhan N, Altman J (1990) Breaching the blood–brain barrier. New Scientist, 24 Nov.

Schold S (1994) Chemotherapy of central nervous system tumors. In Rengachary SS, Wilkins RH (Eds) Principles of Neurosurgery. London: Wolfe, pp 1–43.1.

Shapiro WR, Shapiro JR, Walker RW (1995) Central nervous system. In Abeloff MD, Armitage JO, Lichter AS, Niederhuber JE (Eds) Clinical Oncology. New York: Churchill Livingstone, pp 851–913.

Steward WP, Cassidy J, Kaye SB (1995) Principles of chemotherapy. In Price P, Sikora K, Halnan KE (Eds) Treatment of Cancer. London: Chapman & Hall Medical, pp 91–108.

Tait DM, Thornton-Jones H, Bloom HJG, Lemerle J, Morris-Jones P (1990)

Adjuvant chemotherapy for medulloblastoma: the first multi-centre control trial of the international society of of paediatric oncology (SIOP I). European Journal of Cancer 26(4): 464–9.

Tortorice PV (1997) Chemotherapy: principles of therapy. In Groenwald SL, Goodman M, Hansen-Frogge M, Henke-Yarbro C (Eds) Cancer Nursing Principles and Practice, 4th edn. Boston: Jones and Bartlett, pp 283–316

Winograd B (1995) New drug development. In Peckham M, Pinedo H, Veronesi U (Eds) Oxford Textbook of Oncology, Volume 1. Oxford: Oxford University Press, pp 486–95.

Workman P, Lewis AD, Cassidy J (1995) In Peckham M, Pinedo H, Veronesi U (Eds) Oxford Textbook of Oncology, Volume 1. Oxford: Oxford University Press, pp 495–511.

Yarbro JW (1996) The scientific basis of cancer chemotherapy. In Perry MC (Ed.) The Chemotherapy Source Book, 2nd edn. Baltimore: Williams & Wilkins, pp 3–18.

Further reading

Perry MC (Ed.) (1996) The Chemotherapy Source Book, 2nd edn. Baltimore: Williams & Wilkins.

Chapter 8 Medication used in the symptom management of CNS tumours

Christopher Evans and Douglas Guerrero

Introduction

At times, drug overusage and drug interactions can be mistaken for tumour progression or recurrence. This chapter aims to provide nurses with a broader overview of specific medication most commonly used in the symptom management of CNS tumours. It will highlight drug usage, administration and potential problems that can be experienced by patients.

Medications will be discussed in relation to those symptoms most common in this group of patients. These will include headaches, dyspepsia, epilepsy, nausea and vomiting, constipation and candidiasis.

Headaches

Headaches are common in patients with brain tumours. Not all headaches result from raised intracranial pressure. However, all headaches require assessment and evaluation to ascertain the cause. The most frequent causes are often raised intracranial pressure, direct effect of the tumour or treatment. Patients with brain tumours also experience stress headaches.

Raised intracranial pressure

Raised intracranial pressure is a potentially life-threatening condition and as such needs to be taken very seriously. There are several categories of disease process that may lead to an increase in raised intracranial pressure. These include neoplasms, haematomas, abscesses, cerebral oedema and hydrocephalus (an abnormal accumulation of CSF).

Raised intracranial pressure can cause symptoms of headache, nausea and vomiting. The aim of treatment is to improve symptoms of raised intracranial pressure as well as reversible neurological deficits.

The two main methods of reducing raised intracranial pressure pharmacologically are by using high-dose corticosteroids, that is dexamethasone, or a cerebral dehydrating agent such as mannitol.

Steroids

It is normal practice to routinely commence patients on steroids preoperatively to reduce the risk of surgical oedema. Steroids are also frequently used at other times for the symptomatic treatment of:

- surgically unrelated raised intracranial pressure giving rise to headache, nausea and vomiting;
- reversible steroid-responsive neurological deficit induced by tumour or treatment.

Steroids have both glucocorticoid (anti-inflammatory) and mineralocorticoid (water and mineral) effects. Steroids are among the most frequently used drugs in patients with cancer (Batchelor et al, 1997), primarily for the control of brain and spinal cord oedema and for the relief of spinal pain (Posner, 1996).

Dexamethasone

In neuro-oncology, the most widely used steroid is dexamethasone. Dexamethasone has high glucocorticoid activity in conjunction with insignificant mineralocorticoid activity. This makes dexamethasone the most appropriate steroid for high-dose therapy in the treatment of cerebral oedema.

There are two tablet strengths: 0.5 mg (500 mcg) and 2 mg. Doses can vary significantly from 16 mg daily to 0.5 mg on alternate days (depending on symptom severity). The highest dose is usually 16 mg daily; however, the best dose is the lowest dose possible that keeps the patient comfortable with minimal side-effects.

Too rapid a reduction of medication following a prolonged course of longer than 7 days can lead to adrenal insufficiency (Addisonian crisis). Withdrawal must therefore always be gradual, depending on symptoms, drug dosage and duration of therapy. An alternate-day dosing regimen may reduce the incidence and severity of adrenal insufficiency.

Dexamethasone may mask signs of infection and decrease patients' natural resistance. As such, any significant intercurrent illness, infections, stress or a relapse in the patient's general condition may require a temporary increase in dosage or a recommencement of dexamethasone.

Patients should be advised to avoid those with colds and other infections such as chicken pox and measles. Any problems with slow wound healing, prolonged inflammation, persistent fever or sore throat should be reported.

Side-effects

It is the responsibility of professionals to discuss potential side-effects with patients. Side-effects are minimised by using the lowest effective dose for the minimum period possible. Side-effects can be unpleasant, and nurses must reassure patients that these are often temporary and usually reversible on completion of therapy. Some side-effects, however, may take weeks or months to improve.

The most common side-effects of steroids are salt and water retention, and increased appetite. However, other side-effects are also evident in many patients, and as such nurses need to be familiar with these.

Gastrointestinal

Gastrointestinal side-effects include dyspepsia, peptic and oesophageal ulceration and candidiasis. It is usual practice for patients on steroids to be taking a prophylactic H_2 antagonist to prevent dyspepsia.

Musculoskeletal

Musculoskeletal effects are numerous and can include proximal myopathy and osteoporosis. Symptoms of persistent back ache and chest pain should be acted on as these may indicate the presence of rib or vertebral fracture.

Steroid myopathy is a common complication among cancer patients receiving dexamethasone (Batchelor et al, 1997). Its presentation is rapid, and it is potentially very disabling. Patients present with muscle weakness restricted to the proximal muscles of the extremities and the neck flexors. This makes it difficult for patients to manage stairs or raise themselves from a sitting position.

Respiratory muscle weakness is also common with steroid therapy and may be accompanied by respiratory symptoms. Patients may experience a significant decline in respiratory function, leading to symptomatic dyspnoea (Batchelor et al, 1997). Steroid myopathy is reversible and resolves over time once the dexamethasone has been discontinued.

The long-term use of corticosteroids can lead to osteoporosis as well as osteonecrosis. Osteoporosis can give rise to vertebral fractures, whilst osteonecrosis can occur in the shoulders, wrist, clavicle or vertebral body and may be confused with spinal cord compression or peripheral neuropathy (Posner, 1996).

Endocrine

Endocrine effects include adrenal insufficiency (Addisonian crisis). The symptoms of adrenal insufficiency are nausea, dyspnoea, fever, hypotension, myalgia and hypoglycaemia. To reverse the symptoms of adrenal insufficiency, the patient needs to be recommenced on dexamethasone, otherwise death can occur.

Steroids can also affect menstrual cycle, so female patients should be informed about the possibility of menstrual irregularities.

Cushing's syndrome is a complication of steroid therapy. The clinical manifestation of this syndrome includes trunkal obesity, a moon face and a buffalo hump. These characteristics result from fat redistribution from the extremities to central body regions such as the abdomen, face and upper back. The increase of central subcutaneous fat deposits stretches the skin, which can rupture subdermal tissue, causing the formation of purple striae. Corticosteroids increase appetite and weight, often considered by many patients to be undesirable side-effects.

Some patients experience hirsutism. This is particularly distressing for females. Such altered body image changes often give rise to depression. If appropriate, nurses should discuss referral for psychological support.

Dexamethasone can cause decreased carbohydrate tolerance, leading to raised blood glucose levels. This can give rise to steroid-induced diabetes. As such, nurses should, at least on a weekly basis, test patients' urine for glucose while they are on steroids. Diabetic patients may require a commencement of or increase in their insulin dose, particularly if the dose of steroid is increased. It is also advisable to refer such patients to a dietitian.

Neurological

Neurological side-effects can include euphoria, depression, insomnia and psychosis. With dexamethasone, steroid-induced psychosis is rare, although it can occasionally be observed (Malseed et al, 1985).

Ophthalmic

Ophthalmic complications include glaucoma, cataracts and corneal thinning as well as an exacerbation of viral or fungal eye disease.

Other side-effects include fluid/electrolyte imbalance, acne, hypertension and cardiac arrhythmias.

Points to note

1. Patients with CNS tumours may require an increase or a decrease in dexamethasone dosages at different stages of their illness. Nurses must therefore inform patients that their steroids requirements may alter from time to time.
2. Patients should be advised to take their dexamethasone with food or a milky drink as this reduces the chance of indigestion.
3. If patients cannot swallow their dexamethasone tablets, these should be crushed and taken with a small amount of liquid. A suspension form is also available.
4. It is usual practice to divide the dexamethasone total dose into two, the first dose being taken with breakfast and the second with lunch or in the early afternoon.
5. The last dose of dexamethasone should be taken before 6 pm in order to avoid steroid-induced insomnia.
6. Families/carers should be involved and also provided with appropriate advice and instructions regarding steroid therapy.
7. Patients should carry a steroid card that should provide information and details of drug, dosage and duration of treatment.
8. Phenytoin increases the metabolic clearance of steroids and may decrease their therapeutic effect.

Mannitol

It may occasionally be necessary for some patients to be admitted to hospital to treat an acute exacerbation of cerebral oedema. The main osmotic dehydrating agent used to reduce raised intracranial pressure is mannitol (Speight and Avery, 1987).

Mannitol is not metabolised and does not cross the blood–brain barrier. Mannitol reduces brain oedema, decreases the production of CSF and is also rapidly excreted by the kidneys. The pressure of mannitol in the circulation draws fluid from the tissue into the blood, thus raising plasma osmotic pressure and decreasing intracranial pressure.

Dosage

In neuro-oncology, the usual dosage is 100 ml, 20% mannitol over 30 minutes repeated two or three times daily.
Its effectiveness is usually restricted to 48–72 hours.

Points to note

1. As intravenous mannitol produces osmotic diuresis, it may at times be necessary to use a conveen or catheterise those patients with major physical disabilities prior to drug administration.
2. Patients may complain of a dry mouth and thirst due to diuresis, so oral fluids and mouth care may be necessary.
3. A fluid chart should be maintained in order to monitor the patient's intake and urinary output.

Analgesics

For the symptomatic relief of headaches not resulting from raised intracranial pressure, the following analgesic stepladder is recommended.

Paracetamol

The usual paracetamol dose recommended is 1–2 tablets four times a day. Patients should be advised not to take more than two tablets at any one time and not more than eight tablets in 24 hours. Overdosage of paracetamol can cause hepatotoxicity.

Co-dydramol and co-proxamol

The recommended dosage for both co-dydramol and co-proxamol is 1–2 tablets four times a day (no more than two tablets at any one time) and not more than eight tablets in 24 hours. Side-effects may include drowsiness, which may be exacerbated by alcohol consumption. Overdosage of co-proxamol tablets is complicated by respiratory depression and heart failure because of the dextropropoxyphene, and by hepatotoxicity from the paracetamol. As such, overdosage may require treatment.

Dihydrocodeine and codeine

Dihydrocodeine and codeine are both mild opiates. The oral dosage of dihydrocodeine and codeine is 30 mg up to six times in 24 hours, to a total dose not exceeding 240 mg. Patients should not generally receive an oral dose of dihydrocodeine 60 mg as this does not carry twice the analgesic effect of a 30 mg dose but can cause twice the side-effects of a 30 mg dose. However, some patients do benefit from a 50 mg/60 mg intramuscular/oral dose of dihydrocodeine, depending on at what point the dose/response curve plateaus for that individual patient. Nevertheless, the 90 mg doses of dihydrocodeine used at some centres are not justified.

Equivalence quoted between dihydrocodeine and codeine varies from source to source, but they are generally regarded as interchangeable. Dihydrocodeine and codeine are also available in oral syrup form.

Side-effects

Side-effects for both dihydrocodeine and codeine include drowsiness, which may be exacerbated by alcohol consumption. Constipation is often a common side-effect and patients may require laxatives. Lightheadeness, dizziness and nausea are occasionally experienced by some patients.

Strong opiates

The use of mild opiates (dihydrocodeine and codeine) is often preferable in neuro-oncology over strong opiates such as morphine for the following reasons. Dihydrocodeine and codeine initially cause less drowsiness than morphine, and codeine causes less pupillary reaction than morphine. These are important considerations, especially if undertaking neurological assessements (see Chapter 2).

However, at the terminal stages of disease, strong opiates may be recommended to improve the patient's comfort.

Points to note

1. Patients may benefit from therapeutic massage and/or aromatherapy, especially if the headaches are the result of psychological stress.
2. Explain to patients that the best analgesic effects are gained if analgesics are taken regularly prior to the commencement of the headaches.
3. Reassure patient about constipation. Explain that this is a common problem with the repeated administration of analgesics. Provide a suitable laxative and refer the patient to a dietitian.

4. Monitor headaches as a change in severity, any development of neurological deficit, changes in the level of consciousness or other symptoms will require immediate medical referral.

Dyspepsia

Dyspepsia is a common discomfort often described as indigestion, a feeling of fullness or pain that is often gnawing or burning in nature and is localised to the upper abdomen or chest.

The use of pharmacological doses of corticosteroids may cause dyspepsia and, rarely, gastrointestinal bleeding. This is because dexamethasone, like other glucocorticoids, stimulates acid and pepsin secretion and inhibits the production of protective mucus.

Histamine plays a major role in gastric acid secretion. The H_2 antagonists effectively block the secretion of gastric acid and reduce acidity and pepsin activity. As such, H_2 antagonists have an important role in the therapeutic management of dyspepsia.

The H_2 antagonists include cimetidine, ranitidine and the relatively newly introduced famotidine and nizatidine. In neuro-oncology, H_2 antagonists are used prophylactically to prevent or alleviate the discomfort of oesophagitis and gastritis associated with steroid therapy.

Ranitidine

Ranitidine is the most common H_2 antagonist prescribed to neuro-oncology patients. It has a good safety profile, that is, it has been used in clinical practice in tens of thousands of patients for many years. Ranitidine is a potent hydrochloric acid secretion inhibitor and reduces daytime and nocturnal gastric acid secretion. The usual prescribed dose is one 150 mg tablet twice a day. Peak serum level occurs 2–3 hours following oral administration, and the drug effect persists for between 8 and 12 hours. Absorption is not affected by food consumption.

Ranitidine is only taken during dexamethasone administration (its dose remaining constant regardless of the steroid dose) and is discontinued on completion of dexamethasone therapy unless the patient has a history of gastric problems. Ranitidine is also available as effervescent tablets, syrup and an injection.

Side-effects

Possible side-effects include headaches, dizziness, constipation, nausea, abdominal pain, rash and malaise as well as transient and reversible changes in liver function tests. It should therefore be used with caution in those patients with a history of impaired renal and hepatic function. Ranitidine should also be used with caution in pregnant women and nursing mothers as well as children.

Points to note

1. Instruct patient and family on the proper administration of ranitidine tablets, that is, 150 mg twice a day.
2. Remind patients that ranitidine will be taken during steroid administration and discontinued on the completion of steroid treatment.
3. Be aware that false-positive tests for urine protein may occur during ranitidine therapy. This is important as patients undergoing steroid treatment will have their urine tested for sugar and may test positive for protein.
4. Be alert for side-effects of treatment and do not confuse ranitidine-induced headaches with headaches resulting from raised intra-cranial pressure.
5. If dyspepsia symptoms are not alleviated with ranitidine therapy, proton pump inhibitors such as omeprazole, lansoprazole and pantoprazole should be considered.

Cimetidine

Cimetidine is not recommended for use in neuro-oncology patients as it can precipitate confusion and reduces the liver metabolism of certain drugs, such as phenytoin and diazepam. It should also be avoided in those patients undergoing warfarin treatment.

Epilepsy

Epilepsy (seizures, fits, convulsions) is the clinical manifestation of a sudden, transient, abnormal neuronal electrical discharge in the brain (see Chapters 3 and 5). Most forms of epilepsy are idiopathic in nature, although approximately 40% of patients with brain tumours present with seizures (Thomas and Graham 1980; Cascino 1990; Guerrero 1995).

Often, prior to neurosurgery, patients with suspected supratentorial tumours and no history of epilepsy are commenced on antiepileptic drugs as a prophylaxis against seizures. This is because there is always a small risk of experiencing a seizure as a consequence of neurosurgery.

Considerations with anti-epileptic drugs

The objective of treatment with anti-epileptic drugs is to prevent the occurrence of seizures by maintaining an effective plasma concentration of the drug while at the same time minimising the risk of side-effects.

The drug and dose must be individualised according to individual patients' needs. Some anti-epileptic drugs are not only ineffective in certain types of seizure disorders but may actually worsen them. Successful therapy therefore depends upon accurate diagnosis, careful selection of the drugs and critical dose adjustment (Malseed et al, 1985).

Therapy is usually initiated with a single agent (monotherapy), but complete control of some seizure types may require the addition of a second and sometimes a third drug (combination therapy). However, frequent dosage alterations or too rapid a shifting between anti-epileptic drugs should be avoided.

The ideal pharmacokinetics of an anti-epileptic drug are good oral bioavailability with a drug half-life of 12–24 hours (allowing for once to twice daily administration), lack of metabolism and no drug interaction; unfortunately, no such drug exists (Walker and Patsalos, 1995).

Stabilisation of the patient can be a difficult task. Once it has been attained, the patient should be advised of the dangers of altering the prescribed drug regimen or subjecting themselves to physical and emotional stress that might compromise their stable condition (Malseed et al, 1985).

Patients should be asked to report any unusual symptoms that occur during therapy as this may indicate an early manifestation of serious toxicity (Malseed et al, 1985).

Any alterations to or discontinuation of anti-epileptic drugs must be carried out slowly over a period of weeks. Abrupt alterations or discontinuation could precipitate repetitive seizures (status epilepticus), which can be fatal (Malseed et al, 1985).

Anti-epileptic drugs can interact with other prescribed medications, the effect of either being increased or decreased. Therefore monitoring of the blood level of anti-epileptic drugs should be undertaken as is deemed appropriate.

If the patient misses a dose of anti-epileptic drug, he or she should be advised to take the next dose when it is due. If a dose is missed on two consecutive days, medical opinion should be sought.

Phenytoin

Phenytoin (Epanutin) is not a CNS depressant and is the drug of choice in patients with tonic-clonic and partial seizures.

The adult oral dose is initially150–300 mg daily increased gradually as necessary up to a total of600mg per day. Any increase in dosage should be made gradually in 50 mg increments in order to avoid marked changes in plasma concentration that can result in the patient experiencing unpleasant side-effects. Phenytoin is available as capsules, infatabs (chewable tablets), a suspension and intravenous injections. A 100 mg capsule is bioequivalent to 90 mg suspension, which equates to a volume of 45 ml.

Intravenous phenytoin must be given as a slow bolus at a maximum rate of 50 mg per minute in order to avoid bradycardia and hypotension. It is advisable to monitor blood pressure and respiratory rate as well as carrying out an ECG during its administration.

The intravenous line should be flushed with sodium chloride 0.9% injection both before and after drug administration in order to avoid local venous irritation caused by the alkalinity of the phenytoin preparation. Flushing is also important to avoid precipitation with other drugs in the intravenous line.

Plasma levels

There are two quoted therapeutic (target) ranges for phenytoin: 10–20 mg/l and 40–80 mmol/l. CNS side-effects are related to serum concentration and usually develop at concentrations greater than 20 mg/l or 80 mmol/l. As the drug concentration increases, so do the severity and frequency of the side-effects.

There are various indications for when plasma levels should be monitored. These include:

- uncontrolled seizures;
- a sudden increase in seizure frequency;
- drug-induced toxicity;
- when in doubt about the patient's compliance;
- when adding or stopping other anti-epileptic drugs;
- in situations where the absorption of the drug might be affected;
- during pregnancy.

Side-effects

Side-effects are dose related. Nystagmus, blurred vision and drowsiness are usually the earliest symptoms detected, beginning at concentrations of between 15 and 30 mg/l, or 60 and 100 mmol/l. Ataxia occurs with plasma levels above 30 mg/l, or 100 mmol/l. Mental changes, including alterations in the patient's consciousness, can occur above 40 mg/l, or 120 mmol/l.

Other common side-effects include nausea, dizziness, headaches and insomnia.

Reversible cosmetic side-effects include gum hypertrophy, acne, hirsutism and facial coarseness. These effects often cause psychological distress to patients.

Haematological side-effects are rare but include megaloblastic anaemia, leucopenia and thrombocytopenia. It is therefore important that symptoms such as sore throats, fever and mucosal ulceration are taken seriously as these may be the early signs of blood dyscrasias.

Points to note

1. Phenytoin has a long half-life, and the total dose can therefore be taken once a day.
2. Phenytoin is alkaline and should be taken after food to minimise gastric irritation.
3. The effects of phenytoin may be diminished by alcohol, so patients should be advised to drink alcohol in moderation.
4. Phenytoin increases the metabolism of oral contraceptives, causing a reduced contraceptive effect.
5. Phenytoin reduces the anticoagulant effect of warfarin because of its enzyme induction effect. It is therefore important to monitor the prothrombin time when the patient is taking both warfarin and phenytoin.

Carbamazepine

Carbamazepine (Tegretol) is the drug of choice for simple and complex partial seizures and for tonic-clonic seizures. It generally has fewer side-effects than phenytoin. In adults, treatment with carbamazepine should be initiated at low doses of 100–400 mg daily in order to allow the CNS tolerance of side-effects. The dose is increased by increments of 100–200 mg every 2 weeks until a usual dose of 800–1200 mg is reached. The maximum dose is 2000 mg per day.

Carbamazepine is available as tablets, chewtabs, liquid and suppositories. A 125 mg suppository is equivalent to a 100 mg tablet. It is usually recommended that suppositories are not used for longer than 7 days; however, in practice they are often used for longer. The reason for such a recommendation is that all clinical trials involving carbamazepine suppositories have lasted no longer than 7 days.

Plasma levels

The plasma concentration for optimum response is 4–12 mcg/ml (<42 mmol/L) for monotherapy and 4–9 mcg/ml when carbamazepine is part of multiple therapy. (For indications of monitoring plasma concentration, see phenytoin.)

Side-effects

Dose-related side-effects include diplopia, dizziness, headache and nausea. Symptoms are often worst 2 hours after administration, corresponding to peak plasma levels. Symptoms can be alleviated by dividing the total daily dose into two or three doses per day or by using the controlled-release (retard) formulation.

Ataxia, unsteadiness and diplopia are seen at levels above 12 mcg/ml. Lethargy, severe sedation and increased seizure frequency are seen at levels above 20 mcg/ml (Brodie and Dichter, 1996).

The most common idiosyncratic side-effect is urticarial rash, which develops in approximately 10% of patients. Less common skin side-effects include erythema multiforme, which often occurs on the extensor surfaces of limbs, and Stevens–Johnson syndrome, which incorporates erythema multiforme involving the mucous membranes of the mouth, throat, eyes, urethra and vagina, as well as photosensitivity.

Serious haematological problems occur in approximately 1% of patients. The most common blood dyscrasia is leucopenia, usually transient, the white cell count reverting to normal during or after the discontinuation of carbamazepine. The early detection of blood dyscrasias is vital as, in some patients, aplastic anaemia may be irreversible.

Carbamazepine can have an antidiuretic hormone-like action; the resulting hyponatraemia (low sodium level) is usually mild and patients asymptomatic, but if the sodium falls below 120 mmol/l, confusion, peripheral oedema and decreasing control in seizures can be present (Brodie and Dichter, 1996).

Points to note

1. It is advisable to monitor the patient's haematology and liver

function tests at the onset of therapy, after dosage adjustments and thereafter every 3 months.
2. Patients should be told to report any signs of sore throat, mucosal ulceration or bruising as these could be early signs of haematological toxicity.
3. Carbamazepine is a powerful enzyme inducer, accelerating its own metabolism and decreasing the effect of other anticonvulsants.
4. Carbamazepine is highly protein bound and may potentiate the effect of other protein-bound drugs such as salicylates, oral hypoglycaemics, anticoagulants and anti-inflammatory drugs by displacing them from protein-binding sites (Malseed et al, 1985).
5. Drugs that inhibit the metabolism of carbamazepine sufficiently to cause adverse CNS side-effects include cimetidine, dextropropoxyphene (found in co-proxamol), erythromycin, diltiazem and verapamil (both diltiazem and verapamil are calcium-channel blockers used in the treatment of angina and hypertension) (Brodie and Dichter, 1996).

Sodium valproate

Sodium valproate (Epilim) is effective in controlling tonic-clonic seizures. Controlled trials in partial epilepsy suggest that it has an efficacy similar to that of carbamazepine and phenytoin, but more evidence is awaited (British National Formulary, 1997).

The starting dose for adults is 600 mg daily given in two divided doses (preferably after food), increasing by 200 mg a day at 3-day intervals to a maximum of 2.5 g daily in divided doses. The usual maintenance dose is 1–2 g daily.

Sodium valproate should be avoided in children under 3 years of age, patients with pre-existing liver disease and those with a family history of childhood hepatic disease. It must not be used concurrently with salicylates and should be stopped in those patients who develop nausea, vomiting, lethargy, oedema or jaundice.

Sodium valproate is available as tablets, liquid and an injection.

Plasma levels

There is no clear-cut relationship between the plasma concentration of sodium valproate, its effects and its toxicity. The daily variation in plasma concentration is wide, so the routine monitoring of plasma levels is generally unhelpful. Monitoring of plasma levels can be carried out if toxicity or a lack of clinical response because of non-compliance is suspected. The accepted therapeutic range is a pre-dose concentration of 50–100 mg/l.

Side-effects

Dose-related side-effects include nausea, vomiting, weight gain (from appetite stimulation), tremor and menstrual irregularities including amenorrhoea. Sedation, memory impairment and lethargy are rare.

Approximately 20% of patients experience hyperammonaemia (raised ammonia levels in the blood) without hepatic damage; this is usually asymptomatic but may cause confusion, nausea and vomiting. Fatal hepatic failure is rare but can occur during the first 6 months of treatment.

Points to note

1. Advise the patient to report any visual disturbances as ocular toxicity has been noted (Malseed et al, 1985).
2. Sodium valproate is excreted in the urine as a ketone-containing metabolite so urine may test positive for ketones.
3. Liver function tests should be undertaken prior to the commencement of therapy and at intervals during therapy in order to monitor for hepatic disturbances.
4. Sodium valproate may potentiate the effects of other CNS depressant drugs such as alcohol and opiates.
5. Be aware that carbamazepine, phenobarbitone and phenytoin induce hepatic microsomal enzymes and increase the clearance of sodium valproate. This may necessitate a dose increase of sodium valproate.
6. Sodium valproate interferes with platelet aggregation and may therefore enhance the action of anticoagulants and salicylates.
7. Sodium valproate does not interfere with the action of oral contraceptives (Malseed et al, 1985).

More recent anti-epileptic drugs include vigabatrin (Sabril), lamotrigine (Lamictal) and gabapentin (Neurontin). These are not at present commonly used in neuro-oncology. Side-effects are varied and include headache, nausea, vomiting, dizziness, dyspepsia, ataxia and occasionally a generalised body rash.

Nausea and vomiting

It is imperative to assess whether nausea and vomiting result directly from raised intracranial pressure, because of treatment or the patient's anxiety due to the tumour, as its aetiology will dictate the appropriate treatment for the patient. For example, nausea and vomiting due to raised intracranial pressure will necessitate steroid and/or mannitol treatment, whilst nausea and vomiting resulting from cytotoxic chemotherapy will require appropriate anti-emetic therapy. Anxiety may occasionally predispose some patients to experience the feeling of nausea. This can often be treated with appropriate psychological support and/or referral to a practitioner of a complementary therapy such as aromatherapy or massage.

Anti-emetic drugs used in the treatment of nausea and vomiting include cyclizine (which has fewer sedating effects than some other antihistamines and acts directly on the vomiting centre), metoclopramide (which acts selectively on the chemoreceptor trigger zone as well as having a peripheral action in the gut) and domperidone (which has a similar action to metoclopramide but is less sedating as it does not readily cross the blood–brain barrier). As both metoclopramide and domperidone act on the chemoreceptor trigger zone in the medulla, they are not effective in patients suffering from motion sickness and other vestibular disorders.

Dose

To accompany chemotherapy treatment of low emetogenicity (sickness-inducing potential), the use of domperidone 20 mg orally every 6 hours for 3–5 days is recommended. For moderate emetogenicity, dexamethasone 8 mg intravenously as pre-treatment followed by dexamethasone 4 mg orally 8-hourly for 2 days, in combination with domperidone 20 mg orally 8-hourly for 3–5 days, is recommended. For chemotherapy regimens of high emetogenicity, the recommendation is dexamethasone 8 mg intravenously in combination with a $5HT_3$ antagonist such as granisetron 3 mg intravenously or ondansetron 8 mg intravenously given as pre-treatment followed by dexamethasone 4 mg orally 8-hourly for 2–3 days and domperidone 20 mg orally 8-hourly for 3–5 days.

Granisetron and ondansetron are specific ($5HT_3$) serotonin antagonists and are used on patients whose nausea and vomiting are not controlled by other drugs. It is worth noting that the $5HT_3$ antagonists are not very effective in controlling delayed emesis, that is, emesis after 24 hours, and are therefore usually given as a single intravenous dose prior to the administration of cytotoxic chemotherapy.

Side-effects

Side-effects of cyclizine include dry mouth, drowsiness and blurred vision. Cyclizine may aggravate severe heart failure and counteract the haemodynamic benefits of opioids. Cyclizine is available as tablets, suppositories and an injection.

Side-effects of metoclopramide include extrapyramidal effects (more so in the younger patient), drowsiness, restlessness, diarrhoea and depression. Caution must be taken if used in patients with hepatic and renal impairment, or during pregnancy and breastfeeding. Metoclopramide is available in tablet, syrup and injection forms.

The side-effects of domperidone include raised prolactin concentrations, possible galactorrhoea, that is, lactation not associated with breastfeeding, gynaecomastia (the enlargement of one or both breasts in men), reduced libido and rashes. Caution must be taken if used in patients with renal impairment or during pregnancy and breastfeeding. Domperidone is available in tablet, suspension and suppository forms.

Side-effects of granisetron include constipation, headache, rash and transient increases in liver enzymes. Caution must be taken if used during pregnancy and breastfeeding. Granisetron is available as a tablet, injection and liquid.

Side-effects of ondansetron include occasional transient visual disturbances, chest pain and arrhythmias (following intravenous administration). Other less severe side-effects include constipation, headache, a sensation of warmth or flushing in the head and over the stomach. Caution must also be taken if used in patients with a history of hepatic impairment, or during pregnancy and breastfeeding. Ondansetron is available as a tablet or an injection. It is worth noting that the efficacy of granisetron and ondansetron is enhanced if each is used together with dexamethasone.

Constipation

The use of analgesia coupled with decreased mobility may cause constipation. The prophylactic use of laxatives may prevent or alleviate the discomfort associated with constipation and improve the patient's comfort and quality of life. In the absence of further complications co-danthramer can be used to prevent and treat constipation.

Co-danthramer

Co-danthramer is a stimulant laxative and works by increasing intestinal motility.

The usual dose of co-danthramer is 1–2 capsules or 5–10 ml at night time. The dose is dependent on the degree of constipation as well as the frequency and consistency of the stool. Co-danthramer is available in capsule (ordinary and strong) and suspension (ordinary and strong) forms.

Side-effects

Abdominal cramp as well as urinary discolouration (red to yellow brown) may occur. The prolonged use of co-danthramer may precipitate the onset of an atonic non-functioning colon and hypokalaemia (low potassium) (British National Formulary, 1997).

Co-danthramer should be avoided in children and during pregnancy and breastfeeding. Studies in rodents indicate a potential carcinogenic risk.

Points to note

1. Ascertain the patient's normal bowel habit.
2. Ensure that the constipation is not secondary to an underlying undiagnosed complaint.
3. Provide dietary advice, including that on adequate fluid and fibre intake, and/or refer to a dietitian as appropriate.
4. Instruct the patient on the proper method of administration of co-danthramer capsules or suspension.
5. Inform patients that medication takes 6–12 hours to act so that administration in the evening should ensure morning bowel evacuation.
6. Inform the patient that discolouration of the urine may occur.
7. Patients with bowel and/or urinary incontinence are at risk of co-danthramer burns as danthron is excreted in urine and faeces.
8. Adjust the dose of co-danthramer to provide regular, but not excessive, bowel action.
9. Reduce or discontinue medication when regular bowel action has been achieved or when the patient discontinues analgesic medication, if appropriate.
10. Be aware of the excessive use of co-danthramer as abuse may lead to hypokalaemia and an atonic, non-functioning colon.

Candidiasis

Oral candidiasis can at times be present in patients taking corticosteroids. Signs of oral candidiasis include white patches in the oral cavity, a sore throat on swallowing, a coated tongue and a dry mouth. Patients should be commenced on an antifungal preparation in order to reduce the discomfort associated with oral candidiasis and prevent the spread of infection to perioral and oesophageal sites. The antifungal drug nystatin is usually the first drug of choice.

Nystatin

Nystatin is not absorbed from the gastrointestinal tract. It is active against a number of yeasts and fungi but is principally used for *Candida albicans* infections of skin and mucous membranes. It is also used in the treatment of intestinal candidiasis (British National Formulary, 1997). Nystatin is available in oral suspension and pastilles. The recommended dose is 1 ml (100 000 units) 6-hourly or 1 pastille 6-hourly for 7 days, continued for 48 hours after the lesions have resolved.

Side-effects

These include nausea, oral irritation and sensitisation.

Points to note

1. Weekly examination of the oral cavity should be carried out during the patient's treatment with an antifungal preparation or while he or she is on corticosteroid therapy.
2. Advise the patient on oral hygiene during radiotherapy and/or chemotherapy treatment, particularly during the administration of corticosteroids.
3. Advise patients on the proper use of nystatin, including the treatment of dentures to prevent cross-infection.
4. Assess and advise the patient on dietary intake and, if appropriate, referral to the dietitian and/or oral hygienist.
5. Review the effectiveness of treatment weekly by oral examination and consider the use of a stronger antifungal preparation if no response is observed.

Conclusion

Symptom management is a prerequisite of expert patient care. Those nurses who take an active role in the management and anticipation of symptoms in patients with CNS tumours are playing an important role in the improvement of the quality of life not just for patients, but also for their carers. An understanding of common medications used and drug interactions should also make nurses alert to potential drug-related problems. Such knowledge will help nurses to reassure patients and whenever possible allow for appropriate interventions in order to minimise unpleasant drug side-effects.

References

Batchelor TT, Taylor LP, Thaler HT, Posner JB, DeAngelis LM (1997) Steroid myopathy in cancer patients. Neurology 48: 1234–8.

British National Formulary (1997) No. 33 (March). London: British Medical Association/Royal Pharmaceutical Society of Great Britain.

Brodie M, Dichter M (1996) Antiepileptic drugs. New England Journal of Medicine 334(3): 168–75.

Cascino GD (1990) Epilepsy and brain tumors: implications for treatment. Epilepsia 31 (supplement 3): 37–44.

Guerrero D. (1995). A retrospective analysis investigating the prevalence of epilepsy in patients with glioma. MSc Clinical Neuroscience thesis, University of Surrey.

Malseed RT, Malseed ZK, Grimus F (1985) Pharmacology, drug therapy and nursing considerations, 2nd edn. Philadelphia: JB Lippincott.

Posner J (1996) Neurologic complications of cancer. Philadelphia: FA Davis.

Speight TM, Avery GS (1987) Avery's drug treatment, 3rd edn. Auckland: Adis Press.

Thomas DGT, Graham DI (1980) Brain Tumours: Scientific basis, Clinical Investigations and Current Therapy. London: Butterworth.

Walker M, Patsalos P (1995) Clinical pharmacokinetics of new antiepileptic drugs. Pharmacology and Therapeutics 3: 168–75.

Chapter 9 Multidisciplinary teamwork

Sarah N Fisher

Introduction

The purpose of this chapter is threefold; it aims to:

1. familiarise the nurse with the concept of good multidisciplinary teamwork and how such teams, when used effectively, can enhance care by the provision of an integrated care package for the neuro-oncology patient;
2. indicate key members of the multidisciplinary team who play a pivotal role in the management of the neuro-oncology patient and highlight their contribution to care;
3. emphasise the major role of patients and families when planning care, not only treatment and rehabilitation programmes within the hospital setting, but also the package of care required to enable them to function optimally at home and into the palliative care stage of the disease.

Nurses must be continuously motivated to utilise professional skills through genuine teamwork in order to offer a high-quality integrated service to the patient and family.

A diagnosis of a CNS tumour is devastating for the patient and his family, and is likely to be viewed with fear and dread: 'Fears of pain, prolonged aggressive treatment and a sentence of death' (David, 1993). To be faced with the anticipation of dying from cancer is to be struck with one of the ultimate painful emotional events of life (Singer, 1984). In addition, there is, for neuro-oncology patients, the immediate fear that they will be disabled by their disease and lose the ability to function physically, cognitively and intellectually. Robinson (1992a) comments that the widespread fear response has multiple origins, not necessarily related to fact or logic. Fear may arise, in part, from an awareness that the incidence of cancer in general is high. A second basis for this fear may be that cancer spares no age, sex, ethnic or economic group and is not confined to the devalued or marginal members of society. The fear response may also be influenced by the extensive media coverage of cancer in its various forms and stages as 'news'. Finally, there is a widespread perception that cancer treatment is disfiguring, painful, protracted, expensive and often fruitless.

The inherent fear of cancer, with its consequent stigmatisation, is probably the most difficult problem that cancer survivors and their rehabilitators have to overcome. The concept of rehabilitation in cancer care is not new, nor is the concept of a team approach to rehabilitation. In 1971, Raven described rehabilitation as 'a programme of total care which should be planned when the patient is first seen and is designed for his restoration to as near normal a life as possible' (Raven, 1971). In 1978, Downie, in *Cancer Rehabilitation: An Introduction for Physiotherapists and the Allied Professions*, discusses teamwork in rehabilitation, including the psychological and nutritional needs of patients as well as the treatment of lymphoedema and the use of massage (Downie, 1978). Given the complex and multifaceted nature of the problems faced by the neuro-oncology patient, few would dispute that the needs of such patients and their families are likely to be best met by the team approach to care.

Why teamwork?

Multidisciplinary teamwork is a cornerstone of rehabilitation therapy. By using a patient-centred approach, rehabilitation professionals strive to collaborate and share information in order to promote rehabilitation and self-care in patients (Boroch, 1976). Teamwork is a concept that has been acclaimed in the management literature as bringing benefits to both the organisation and the individual. Over the years, it has played an increasing part in health care delivery, as advances in knowledge and technology have brought a range of new and varied health disciplines into the hospital environment. A major reason for its continued growth is the belief of many health care professionals that a high-quality service will involve collaborative effort across professional boundaries (Embling, 1995).

The reason for the continuing growth of the teamwork movement is easy to identify. The very commitment of health care professionals to a philosophy of helping and caring reinforces the ethic of collaborative working, especially when the good of the patient depends upon it. Similarly, professionals' own concepts of high-quality service have tended to involve a collaborative effort across professional and specialist boundaries. As various disciplines have tried to grapple with increased specialisation and the potential fragmentation of patient services that it may bring, co-operative endeavour has been widely advocated. Many professionals are acutely aware that the problems experienced by patients are often interconnected and that the expertise required for effective intervention may elude a single profession.

Teamwork – the myth

A rosy picture of multidisciplinary teamwork has been painted by the management literature: a team recognises itself as a team because members describe how they share a common purpose requiring the unified efforts of all the members to achieve that purpose (Richardson, 1992). While a team may have a shared direction of purpose, members do not 'shadow' each other or need total involvement in every decision. Effective communication is therefore an essential component of the team's ability to function efficiently and effectively. A team's leader develops the leadership qualities of team members. In addition, team members are able to support and buffer one another against the stresses of the workplace. The sense of involvement created helps to motivate people creatively, thereby reducing the opportunities for feelings of hurt and paranoia, and the destructive waste of energies that can otherwise be directed towards back-stabbing and in-fighting. The recognition of a mutual responsibility towards common objectives is enhanced, the barriers of rivalry and jealousy are decreased and there is increased awareness among members of each other's pressures and problems.

The effective team knows where it is going, sets realistic targets, uses resources energetically and imaginatively, has a wide range of alternatives for action and will investigate coping strategies as necessary. In such a team, members will trust each other to pursue their bit of the common task. In dealings with the outside world, teams will behave sensitively and assertively (Richardson, 1992). However, in practice, it appears that effective multidisciplinary teamwork is often difficult to achieve.

Teamwork – a definition

Teamwork is defined in the *Concise Oxford Dictionary* (1982) as 'a combined effort or organised co-operation'. Blake and Mouton (1964) state that the word 'team' is likely to be used to refer to any set of individuals who co-operate in accomplishing a single, overall result. They explain that a good team has task specialisation and a division of labour, but that the division of effort is merged into a single co-ordinated result in which the whole is more than, and different from, the sum of its individual parts.

Features of effective teamwork

Zenger and Miller (1974) consider shared goals and mutual respect to be necessary if there is to be teamwork that really counts in an organisation. Rubin et al (1976) maintain that 'if the basic mission or job requires that you and others must work together and co-ordinate your activity with each other, then you are a team even though you may not formally call yourself a team'. Thus a salient feature of a team is an element of interdependence, that is, the job cannot be done by just one person (Lynch, 1981). This implies that effective multidisciplinary teamwork cannot be achieved when health care professionals apply their skills sequentially rather than collaboratively (Embling, 1995). The range of professionals represented within a multidisciplinary team is also vital. If decisions about overall patient plans are to be reached, it is essential that all relevant disciplines contribute fully to them (Embling, 1995). Experience suggests that simply establishing a team does not ensure that effective decisions are made. Multidisciplinary team decision-making brings a greater sum total of knowledge, information and approaches to problems and results in a better understanding and increased acceptance of the final decision (Fargason and Haddock, 1992).

In summary, a team can be defined by the following characteristics (Lynch, 1981; Embling, 1995):

- shared goals;
- interdependence;
- co-operation;
- co-ordination of activities;
- task specialisation;
- division of effort;
- mutual respect.

Mutual respect within teams does not require agreement on every issue. However, it does require a willingness to trust each other's skills and expertise.

Handy (1976) describes the organisational uses of teams and considers them to be a way of:

- distributing work;
- problem-solving and decision-making;
- information- and idea-collecting, and information-processing;
- co-ordinating and liaising between individuals in groups and between groups;
- managing and controlling work;
- testing and ratifying decisions;
- increasing commitment and involvement.

Teams also have a purpose for individuals in the organisation (Handy, 1976), providing a means of:

- satisfying social need and gaining a sense of belonging;
- establishing a self-concept;
- gaining help and support;
- sharing and helping.

It can be seen from these functions that the dynamics of teamwork can be highly complex, and getting a team to work effectively is likely to take time. The prerequisites for satisfactory integration of a team (Giguere and Lewis, 1994) are:

1. common objectives for the team, accepted and understood by all members;
2. a clear understanding by all team members of their roles, functions and responsibilities;
3. a clear understanding by each team member of the roles, functions, skills and responsibilities of the other team members;
4. mutual respect for the role and skills of each member, allied to a flexible approach.

Conflict

Professional roles are cited as problematic for achieving collaboration within multidisciplinary teams. Although medicine, the traditional health care profession, is founded on a pathophysiological paradigm, nursing and other health care professions tend to focus on a holistic problem-solving framework. Whilst these approaches are not fixed, the ideologies are indoctrinated into professionals early on in their careers. The complexity of uniting groups of professionals, each with their different value systems, is certainly a challenge. Teamwork implies co-operation rather than conflict, so awareness of the historical differences between professions and their ideologies can lead to a greater understanding and respect for differences.

At the same time, recognising the potential for non-defensive approaches to changing practices is important in order to benefit the patient. Conflict *per se* is neither good nor bad but neutral. It is the individual's interpretation and the outcome of conflict that often gives conflict a negative connotation. However, conflict appropriately channelled can act as a motivator and stimulator for ideals and proposals within the team (Rowe, 1996).

Team leadership

An important issue arising in discussions of multidisciplinary teamwork is that of team leadership. Leadership is a vital process within any organisation, and whilst it has been mooted that a well-motivated team of professionals should be able to tackle problems systematically without a leader, this appears not to be true in practice. Handy (1976) states that 'there is a need in all organisations for individual linking pins who bind groups together'. Whatever they are called – leaders, co-ordinators or facilitators – their role would seem to be of the utmost importance in procuring good teamwork. The need for an appropriately skilled team leader is widely documented in the management literature.

Whilst leadership styles may vary, a leader must clearly possess skills that effectively facilitate teamworking. Although any brief summary of such skills cannot do justice to the complexity of interactions between a leader and his team, examples include (Handy, 1976):

- the ability to listen and communicate effectively with team members;
- the ability to problem-solve in a circumspect manner;
- a positive attitude towards other team members;
- the ability to optimise the contribution and abilities of team members.

- Explorer-promoter – an outgoing person, looks for new opportunities to sell the team's strengths and skills, brings ideas encountered back to the team (broadly similar to Belbin's resource investigator).
- Concluder-producer – ability to ensure that the team's projects are fully processed to completion (broadly similar to Belbin's company worker with an element of completer finisher).
- Upholder-maintainer – essentially has the sensitivity and optimism to motivate the team and mediate conflict between members, helps to prevent burnout (broadly similar to Belbin's teamworker).
- Assessor-developer – quite a critical-minded person able to assess and identify the most promising idea; also has an aptitude for developing the less practical ideas, for example from the creator-innovator, towards a workable option (broadly similar to Belbin's monitor-evaluator).
- Controller-inspector – mindful of detail and exactitude (similar to Belbin's completer-finisher); focuses the team upon its standards of work and achievement.
- Reporter-advisor – to some extent, everyone has to perform in this function, reporting on their own contribution, but the team will usually need a member who has a distinct flair for the delivery of reports.
- Linker – draws together the efforts of the team; is often the chairperson (broadly similar to Belbin's chairman).

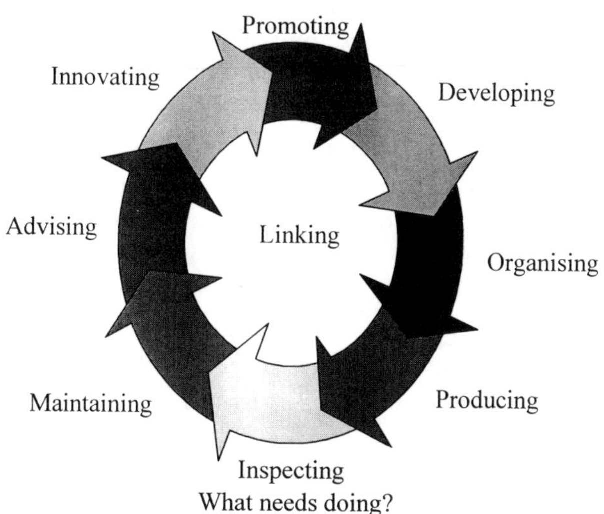

Figure 9.1 Major work functions. Team building adapted from Margerison and McCann (1985, 1989).

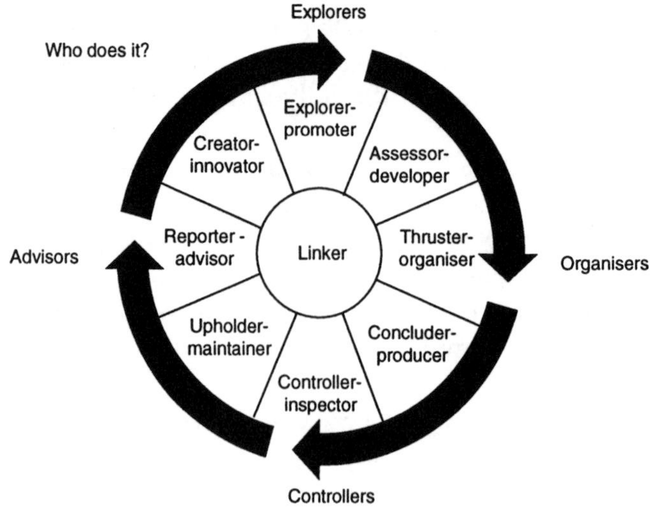

Figure 9.2 Team management wheel. Adapted from Margerison and McCann (1985, 1989).

There are some clearly recognisable overlaps between Belbin's management team roles and Margerison and McCann's team management resource (Figures 9.1 and 9.2), but these are not exact overlaps.

Adair (1986) mistrusts the attribution of personality qualities to roles in the team and advises that a team needs a mix of skills spread around its members. Those skills should be for analysis, reasoning, synthesis, holistic thinking, valuing, intuition, memory, creativity and numeracy. All members must, however, have a general ability to work in teams, and upon this point all the investigators agree.

Team leaders rarely have the luxury of picking the team members to create a balance of resources. There is often the inheritance of an existing team, with its inherent problems, strengths and weaknesses (Richardson, 1992), or a professional is selected to be a member of a team by a departmental or professional manager who is remote from the team and thus not fully aware of its needs (Embling 1995). However, Belbin (1981), Margerison and McCann (1985, 1989) and Adair (1986) offer models that can be used to inform team discussions about its strengths and weaknesses, with a view to improving, where necessary, the balance of the team's skills and performance.

The value of teamwork

In the health care services today, many professional personnel continue to consider that multidisciplinary teamworking is a valuable approach to patient care. For example, the Code of Professional Conduct issued by the United Kingdom Central Council for Nursing, Midwifery and Health Visiting (UKCC) states that 'each registered nurse ... shall work in a collaborative and co-operative manner with health care professionals and others involved in providing care and recognise and respect their particular contributions within the care team' (UKCC, 1992).

The advantages of multidisciplinary teams (Øvretveit, 1990) are listed below:

1. A better service: the main function of multidisciplinary teams is to ensure that patients get a better service than they would otherwise receive from independent professional and agency help.
2. Easier workload management: teams also make it easier to manage workload and to establish common priorities across professions. Given the time and skills available, difficult decisions have to be made about priorities, but teams allow practitioners to share the work, each member undertaking a fair share of unpopular as well as popular work.
3. Colleague support: practitioners often receive vital support and advice from other team members in dealing with complex cases. Certain types of technical advice can, of course, only come from a member of the same profession, and regular contact is necessary to keep up to date in profession-specific skills and knowledge. Emotional support is also important in stressful work with patients, and team members can be of great help to each other.

Teamwork and team management concepts offer a framework for the management of complex issues and constant change that face the neuro-oncology patients and their families, by creating the dynamic problem-solving required in the delivery of quality care. Kane (1975) and Lowe and Herranen (1978) suggest that the collaboration of professionals enhances the capabilities of health services to arrive at a comprehensive understanding of patients, solves complex problems and develops and implements plans. To this end the multidisciplinary team must be fluid, with merging and changing borders, and specialists must remain as individuals within the team (David, 1993). Figure 9.3 summarises the essential components of effective team functioning.

Summary

In conclusion, the essence of effective multidisciplinary teamwork for the neuro-oncology patient is the dynamic process (facilitation)

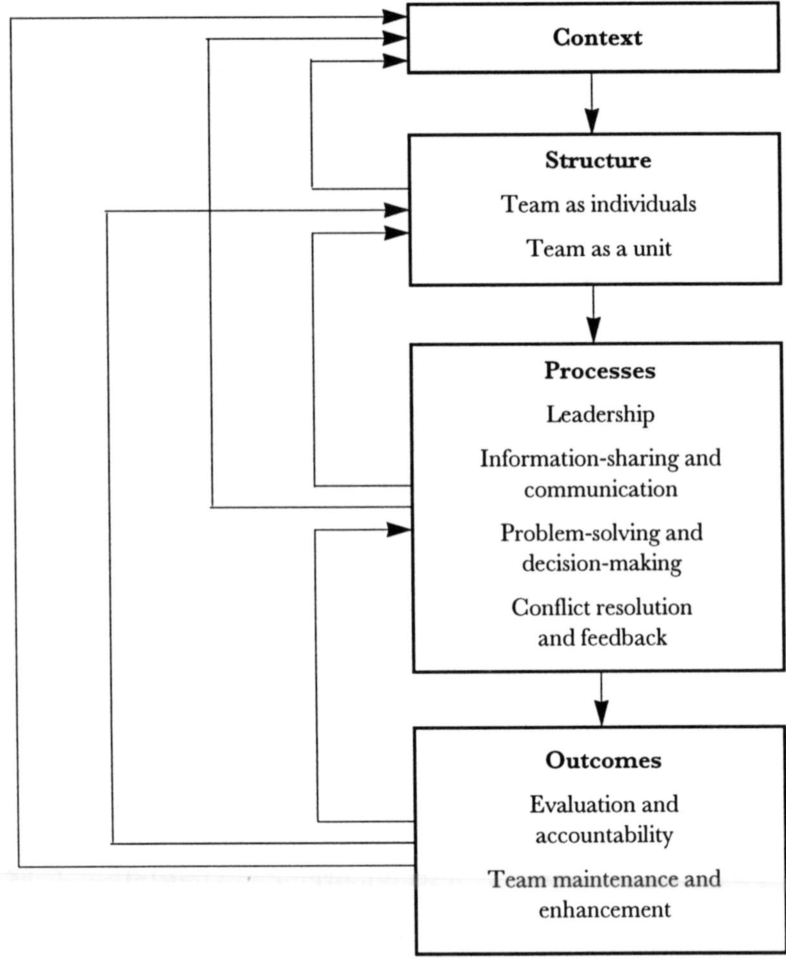

Figure 9.3 Essential components of effective team functioning. Adapted from Saltz (1992).

directed toward the goal of enabling the patient to attain his or her optimal quality of life within the limitations imposed by the disease or disability in terms of his or her physical, mental, emotional, social and economic potential. The initial goal of rehabilitation is the elimination, reduction or alleviation of disability, whilst the ultimate goal is the establishment of patients as functional individuals in their own environment (Dietz, 1981).

Rehabilitation is most successful when it begins early and has been preceded by and co-exists with effective preventative measures. The prevention of unnecessary loss of function often shortens the period of rehabilitation and maximises outcome. A wide range of professional roles and expertise may be required to assist the patient to achieve these goals. No one professional intervention would be wholly effective in isolation. The impact of disease on an individual's life can only be understood when viewed within the context of the patient's goals, values and needs, and the styles of life developed to pursue them (Dudas and Carlson, 1988). The holistic approach afforded by an effective multidisciplinary team plays a vital role in helping patients to adjust to the major life changes they are likely to experience upon diagnosis of a CNS tumour.

Specific roles of team members

It is impossible to view the care and neurological rehabilitation of the neuro-oncology patient in professional isolation. The combined efforts of all team members are essential in assisting patients to attain their goals. The role of the medical staff lies in determining the diagnosis and subsequent medical management, and the role of the nurse is pivotal in providing care throughout all aspects of treatment.

It is recognised that other professionals involved in the care of neuro-oncology patients, for example the clinical nurse specialist, social worker and clinical psychologist, warrant attention being paid to their specific roles. A lack of emphasis here in no way reflects any lack of recognition of their importance in the total picture of care delivered to this patient group. However, the role of three key professions – occupational therapy, physiotherapy and speech and language therapy – are discussed briefly.

The role of the occupational therapist in neuro-oncology

Occupational therapy is the treatment of physical and psychiatric conditions through specific activities in order to help people to reach their maximum level of function and independence in all aspects of life. The aim of occupational therapy intervention is to promote optimal functional independence, and it uses a problem-solving approach to manage physical and cognitive difficulties with which the patient presents. The occupational therapy process involves assessment, planning, implementing treatment, monitoring progress and evaluation. The patient's and carer's involvement is integral to this process.

There are no clear boundaries between the following difficulties: they often overlap, and all have the potential to result in functional and social problems. Possible difficulties may include temporary, permanent or progressive impairment in cognition, perception, vision, physical state, for example hemiplegia, function and psychosocial areas. The occupational therapy role includes assessment and treatment in relation to:

- physical factors, for example muscle strength, joint range of movement, muscle tone, sensation and pain;
- functional factors such as self care, mobility, perceptual abilities, domestic activities, work/school activities and leisure and recreational activities;
- psychological factors, for example insight into illness, motivation for rehabilitation and cognitive abilities;
- social factors, for instance the patient's home situation, the available support systems and the carer's insight and abilities;
- educating and supporting patients and carers in coping with disabilities.

The presenting symptoms and dysfunctions may be caused by the tumour itself or may result from treatment, often giving a very complex picture, including fluctuations in the patient's condition, with which the patient has to deal. Early referral to the occupational therapist is essential in planning ahead if deterioration is expected. For example, issues related to discharge planning, access and home visits, arranging equipment to aid independence, housing and so on can be anticipated and organised.

Key areas of interest to the occupational therapist are cognition, function (activities of daily living) and relaxation.

Cognition

Changes in cognition can be a major influencing factor in the rehabilitation of a patient (Cooper, 1997). Normal cognition enables individuals to isolate relevant features of a task, formulate a plan, break a task down into steps, perform actions and behaviours in the correct sequence and modify the response when appropriate. Occupational therapy intervention aims for maximum recovery, but if recovery is limited, compensation and adaptation techniques are employed.

Cognitive skills of concern to the occupational therapist are attention, short-term memory, planning and problem-solving, which are all essential in functional independence. Grieve (1993) states that 'attention is closely linked to perception in all human occupation'. She distinguishes between:

- focused attention: the ability to process one input and ignore others;

- attention capacity: the ability to shift attention from one task to another and to do two things at the same time;
- automatic and controlled processing: automatic processes are fast, do not require attention and are difficult to modify; controlled ones are slow and demand attention but are flexible when circumstances change.

Shifts of attention are important for flexibility in behaviour and action. Attention is closely linked to memory, and severe memory impairment presents as the inability to learn and retain new information. This can cause difficulties in planning, sequencing and carrying out activities. In extreme cases, patients forget what they are doing.

Cooper (1997) states that rehabilitation of the patient with cognitive impairment related to a CNS tumour may involve functional and compensatory techniques. Different methods of performing activities of daily living should be assessed so that patients can maintain their skills. Repetitive practice, setting up a routine and teaching cognitive cues can assist. Spatial and body scheme problems may still exist that can affect safety, and this impairment has implications for arranging discharge planning, resettlement into the community and psychosocial adjustment.

Function

Assessment of daily living activities will identify problem areas and provide a baseline for appropriate intervention. If equipment to aid daily living, for example, one-handed items to assist in the kitchen and bathroom or with dressing and toileting, is provided, re-evaluation is needed as the patient's condition is likely to change. The safety of using such items must therefore be checked as, for example, with bathing aids if the patient's transfers and stability deteriorate. It is important for the occupational therapist to be selective in providing equipment and not to clutter patients and their homes with too many items. This will just add further confusion to the situation and is likely to reinforce feelings of being disabled.

Relaxation

Relaxation and stress management techniques can be used to help the patient and carers deal with the anxiety of the diagnosis and treatment. The patient has to have the concentration skills to be able to carry out the exercises, and careful assessment of the patient's ability to participate in, and benefit from, this intervention is required.

In describing her work with cognitive disorders, Villemoes (1995) wrote:

> at the end of rehabilitation the Occupational Therapy intervention is directed towards:
>
> - stabilisation of the relearned functions and skills
> - compensation of dysfunctions
> - supporting the patient in making realistic plans for the future
> - supporting the patient and the relatives to cope with the altered person
> - supporting integration of the relearned functions, skills and compensation techniques in the patient's daily life in relation to activities of daily living, work, leisure and social life.

Occupational therapy has a clear role in the treatment of patients with CNS tumours, in both the acute and the palliative stages. It may include techniques used in other areas of neurology, but the therapist needs to be aware of potential difficulties because of fluctuations in the patient's performance.

The role of the physiotherapist in neuro-oncology

The role of the physiotherapist in the management of a patient with a CNS tumour is multifaceted and frequently begins at diagnosis. There are three common presentations that will bring about referral to a physiotherapist:

1. following surgery, either stereotactic biopsy or debulking of the tumour (see Chapter 5), when the patient may present with acute neurological symptoms and post-anaesthetic respiratory problems;
2. a slow onset of physical symptoms, such as hemiplegia or unsteady walking;
3. a sudden onset of physical symptoms, for example following an epileptiform seizure.

In the postoperative patient, the key elements of physiotherapy intervention involve:

- the maintenance of respiratory function, especially important in the prevention of secondary brain damage as a result of anoxia;

- the maintenance of joint range of movement and muscle length;
- the positioning of the patient to maximise both of the above.

These interventions are essential in maintaining the patient in an optimal physical state in preparation for more active rehabilitation when his or her medical status allows.

Physiotherapy assessment

Assessment of the neurologically damaged patient is complex and time-consuming. The patient may fluctuate greatly from day to day and within a 24 hour period. Flexibility on the part of the therapist is therefore vital, and simultaneous assessment by more than one professional may be required and indeed useful in giving the broadest picture of the patient's capabilities. For example, combined sessions between the physiotherapist and occupational therapist may enhance the assessment and treatment process.

Assessment comprises an evaluation of the following elements:

- the quality and amount of movement of the head, trunk and limbs, both in isolation and in relation to each other;
- the posture when lying, sitting and standing;
- the muscle tone and reflexes;
- sensation and proprioception;
- co-ordination;
- balance;
- functional ability, for example rolling, moving from lying to sitting and sitting to standing, and walking.

None of these components can be evaluated in isolation. They are intrinsically linked and, in an undamaged nervous system, equip the person with the basis for normal movement and function. Analysis of normal movement is recognised as an essential prerequisite for the assessment of patients with an impairment of movement. It is this analysis which provides the basis for the problem-solving approach to treatment. Improved understanding and awareness of movement enables the physiotherapist to identify how a posture or movement differs from the normal and why an individual may have difficulty with functional skills (Edwards, 1996).

Normal movement

Normal movement has been described by many authors as a basis for treatment of the neurologically damaged patient (Carr and Shepherd, 1986; Bobath, 1990). A wide range of different clinical presentations exist in patients with neurological dysfunction, and different aspects of movement impairment will consequently be demonstrated; for example, a patient with an intracranial tumour may present with spasticity, ataxia or indeed a combination of the two. Clinical presentation and appropriate treatment intervention may only be accurately assessed on the basis of an extensive knowledge of normal movement. The main remit of the physiotherapist is to enable patients to attain their optimal level of function with regard to effectiveness and economy of movement (Edwards, 1996). The implications of behavioural, perceptual, cognitive or memory dysfunction on movement cannot be considered to be a separate entity from these aspects.

Neurological damage is often manifested by diverse physical disabilities. In some conditions, CNS tumours included, the presence of abnormal tone dominates the picture. The differing types of abnormal tone are determined by the site and extent of the lesion. Environmental factors such as correct positioning and movements to maintain, and where necessary regain, joint range are essential to maximise the level of function for each individual. The physiotherapist must recognise that restoration of normal movement is often an unattainable goal and work with the patient to ensure the optimal functional outcome. There should be a balance between the re-education of more normal movement patterns and the acceptance and promotion of necessary and desirable compensation to obtain optimal function (Edwards, 1996).

Posture and positioning

The control of body posture includes the alignment of body segments to each other and to the supporting surface. It requires a fixed, or reference, point around which movement can occur. The choice of position, both for support and for the performance of movement, must be considered with respect to prevailing abnormal tone, the influence of gravity, the potential structural deformities and the preservation of tissue viability (Pope, 1992).

Movements are regularly performed on patients who are unconscious, paralysed or have hypertonus, in order to maintain muscle and joint range. Emphasis is placed on functional movements, ensuring an appropriate response throughout the whole body rather than movements of an isolated part. Early mobilisation of the patient is encouraged as and when the medical condition allows. Movements of the limbs while the patient is confined to bed are difficult in terms of facilitating activity within the trunk. Where bed rest is unavoidable, it is essential to maintain mobility and to stimulate postural adjustments when moving the limbs. Patients who are unable to move or who are dominated by spastic stereotyped postures are in as great a danger of developing shortening of neural structures as they are loss of range of the musculoskeletal system (Edwards, 1996). Davies (1994) advocates the use of specific tension tests for the maintenance or restoration of adaptive lengthening of the nervous system. Positioning in a variety of postures is recommended, particularly for patients dominated by severe hypertonus. Many patients with increased tone demonstrate a degree of asymmetry that, without treatment, may lead to contracture within the spastic pattern. Treatment of the patient in the sitting position provides an opportunity for the physiotherapist to mobilise the trunk and facilitate the correct alignment with proximal control and stability. Slow, rhythmical movements, while providing full support from behind the patient, are more effective in reducing tone and increasing mobility. Smaller-range movements with less support and intermittent pressure as required to gain a 'holding' response are more effective in stimulating activity (Edwards, 1996).

Patients with hemiplegia develop compensatory strategies to contend with their asymmetry. Those with low tone may develop excessive activity of the 'unaffected' side as they struggle to support the weight of the flaccid hemiplegic side. It is often overactivity of the sound side that precludes any activity of the affected side. Hemiplegic patients with spasticity may develop shortening of the trunk side flexors of the affected side. Although hemiplegia is by definition a condition affecting half of the body, the consequences of motor and sensory impairment of one side inevitably affect all aspects of movement (Edwards, 1996).

Treatment progression

The long-term goal may be that the patient will walk independently, but it is important to provide stepping stones along the way, in the form of short-term goals, to enable the patient to realise that perhaps only small, but substantial, progress is being made. Family and friends must also be involved in the treatment programme. This is especially important in the rehabilitation of patients with a cognitive deficit. These patients may not be able to comply actively with treatment and it is often through the more constant input of carers that positive changes can be implemented (Edwards, 1996).

The majority of patients with neurological disability demonstrate a complex and varied picture that is potentially changeable depending on the existing pathology and the environment in which they function. The purpose of rehabilitation is to enable the patient to experience as normal a lifestyle as possible and to minimise the effects of abnormal tone in terms of function.

It is also important to recognise the role of the physiotherapist in assisting the patient and family to adjust to the patient's changed physical status. A particularly sensitive time is when the patient is deteriorating because of progressive disease and both patient and carers are learning to cope with a more dependent physical picture. The physiotherapist is able to offer advice, practical assistance and support in managing the deterioration.

The role of the speech and language therapist in neuro-oncology

Acquired communication and swallowing disorders are identified areas in which a speech and language therapist is involved with assessing and managing. As these are neurological functions, primary intracranial tumours of the dominant cerebral hemisphere and brain stem are those which most frequently initiate referral to a speech and language therapist. Metastatic brain disease and CNS lymphomas may also disrupt a patient's communication and/or swallowing abilities. It is rare for extracranial tumours to cause a language disturbance (Murdoch, 1990). As the majority of patients with CNS tumours referred to a speech and language therapist present with a communication disorder, that will be the initial focus. The role of the speech and language therapist with communication-impaired patients is to:

- differentially diagnose communication impairment;
- assess the type and degree of communication impairment;
- identify any retained abilities;
- reduce language impairment;
- help patients and those around them to develop strategies for maintaining communication;
- help the patient and family to understand the condition;
- advise the hospital and community multidisciplinary teams on how to communicate most effectively with the patient;
- assist the patient's reintegration into the community.

The majority of right-handed people are left hemisphere dominant for language. Whilst many areas of the brain are involved in language processing, different areas and tracts have different roles, and the complex relationship between structure and function is not fully understood (Caplan, 1987). The structures involved are the frontal, temporal and parietal lobes of the cerebral cortex, and although the role of the subcortical structures (thalamus and basal ganglia) and language is increasingly acknowledged, it is ill defined (see Chapter 1). Patients with CNS tumours have further complicating factors that can contribute to the variety, type and combination of communication problems:

- the site and size of the tumour;
- the grading of the tumour;
- the existence of surrounding oedema;
- any surgical intervention and/or radiotherapy treatment (see Chapters 5 and 6);
- the use of medication (see Chapter 8).

It is important to note that distortion and/or compression of the cerebral tissue can occur at a distance from the tumour. As a consequence, a communication disorder may have no direct relationship to the location of the tumour (Murdoch, 1990).

Communication – language and speech

The value and complexity of communication often only becomes apparent when it is disrupted. Speech and language shape our thoughts and dreams, and permit interaction with others. They are intrinsic and essential to our well-being. When a person is faced with the diagnosis of a CNS tumour and has a resulting communication disorder, the sense of loss is often described as a devastating experience. Intracranial tumours may disrupt communication at any level, ranging from an occasional hesitancy in word-finding to a complete loss of language-processing in all modalities.

A brief overview of a speech and language therapist's terminology includes:

1. Dysphasia: a complex disorder of language-processing that may also include:
   dysgraphia: a disorder of writing;
   dyslexia: a disorder of reading.
2. Dyspraxia: a sensorimotor disorder causing difficulty with initiating and sequencing purposeful and/or voluntary movements. For example, in oral dyspraxia, the patient is unable to protrude the tongue when asked but is able to lick an ice cream. In verbal

dyspraxia, the patient automatically says 'Hello' in greeting but is unable to articulate 'h' in therapy tasks.

3. Dyscalculia: a disorder of numeracy.
4. Dysarthria: a neuromuscular disorder of speech caused by weakness or paralysis of the relevant muscles, that is, muscles of respiration, phonation and articulation. The type of dysarthria will depend on the site of the lesion and may present as flaccid, spastic, ataxic or mixed dysarthria. For example, in spastic dysarthria, there is slurred, imprecise and effortful speech with a slowed rate (Darley et al, 1975).

There are additional features that differentiate the dysphasia within this patient group from those dysphasias exhibited by people who present following a cerebrovascular accident. It generally has a fluctuating and progressive pattern that can be further complicated by the side-effects of radiotherapy, some of which, such as somnolence, are transient (see Chapter 6). The cognitive deficits may include:

- poor memory ;
- reduced concentration;
- increased distractibility;
- shorter attention span;
- generalised fatigue.

These additional features have an obvious detrimental impact on language function and may be treatment or disease related.

Referral to the speech and language therapist may be at any stage of overall patient management. Intervention is governed by factors such as:

- the stage of the disease;
- the type of treatment;
- the rate of disease progression;
- the patient's reaction to the diagnosis and consequent deficits;
- individual psychosocial needs;
- coping styles;
- experiences;
- communication style.

The individual differences are highly relevant and need to be acknowledged when assessing a patient's communication. The timing of the intervention is paramount when deciding on the type of assessment and management. Patients may be experiencing some of the fluctuations and features described above; their overall prognosis may be poor, thus precluding a lengthy formal assessment. An informal language assessment will help to guide the therapist towards further appropriate assessment and management. Detailed information about the level of communication breakdown enables intervention to be tailored to individual needs. Regular review and monitoring of the patient's communication function are therefore essential.

Treatment strategies

By identifying the patient's abilities and level of impairment, compensatory strategies may be used to determine the easiest way of achieving effective and successful communication. For example, a patient's writing may be more reliable and accurate than his or her ability to speak. Other people's reactions to dysphasia can be a potential barrier, and these need to be acknowledged. The onus, or balance, of the conversation may have to change for it to be successful. The conversation partner may need to learn and develop skills to elicit and interpret the patient's communicative intent, for example by:

1. allowing extra time for the patient to process information ;
2. limiting the amount of information that is given to the patient;
3. when verbal expression is limited to single words, using closed questions to elicit a yes/no response.

Such strategies can help to reduce any feelings of inadequacy or embarrassment for both parties.

Quality of Life

The patient's quality of life is of paramount importance so support and maintenance of the optimum level of communicative function is central to the speech and language therapist's role. Intrinsically linked to quality of life are the psychosocial effects of dysphasia. There are the social changes, for example, role changes within the family (Le Dorze and Brassard, 1995; Parr, 1995), possible unemployment and an increased chance of social isolation. These changes impact not only on patients' emotional and psychological well-being, self-image and relationships with others, but also on their motivation to communicate.

The speech and language therapist can alleviate patients' and carers' anxieties by providing clear, pertinent verbal and written information about the nature of the dysphasia, and reassurance can be given that dysphasia does not imply mental incapacity.

Communication aids

When there is a severe level of either receptive and/or expressive dysphasia, a communication aid (for example picture chart, book or electronic device) may prove useful. No matter how simple or sophisticated the aid, once it is introduced, the communication is no longer two way but three way. Using a communication aid may facilitate communication but it will require planning and extra concentration, listening and watching, and interpretation by both the patient and the conversation partner. Acknowledgement of these factors ensures more realistic expectations of the aid, thus avoiding disappointment.

Posterior fossa tumours

Posterior fossa tumours involving the brain stem, cerebellum and cranial nerves may cause dysarthria and/or dysphagia.

Speech

The approach and role of the speech and language therapist to the management of patients with CNS tumours who present with dysarthria is essentially the same as for cranial nerve deficits of any other aetiology. The pattern and course of the disease will influence the outcome. For example, fluctuating abilities and side-effects of treatment such as radiotherapy may mean that it is more appropriate for a communication aid to be used prior to any work on orofacial and articulatory exercises. The aim of intervention is again to maintain the patient's optimum level of communication.

Swallowing

Dysphagia is the term for swallowing disorders caused by damage to or disease of the relevant cranial nerves and anatomical structures. The swallowing process is an extremely complex and rapid action that includes voluntary and involuntary components. It refers to the entire act of deglutition, from the placement of food in the mouth, until it passes into the oesophagus.

Dysphagia necessitates careful initial assessment and monitoring by the speech and language therapist. Assessment may be informal, using a subjective 'bedside' clinical assessment, or formal, using videofluoroscopy (a modified barium swallow). Both types of assessment are often used to complement one another. It is the oropharyngeal stages of the swallowing process that will be the focus of the speech and language therapist's intervention. Close liaison with the patient and carers as well as the nursing, medical and dietetic teams is important once the level and nature of the dysphagia has been assessed and identified. Intervention can be divided into two categories:

1. compensatory techniques such as modifying food consistencies or changing posture when swallowing;
2. therapy procedures that aim to alter the physiology of swallowing, for example the supraglottic swallow (voluntary airway protection).

Liaison enables a carry-over of identified strategies and/or therapy procedures. The purpose of intervention by the speech and language therapist is ultimately to assist the patient to swallow safely (that is, without food or drink being aspirated into the airway) whilst maintaining adequate hydration and nutrition.

Summary

Therapists' roles are complex, involving many different assessment methods and types of intervention. What is clear is that no one role is of greater importance. Each therapist has a significant role in the patient's management which only that profession can provide. However, it is the combined efforts of all professional groups that will afford the patient the best possible outcome.

The role of the patient and family

The diagnosis of a CNS tumour affects the entire family. It generates great anxiety within a family and alters communication patterns, roles and relationships among its members (see Chapter 11). This results in stressful outcomes both for the person who has the tumour and for the other members of the family. Moreover, families play a significant role during the time of illness, and their reactions contribute to the patient's response to their condition. Rather than being passive observers, family members are active, vital participants in the patient's treatment and care (Lewandowski and Jones, 1988; Woods et al, 1989). It is the family rather than the isolated patient who experiences the illness, and therefore families should not be treated as bystanders but as an influencing, organising and creative agent (Robinson, 1992a).

CNS tumours, as with any cancer diagnosis, are a potent agent of change. Regardless of the magnitude or direction of change, the diagnosis of a CNS tumour consistently disrupts a family's established patterns of daily living. As patients find themselves facing a life defined by uncertainties, remissions, exacerbations in disease and changes in treatment, the family is similarly confronted with continual change. Each member of the family, the patient included, must deal with the ramifications of the diagnosis for themselves as individuals while attempting to cope as a family with the disease and its treatment (Robinson, 1992a).

Family system theory

The family as a whole is a living system that is distinct from, yet connected to, the life of its individual members. It is a complex, dynamic network of interconnected and interactive relationships. As a system, each family adopts its own unique way for restructuring the roles, relationships and responsibilities that direct its family life. It also has its own system for handling life's differing crises, emotional upheavals, conflicts and demands. Families affirm, protect and define standards of acceptable behaviour, values and beliefs (Robinson, 1992a). Families who make a good adjustment to illness have a clear separation of generations, flexibility in and between roles, direct and consistent communication and, above all, a tolerance of individualism (Johnson, 1988).

The role of family members

By virtue of their relationship to the patient, family members play two distinct and potentially contradictory roles. They function as the patient's first-line emotional support, and are perceived as such and encouraged by health care professionals (Giaquinta, 1977). Simultaneously, they are viewed with the patient as the unit requiring care, equally in need of support. For example, the families of patients with CNS tumours often have to learn new ways of communicating with the patient because of the presence of a language deficit directly resulting from the tumour. This changes the natural communication methods used within the family unit and places an enormous strain on all concerned, often requiring the support of the multidisciplinary team to facilitate an emotionally painful process. Thus problems faced by family members are often described on the basis of clinical observation as being even more stressful than those faced by patients. Families are noted to be 'disrupted and sometimes impaired by a cancer diagnosis, and have been described as functioning in a perpetual limbo' (Cassileth and Hamilton, 1979).

Families have a powerful influence on adjustment. Patients who have less support from their families have a more difficult time adjusting to the CNS tumour and experience more fears of recurrence (Northouse, 1984). Thus the family of the neuro-oncology patient plays an integral role in the patient's care and also in the patient's response to illness. However, family members also have unique needs of their own as they cope with the impact of cancer on their lives. It is important therefore to recognise that, when a patient is diagnosed with a CNS tumour, the family members also become a focus of care.

One of the most important premises in family system theory is that the family is capable of taking in information, changing and growing throughout the course of a patient's illness. Intervention by health care professionals needs to focus on this health aspect of family functioning and facilitate the process. Intervention aimed at teaching the neuro-oncology patient and family must assume a priority position in the family's total care. For example, the family of a physically dependent patient who wish to care for him or her at home will need to be taught appropriate moving and handling techniques in order safely to carry out care tasks such as washing or toileting. They may be required to use items of equipment such as a hoist with which they have never previously come into contact. The family must be confident in carrying out these tasks safely and efficiently, for both themselves and the patient. Such a family should be supported in their caring by the appropriate community services.

Professionals often view the diagnosis of a CNS tumour as constituting a family crisis, requiring psychological adaptation for all members. However, families might need to perceive themselves as being not in a state of crisis but in a life circumstance that they are capable of taking in their stride. Families describe developing adaptive strategies that support the normal rather than the abnormal aspects of their situation (see Chapter 11).

As health care professionals with busy clinical workloads, it is all too easy to deal only with the obvious issues. However, Robinson (1992b) suggests that 'we need to take time to reflect on not only our own working practices and the effect that these have on the patient, but also on the patients' perceptions of their problems, and act on what we are really being told. It is important to make time both to listen to patients' problems and to work out with them their solutions. We need to realise the importance of giving information relevant to the patient's needs, and to develop skills that enable us to assist patients in taking an active role in their problem solving' (Robinson, 1992b).

Being a neuro-oncology patient is extremely difficult. Many feel that their body has been taken over, not only by their disease, but also by the doctors, nurses and therapists who 'do' things to it and with it. This lack of control and general panic may precipitate a passivity in some patients and non-compliance in others. These patients are trying to exert their own wants and needs in the only way they know how, by refusing treatment and help. Not only do neuro-oncology patients have to adjust to suffering from a potentially fatal disease and the realisation of their own mortality, but they may also have to come to terms with disability resulting from the disease itself or from its treatment (see Chapter 10). By allowing patients to determine their most important problems, listening to them and working with them in finding an acceptable solution, it is possible to achieve a high (patient-defined) success rate and a dramatically increased level of job satisfaction for the health care professional (Robinson, 1992b).

Setting treatment plans for patients with CNS tumours will only be successful if the content and context of that agenda are appropriate for each individual and take their priorities for treatment into account. This may require much negotiation as the needs that the health care professional identifies as priorities for patients may be different from those which patients feels are more important for themselves. Defining a treatment programme in conjunction with the patient involves identifying problems and setting goals and objectives. The functions of assessment are for diagnosis of the problems and agenda evaluation, for predicting future success and for assessing attainment. Patients' perceptions of the usefulness of this process will have a significant influence on their ability to learn and make adjustments to a changed view of themselves, physically, psychologically, emotionally and socially. In defining problems and setting goals, patients may come to realise their strengths and weaknesses and therefore be able to decide on an appropriate course of action. In doing so, they retain autonomy and control over their own lives (Robinson, 1992b).

The family as team members

Family members have been referred to as the 'gateway' to the team (Rothberg, 1992) or even, in the rehabilitation literature (for example Anderson, 1984), as team members. However, family caregivers are typically even less likely than patients to be active members of formal team activities, even if patients and/or their families are engaged in providing essential input to or follow-through of team activities (Saltz and Schaefer, 1996). One key underlying assumption in team practice is that drawing upon the expertise of more than one practitioner can enhance the outcome of assessment and intervention with the patients seen in formal health care contexts, especially where multiple problems prevail. Another assumption is that patients, who are widely seen as the focus of the team's efforts, and in many cases their family caregivers, are members of the team.

Team structure plays a major role in the degree of integration of family caregivers. Most team members, especially in health care settings, are professionals with training and experience in a particular discipline. Family members and patients are typically regarded as, at best, 'lay' team members. They usually do not have detailed knowledge of the roles and functions of professionals on a team and may be totally unaware that a treatment team is actually formally working together, especially if patients/families are not directly involved in team meetings or engaged in other mechanisms of team communication. However, families are in fact 'specialists' in providing a wealth of information regarding the patient, for example pre-illness functioning. One or more team members will 'represent' the family in the team context. For example, the team member who has a special rapport with one or more family members may serve as their advocate and even a broker for services on behalf of the family. In many multidisciplinary teams, the professional whose expertise is most pertinent to the patient's major problem becomes the designated care manager. In such instances, family caregivers become 'unseen' members of the team (Saltz and Schaefer, 1996). Assessment, care planning and implementation are major points of contact where family involvement is critical, especially for the patient whose cognitive status is impaired.

Inadequate leadership similarly can lead to alienation and even a lack of co-operation of family caregivers. Information-sharing and communication among team members can be affected by family input, especially in cases where family members selectively share information depending on whom they relate to among the professional team members. If family input is limited during problem-solving and decision-making, formal team activities that make assumptions about family caregivers' perspectives can have a negative effect on planned interventions (Saltz and Schaefer, 1996).

Summary

It can therefore be seen that both patients and their families are pivotal in the delivery of care given by the multidisciplinary team. This is particularly important in neuro-oncology, where illness brings with it major deficits and alterations in lifestyle for both the patient and family. Unless strategies are employed that meet the needs of the family as well as the patient, the team will not be effective.

To conclude this chapter, it is worth noting that each topic has a wealth of literature available to the reader and that an overview has been given here. Readers are encouraged to evaluate the functioning of the team in which they work and strive to facilitate its development for the benefit of the patients, their families and the efficient and effective delivery of valuable services provided by health care professionals in the management of neuro-oncology patients.

Acknowledgements

We are grateful to Helen White, Speech and Language Therapist, and Jill Cooper, Head Occupational Therapist, at the Royal Marsden NHS Trust for their contribution to this chapter.

References

Adair J (1986) Effective Team Building. London: Gower.

Anderson TP (1984) Rehabilitation management and the rehabilitation team. In Basmajian JV, Kirby RC (Eds) Medical Rehabilitation, pp.10–77. Baltimore: Williams & Wilkins.

Barret P (1987) Team building. In Stewart DM (Ed.) Handbook of Management Skills. London: Gower.

Belbin RM (1981) Management Teams: Why They Succeed or Fail. London: Heinemann.

Blake R, Mouton J (1964) The Management Grid. Houston, TX: Gulf Publication Company.

Bobath B (1990) Adult Hemiplegia: Evaluation and Treatment, 3rd edn. London: Heinemann Medical.

Boroch RM (1976) Elements of Rehabilitation Nursing. St Louis: CV Mosby.

Caplan D (1987) Neurolinguistics and Linguistic Aphasiology: An Introduction. Cambridge: Cambridge University Press.

Carr JH, Shepherd RB (1986) Motor Training following stroke. In Banks M (Ed.) Stroke, pp. 56–69. London: Churchill Livingstone.

Cassileth BR, Hamilton JN (1979) The family with cancer. In Cassileth BR (Ed.) The Cancer Patient: Social Aspects of Care, pp. 67–84. Philadelphia: Lea and Febiger.

Concise Oxford Dictionary (1982) 7th edition. Oxford: Clarendon Press.

Cooper J (Ed.) (1997) Occupational Therapy in Oncology and Palliative Care. London: Whurr.

Darley F, Aronson A, Brown J (1975) Motor Speech Disorders. London: WB Saunders.

David JA (1993) A study of the role of the rehabilitation team. European Journal of Cancer Care 2: 129–33.

Davies PM (1994) Starting Again. London: Springer-Verlag.

Dietz JH (1981) Rehabilitation Oncology. New York: John Wiley & Sons.

Downie PA (1978) Cancer Rehabilitation: An Introduction for Physiotherapists and the Allied Professions. London: Faber & Faber.

Dudas S, Carlson CE (1988) Cancer rehabilitation. Oncology Nursing Forum 15(2): 183–8.

Edwards S (1996) Neurological Physiotherapy: A Problem Solving Approach. London: Churchill Livingstone.

Embling S (1995) Exploring multidisciplinary teamwork. British Journal of Therapy and Rehabilitation 2(3): 142–4.

Fargason CA, Haddock CC (1992) Cross-functional, integrative team decision making: essential for QI in health care. Quality Review Bulletin 18(5): 157–63.

Giaquinta B (1977) Helping families to face the crisis of cancer. American Journal of Nursing 77: 1585–8.

Giguere M, Lewis M (1994) The interdisciplinary team component of case management: a positive experience. CONA Journal 16(3): 17–21.

Grieve J (1993) Neuropsychology for Occupational Therapists. Oxford: Blackwell Science.

Handy CB (1976) Understanding Organisations. Harmondsworth: Penguin Books.

Johnson J (1988) Cancer: a family disruption. Recent Results in Cancer Research 108: 306–10.

Kane RA (1975) The interprofessional team as a small group. Social Work in Health Care 1(1): 19–32.

Le Dorze G, Brassard C (1995) A description of the consequences of aphasia on aphasic persons and their relatives and friends: based on the WHO model of chronic diseases. Aphasiology 9(3): 239–56.

Lewandowski W, Jones S (1988) The family with cancer: nursing interventions throughout the course of living with cancer. Cancer Nursing 11(6): 313–21.

Lowe IL, Herranen M (1978) Conflict in teamwork: understanding the roles and relationships. Social Work in Health Care 3: 323–30.

Lynch BL (1981) Team building: will it work in health care? Journal of Allied Health (November): 241.

Margerison C, McCann D (1985) How To Lead a Winning Team. Bradford: MCB University Press.

Margerison C, McCann D (1989) How to improve team management. Leadership and Organisation Development Journal 10(5): 3–42.

Murdoch BE (1990) Acquired Speech and Language Disorders. A Neuro-anatomical and Functional Neurological Approach. London: Chapman & Hall.

Northouse LL (1984) The impact of cancer on the family: an overview.

International Journal of Psychiatry and Medicine 14(3): 215–43.
Øvretveit J (1990) Making the team work!... Professional Nurse 5(6): 284, 286–8.
Parr S (1995) Everyday reading and writing in aphasia: role change and the influence of pre-morbid literary practice. Aphasiology 9(3): 223–38.
Pope PM (1992) Management of the physical condition in patients with chronic and severe neurological pathologies. Physiotherapy 78(12): 869–903.
Raven RW (1971) The concept of cancer rehabilitation and its implications. In Raven RW (Ed.) Symposium on the Rehabilitation of the Cancer Disabled, pp. 21–36. London: Heinemann.
Richardson M (1992) Teams and team management in nurse education. Nurse Education Today 12: 94–100.
Robinson SN (1992a) The family with cancer. European Journal of Cancer Care 1(2): 29–33.
Robinson SN (1992b) The learning needs of cancer patients. European Journal of Cancer Care 1(3): 18–20.
Rothberg JS (1992) Knowledge of disciplines, roles and functions of team members. In Glenview IL (Ed.) Guide to Interdisciplinary Practice in Rehabilitation Settings. Arlington, VA: American Congress of Rehabilitation Medicine.
Rowe H (1996) Multidisciplinary teamwork - myth or reality? Journal of Nursing Management, 4, 93-101.
Rubin IM, Plovnick MS, Fry RE (1976) Improving the Co-ordination of Care. A Programme for Health Team Development. Cambridge, MA: Ballinger.
Saltz CC (1992) A guide to the guide. In Glenview IL (Ed.) Guide to Interdisciplinary Practise in Rehabilitation Settings. Arlington, VA: American Congress of Rehabilitation Medicine.
Saltz CC, Schaefer T (1996) Interdisciplinary teams in health care: integration of family caregivers. Social Work in Health Care 22(3): 59–70.
Singer BA (1984) The psychological impact of cancer on the patient and family. Journal of the Medical Society of New Jersey 81(5): 383–5.
United Kingdom Central Council for Nursing, Midwifery and Health Visiting (1992) Code of Professional Conduct, 3rd edn. London: UKCC.
Villemoes SL (1995) The occupational therapy intervention of patients with cognitive disorders in Denmark. WFOT Bulletin 32: 33–5.
Woods NF, Lewis FM, Ellison ES (1989) Living with cancer: family experiences. Cancer Nursing 12(1): 28–33.
Zenger JH, Miller DE (1974) Building effective teams. Personnel (April).

Chapter 10
Altered body image

Mave Salter

Introduction

The catastrophic effects of altered body image (ABI) in patients with CNS tumours are often trivialised by health care professionals as these changes are deemed inevitable and secondary in importance to medical treatment (Guerrero, personal communication). This chapter will highlight the major altered body image changes to patients with CNS malignancies. It will also discuss the importance of good-quality support and the nurse's role in such care. Additionally, it will assist nurses to be more aware of the changes in body image that these patients may experience as well as increasing the nurse's confidence in supporting this group of patients and their families. Furthermore, it will help to identify ways of monitoring patients in order to minimise body image issues that may be related to treatments and their side-effects (Batchelor et al, 1991).

Individuals being treated for cancer are often faced with distressing alterations to their body structure and function. Depending on the body part affected and the extent and implications of the physical and cognitive alterations, a patient will experience various degrees of body image concern. This can affect how patients feel about themselves and their loved ones, and can ultimately influence the patient's quality of life (Batchelor et al, 1991). This is particularly so for the patient with a CNS malignancy as physical deficits and cognitive problems often occur simultaneously.

As nurses, we can have some 'feeling' of the fears, the sense of stigma, the practical and social problems that are inherent parts of an illness underlying a diagnostic label. Some patients will worry about their job, others will be concerned about the effects of disability on their close relatives and friends, whereas others will be largely worried about their changed body image. Thus diagnosis is a critical time for patients and their families as this may represent a new self-image and identity as a different person, and an identity change that will only become more complicated during progress through the illness trajectory. For patients with CNS tumours, disease and treatment bring with them major changes, both physically and cognitively, which often cause major distress or severe depression (Lindsay, 1989). As such, life for the patient and family will never be the same again (McKeag, 1995).

Body image

Body image is about how we see ourselves and how we feel we appear to others. Wassner (1982) defines body image as the root of identity, self-esteem and self-worth, the bases from which a person functions. Self-esteem is related to the sense of personal value through acceptance and validation as a sexually desirable person (MacElveen-Hoehn, 1985). People who are deformed or disfigured by cancer or its therapies may lose regard for themselves if they feel that important others and society at large do not accept how they look. Body image is therefore to do with how we feel we look, for example well built or slightly built, attractive, unattractive, tall, short and so on. Other factors affecting and impacting on body image formation and dynamics include genetics, socialisation, fashion, culture, race, education and the mass media (Darbyshire, 1986).

Body image includes the space surrounding the body as well as the accessibility to that space (Horowitz, 1966). This therefore has implications for the extensions to their body image that patients may have, for example a prosthesis. Cohen (1991) suggests that clothes, make-up and jewellery as well as aids and accessories such as a walking stick or wheelchair are integrated into body image. The same author suggests that body attributes affecting body image include, but are not limited to, total body size, proportion of body parts, colouration, sexuality, texture of the skin and facial features. Steroids may lead to, for example, an increase in weight, a moon-shaped face and striae on various parts of the body. A patient's sexuality may also be altered because of cognitive deficits.

Societal pressure

Body image issues are of prime importance to the majority of people because of society's pressure regarding how we should look. This affects patients whatever their disease and is even more important in patients with a CNS tumour who may undergo a multitude of body image changes. Illness inevitably blocks some of life's goals, leading to a vicious circle of mood change, depression and unfulfilled hopes. Patients and families may pretend that they are managing when they are not (Salter, 1997). It is therefore important for the nurse caring for this group of patients to assess the meaning of body image change for that particular patient and explore with him or her interventions for coping. For example, patients with physical and/or cognitive deficits may feel that their altered body image no longer renders them an acceptable member of society. However, we can encourage them to enhance their self-esteem by complimenting them on those areas in which they can function appropriately.

Society is very concerned with body image, slimming and keeping fit being multimillion dollar industries. Those people who have to face body image-altering disease and treatment may therefore feel unable to match up to the 'body beautiful' image. Some overeaters feel stressed because they are constantly bombarded by cultural pressures to eat (note how many advertisements display slim people eating and drinking high-calorie food!) or to slim. Thus we receive mixed messages so it is no wonder that we feel a need to 'forgive' ourselves for not looking the way society has coerced us into thinking we should look (Cooper and Cooper, 1996).

This is even more noticeable for those patients who may be continuously hungry, leading to excessive weight gain because of corticosteroid therapy to control symptoms such as raised intracranial pressure.

Altered body image

Patients with CNS tumours experience many losses over varying lengths of time. Some deficits, for example the occasional word-finding difficulty, may initially appear minimal. Family and friends may be attentive, denial high and hope for a cure real. As the patient deteriorates, deficits intensify and it may become increasingly more difficult to re-establish a sense of equilibrium. Types of loss for patients may include loss of control, feelings of worthlessness, changes in role and a desire for life to return to normal (Newton and

Mateo, 1994). Other losses may include changes in short-term memory, gait, strength, endurance, ability to drive and independence. Patients grieve these losses and frequently become angry at their inability to perform the simplest of tasks (Amato, 1991). Furthermore, the ambiguity of the progression of brain tumour and treatment protocols makes it difficult for the patient and family to cope with rapid changes in lifestyle because they feel they have lost control (Newton and Mateo, 1994). This group of patients therefore often become easily frustrated and depressed with their decreased abilities. As such, rehabilitation must be an ongoing process in order to encourage the patient to be as independent as possible. As one husband said to his wife who had a brain tumour, 'I would take you out, but look at your hair [regrowing following surgery]...look at your weight [cushingnoid and heavy from steroids]...look at your gait [her walk was unsteady due to the tumour infiltrating critical brain tissue]'. It is often easy for professionals not to understand how devastated partners may feel when they see how changed their loved one has become. Blame cannot be placed on this husband because he could not cope with his wife's changed body image, and part of his anger was to do with his inability to accept her illness.

Patients with CNS tumours may walk into objects, and be forgetful and inappropriate at times, and may well realise this. So how highly must they rate their self-esteem and how does their partner or family cope with all these changes? A husband may object to having his spouse waiting on him when he feels he should be the breadwinner and head of the family. He may well be fighting for his last bit of independence. Thus nurses must work with carers in finding ways of making things possible. Diplomacy is therefore always needed in nurses' interactions with patients.

Deficits

Sacks (1986) states that neurology's favourite word is 'deficit', denoting impairment of neurological function, including loss of speech, language, memory, vision, dexterity, identity and a myriad of other specific functions and faculties as well as paraesthesia, epilepsy, drowsiness and progressive functional loss. Newton and Mateo (1994) also recognise the devastating effect of speech and language difficulties, visual problems and the long-term effects of treatment and medication. One patient underwent a very traumatic stage of body change because of the cushingnoid effect of steroids; this alteration from her previous attractive appearance to (in her eyes) such a negative body image was a particular cross to bear.

'Life without memory is no life at all' (Bunuel, cited in Sacks, 1986, p 22); 'Our memory is our coherence, our reason, our feeling, even our action. Patients with memory loss have the problem of forgetting in a few seconds what is said, shown or done to them.' As Sacks (p 105) states, 'to be ourselves we must have ourselves'. The ability of patients to learn may be affected by cognitive impairment, memory deficits and/or physical disabilities (Newton and Mateo, 1994).

Children and adolescents

Body image is assumed to be to do with youth, beauty, vigour, intactness and health, and there may be a significant sense of failure in people who do not match up to this ideal (Smitherman, 1981). Children's and young adolescents' judgements of their attractiveness are highly predicative of the global self-worth they see in themselves as people (Harter, 1985). The importance of physical appearance appears to have increased in recent years, with children as young as 6–11 years of age showing concern regarding dieting (Daily Mail, 1996). During normal adolescence, there is a structural, psychological shift in the individual's identity from being bound up with that of the parent to becoming an 'I' (Kuykendall, 1988). However, the ego identify shift and struggle to become independent is too threatening to do alone, so teenagers unconsciously choose to go through the process in the same way as others in their peer group. They change together, the individual becoming a collective 'I'. This impacts on, for example, food (which can adversely affect a diabetic) and clothes. This therefore has implications for the younger patient on steroids who acquires steroid-induced diabetes. Illness impinges on this, and an adolescent who has been fighting for independence may be forced back into a dependent role, leading to aggression or depression. Changed body image for the older child or teenager with a CNS tumour may include deficits that are noticeable to everyone, such as unsteady gait, alopecia or cushingnoid effects. Such youngsters may require psychological support to help them to adapt. One 17-year-old, who presented with personality changes that led to the diagnosis of a brain tumour, was most unhappy on an adult ward, hiding under the bedcovers and behaving covertly. The need for privacy for adolescents in oncology units to develop their social and sexual relationships must thus be respected (Thompson, 1990). Adolescents should not be expected to share rooms with younger children, and parents should be encouraged to give their teenager time to be alone with friends.

Adults

Threats, for example 'I'm not as attractive as I used to be – I am worried that my partner may leave me', are imposed on one's body image throughout the developmental cycle, but these become more numerous in later life (Janelli, 1986, 1993). Ross et al (1989) studied physical changes associated with the ageing process in 60 subjects, 30 of whom were elderly. Regardless of gender, the researchers found that older persons were more concerned with appearance than were the younger group. More time may therefore be necessary to aid adaptation in the older patient.

Body image is closely linked to quality of life. Changes in physical appearance are known to have a negative effect on an individual's quality of life (Die-Trill and Straker, 1992; Mock, 1993). Mulgrew and Dropkin (1991) identified a supportive network of hospital staff as being of great importance in the patient's adaptation to deformity. Thus part of each consultation should be concerned with assessing how the patient is coping with body image changes and intervening as appropriate. For example, one patient would not accompany her children to school because she felt everyone would be focusing on her hair loss and operation scar. She felt it was too hot to wear a wig in summer. Alternatives were discussed and a thin scarf, casually draped over her head and around her neck, appeared fashionable as well as concealing her scar. Acknowledging that hair loss was a problem to her, and therefore important to address, assisted this young wife and mother to adjust more easily to her body image change (see Chapter 11).

Price (1990) suggests that there are three components of body image: body reality (the way our body really is), body ideal (how we would like to look) and body presentation (for example, appearance and dress.) The above example demonstrates those components identified by Price's model. For this young woman, her body ideal and reality did not match, but by the use of a simple scarf, she felt she could go out in public, and her body presentation was now more acceptable.

Altered body image and cancer treatment modalities

Surgery

For those undergoing surgery, the preparation and general anaesthetic will represent a loss of control over body activities. Physical changes after surgery can vary from a small scar to mutilation that is sometimes gross; bodily function may also be altered by surgery (Blackmore, 1988). For patients undergoing craniotomy or spinal surgery, there are very real fears of waking up paralysed or more disabled than prior to surgery (see Chapter 5). Costello (cited in Donovan and Pearce, 1976) suggests that the nursing care of surgical clients with altered body image includes that of assisting patients to:

- accept the operation site;
- touch and explore the area;
- accept the necessity of learning to care for the defect;
- develop independence and competence in daily care;
- reintegrate the new body image and adjust to the possibility of an altered lifestyle.

A person undergoing a neurosurgical procedure will have some shaving of hair, and swelling of the head and facial bruising following surgery. Denning (1982) found that nurses' reactions to deformity or surgery is crucial for the patients' first reactions to their appearance. A nurse with a fear of facial mutilation may find it difficult to support patients with such body image changes. Darbyshire (1986), and Kelly and May (1982) reviewed such adverse reactions by hospital staff. These researchers indicated that the patient with altered body image may also face a communication barrier with those professionals who are still busy dealing with their own feelings about deformity.

Radiotherapy

For those patients undergoing CNS irradiation, fatigue, malaise, anorexia and skin conditions are very real problems (see Chapter 6). Patients receiving radiotherapy may have many fears, such as being burned or becoming radioactive or disfigured (Krumm, 1982). Such fears can have a great impact on body image and quality of life.

Chemotherapy

For patients undergoing chemotherapy, nausea and vomiting, bone marrow depression and thrombocytopenia or neutropenia can be experienced (see Chapter 7). Some patients choose to stop treatment rather than cope with side-effects related to chemotherapy. As such, the decision to continue treatment often depends on the patient's quality of life. For example, if patients experience severe nausea, they are less likely to feel in control of their body, which may already be adversely affected by other factors relating to body image change. Because of cognitive and functional deficits, significant others often assume the role of caretaker when the patient can no longer be independent. Hence lifestyle changes and role reversal occur, and significant others will be affected by the patient's alteration of appearance and functioning. Thus the support of partners and carers is paramount (Newton and Mateo, 1994).

Hair

Throughout history, hair has been symbolic of cultural and social values. In some societies a hairstyle will indicate the social standing, gender, occupation and religious convictions of an individual. It has been stated that the loss of hair as a symbolic loss of self creates an alienation from the self and from others (Freedman, 1994, 1997).

Language

Loss or impairment of speech for any reason is one of the most distressing and frustrating conditions that afflicts human beings. This is because daily life is deeply concerned with communication. Dysphasia is a defect in the use of language, which may occur in comprehension, expression, reading or writing. Dysphasia (expressive and/or receptive) is the result of damage and/or dysfunction in the areas controlling speech. Dysphasic patients may feel that their body has let them down, with implications of body image change and patient frustration and distress with the disability (Lindsay, 1989). This may be made apparent in the 'Does he take sugar?' scenario, when the carer rather than the patient is asked questions, implying that the patient would not understand (see Chapter 9).

Epilepsy

Epilepsy is another category of body image change in the patient with a brain tumour (see Chapters 3 and 5). Lindsay (1989) states that there are many popular misconceptions about the effect of epilepsy on people's lives and people may be refused jobs when it is known that they have epilepsy. Those with epilepsy may be feared because, without warning and in any situation, they may lose control of their movements. We are all afraid of losing control, states Lindsay, and making a fool of ourselves in public, and the person with epilepsy reminds us of this basic fear of reverting to the 'primitive', even losing control of the bladder in public. Furthermore, Lindsay (1989) suggests that a family's 'felt' stigma can lead to eroded self-image. Someone with repeated seizures who begins to lose self-esteem if others continue to reject him or her may become withdrawn from society in order to avoid the unpleasant reactions of others. This can be perpetuated by nurses telling families to keep a close eye on patients in case they have a fit. This then makes families apprehensive about caring for patients at home. In their study of people with epilepsy, Scrambler and Hopkins (1986) found that more unhappiness, anxiety and self-doubt were caused by the fear of stigma than either directly or indirectly through actual stigma.

Mobility problems

Balance is a result of a number of different functions that combine to achieve an integrated, although constantly changing, sensory pattern. Impaired balance may cause patients to fall over, get dizzy spells or be unable to walk with ease. Such mobility restrictions will often make patients very self-conscious, and the introduction of walking aids reinforces the concept of dependency (Lindsay, 1989) (see Chapter 9). Nurses have a vital role to play in assisting the patient's acceptance of aids and other equipment. In the model 'Preserving self: from victim, to patient to disabled person' Morse and O'Brien (1995) suggest that, in striving to regain self and merging the old and the new reality, the major goals were making sense of the event, getting to know and trust the altered body and accepting the consequences of the experience. However, getting to know and trust the new body does not imply that the disabled person likes the new body. This may well be because, as Charmaz (1983) states, there is a loss of self that occurs in chronic illness.

Body image, states Lindsay (1989), 'is about the ability to feel a limb, to appreciate the movements of joints and to appreciate a...place in space and its relationship to the body. Body image is built up by the sense of muscular position, known as proprioception; this sense is dependent on impulses from muscles, joints and tendons by which the body knows itself, and just does this with...perfect, automatic, instantaneous precision the position and motion of all its moveable parts, their relation to one another and their alignment in space.' Disorders of body image may therefore relate to any change of the former. People will need to know that they are no less a person just because of their changed body image.

Impaired continence

Incontinence is still a topic shrouded in embarrassing silence. Simply by being incontinent, having to wear special pants and pads or being catheterised, a person feels less attractive (Lindsay, 1989).

Davis (1997) uses Price's model to assist a patient with loss of continence:

- the need to insert a urinary catheter intermittently for the rest of one's life (body reality);
- the desire for a return to normal continence (body ideal);
- the wearing of sporting/jogging trousers to disguise the need for frequent and easy access for catheterisation (body presentation).

In such situations, nurses can provide basic body image interventions such as concealing catheters and drainage bags wherever possible. In order to preserve patients' privacy and dignity, if at all possible, the bag should be either concealed under the bedclothes or, at the very least, hung opaque side out (Ettinger, 1995).

Stigma

Goffman (1963), in his seminal work on spoiled identity, suggests that containing a stigma needs special timing; thus there is the practice of 'living on a leash' – the Cinderella syndrome. For when a person's differentness is not immediately apparent, he or she then has to decide either to tell or not to tell (Goffman, 1963).

Many patients who are endeavouring to continue to work or fulfil a role in society despite their physical and/or cognitive deficits may be walking such a tightrope. If a stigmatised person is really at ease with his differentness, this acceptance will have an immediate effect upon 'normal' people, making it easier for them to be at ease with patients in social situations. Persons who are ready to admit possession of a stigma may nonetheless make a great effort to keep the stigma from looking large. The individual's objective is to reduce tension, that is, to make it easier for themselves and others and to withdraw covert attention from the stigma (Goffman, 1963). However, this may not always be possible for some patients with a

CNS tumour. Carlisle (1993) spent one day with a facial disfigurement, courtesy of a make-up artist. She concluded that there was 'solicitousness covered up by pity and a desire to have a good stare. I was no longer one of the crowd'.

Stigma is also defined as the disgrace associated with certain conditions, attributes, traits or forms of behaviour. In the case of patients with CNS tumours, this marking may be an obvious deformity, ungainly or unco-ordinated movement or the necessity to use, for example, a stick or wheelchair (Lindsay, 1989). The physically disabled person may feel shame and discomfort, and may then reject and withdraw from encounters with the physically able (Goffman, 1963).

Rating and adjustment to body image

Some body image changes will be obvious to onlookers, but others will be concealed. Some of these changes may be permanent, some temporary. A lack of co-ordination may well be apparent. Thus if a 'normal' person has body image problems, a person whose body image undergoes a change because of disease and/or treatment is even more at risk.

Different people rate body image in a variety of ways. For example, one patient with a brain tumour was, following surgery, never seen in public without his cap on, and even his adult children were prevented from seeing his craniotomy scar. For some, a small change may be more difficult to come to terms with than may a major change in others. Being unhappy with one's body image affects the way in which a person behaves and functions, which in turn rebounds onto others, as for example with a hair cut that has not turned out the way one anticipated. A person who puts on a confident front, will be treated that way, but if a person feels resentful or insecure, people may react to them accordingly. Some patients have a great deal of support from their family, friends or employers, which enables them to adapt well to living their life with a disability. Others may feel much less positive, allowing the altered body image to disrupt their lifestyle; in some extreme cases, the patient may become a recluse.

Others will operate by denial. By ignoring medication regimens and dietary restrictions, neglecting to engage in therapeutic exercise programmes and failing to keep medical appointments, these people attempt to demonstrate to themselves and others that they are neither ill nor limited in any profound way (Wichowski and Kubsch,

1997). It may well be that the patient is too frightened to face the impending reality. Indeed, one patient continued to work on scaffolding despite having epileptic fits, thus denying that he had a problem associated with his CNS tumour.

Sexuality

In our ageist culture, we have negative views of sexuality in the elderly, and the sexual problems of the physically disabled are only beginning to be recognised and discussed. Studies of the chronically ill or disabled have shown that sexual activity is particularly susceptible to change. Whenever illness causes a reduction in physical sensitivity, and even when a good physical recovery occurs, a large proportion of patients reduce their sexual activity. Sexual functioning and drive may not be impaired, but the indirect effects of disability may make intercourse difficult or impossible. These effects include uncontrollable body movements and paralysis. Some people will automatically expect others to withdraw from physical, emotional and social contact because of the new body that they now inhabit, which is 'scarred' by some form of disability; there is a fear of rejection. The patient's personality may also have changed as a result of, for example, a frontal lobe tumour. The nurse may hear spouses say, 'He is not the man I married.' How can they be expected to be intimate with someone who is in effect a stranger? The spouse may now find the physical appearance of the partner repulsive. If the patient has to be cared for by his partner, being, for example washed and dressed, how can the partner look on him as a lover? (Lindsay, 1989). Thus the patient and partner will need counselling to deal with these important issues and may well need to be given permission to express their feelings and concern about alterations in body image (see Chapter 11).

Nursing care

The nurse needs to ensure ongoing support, where appropriate, in the important realm of coming to terms with changes in body image and how this affects activities of daily living, including sexuality. However, nurses should acknowledge that some patients may prefer not to discuss this personal area of their lives (Salter, 1995).

Positive skills and strengths should be stressed rather than emphasising the negative (Lindsay, 1989). Research indicates that nurses can lessen anxiety and therefore reduce pain by listening, by explanation and by recognising that the patient and his relatives are worried and need help (Hayward, 1975). Giving the right information reduces anxiety and also aids a rapid adjustment to stressful events because patients can prepare before they occur, when they are more able to concentrate, rather than when they are in pain (Wilson-Barnett, 1980).

Helping patients to understand and accept their altered body image as a result of disease and treatment is a cancer care priority (Batchelor et al, 1991). Current literature cited in Batchelor et al points out that one-third of all cancer patients suffer from unresolved adjustment to an altered body image. Cancer nurses play an important role in helping cancer patients to adjust to their new body image. The nurse can educate and prepare the patient for body alterations before cancer treatment, teach the patient how to care for him or herself following treatment and help guide the patient through the process of understanding and accepting the new body image after treatment has been completed. Enhancing the nurse's ability to improve the quality of care for patients with an altered body image related to cancer and its treatment is important. For example, nurses need to be available and not hide behind 'task-orientated care' (Table 10.1).

Table 10.1 Nursing interventions to facilitate adaptation in patients undergoing changes in body image – general

- Give advice, information and counselling at appropriate times
- Don't be afraid to admit you don't know the answer, but try to find someone who does
- Be available – don't hide behind 'tasks' or busyness
- Timely relief of pain
- Permit the patient to choose the health care professionals to whom they best relate
- If possible, plan a gradual discharge, for example an afternoon out, an overnight stay, etc.
- Encourage self-care and emphasise what patients CAN do, for example self-medication
- Set short-term and then longer-term goals
- Arrange appropriate support in the community.

Part of the nurse's role is to encourage patients to utilise their social support network. Some patients may be able to adopt a positive outlook, whilst others may feel much less optimistic, allowing the altered body image to disrupt their lives and lead to their becoming isolated. Patients often need support when relatives or friends first see their changed image. Their first outing from hospital is important, and an afternoon away from the ward, extending to a day and then a weekend, if this is practical, is necessary for some people in their gradual letting go of the security of the inpatient world (Salter, 1997).

While in hospital, patients are sheltered from their normal environment, but on their return home, they may wait to see how those around them – family, friends and the primary health care professionals – react. The trend today is for a shorter hospital stay, the patient returning home as soon as possible, so community staff are increasingly having to deal with the physical and psychological effects of body image changes (see Chapter 12). Caring and involved partners play an important role in their spouse's rehabilitation and care, and the nurse can be an active participant in this (Salter, 1997)

Care planning is paramount, especially where there is a disturbance of body image. In such situations, the nursing intervention can be that of encouraging the patient to express feelings about changes in physical appearance or body function. Salter (1997) suggests that incorporating body image into patient care can be developed by using a model of care, whilst Peplau (1969) maintains that a relationship of closeness between the nurse and patient can be a springboard for enabling healthy adaptation to body image changes. Similarly, standards of care (Batchelor et al 1991) may also be used, for example 'The patient will be aware of how to minimise the distress of hair loss and ways of enhancing appearance to distract from hair loss.' Timely referrals to appropriate multidisciplinary team members are also an important part of nursing care (see Chapter 9).

It is important that nurses counsel patients about the measures they should take to prevent further injury and a worsening body image. It may help to enhance other areas of the body, for example by the use of particular clothes, which can detract from the altered body image (Batchelor et al, 1991). Thus the nurse's role is one of communicator, counsellor and patient advocate. Taking a careful history during the assessment, organising patient/family conferences and discharge planning are important aspects of nursing care. Erwin-Toth and Spencer (1991) state that providing quality patient care is the goal of every health care institution. Professional nurses strive to deliver individualised, comprehensive care to their patients, and the aim of nursing interventions is to maximise the health potential of patients in our care (Tables 10.2 and 10.3).

Table 10.2 Nursing interventions to facilitate adaptation in patients undergoing changes in body image – emotional support

- Tailor specific needs and support to the individual
- By liking your patients, their self-esteem improves (Burnard and Morrison, 1990)
- Assess the meaning of loss for the patient and ways of moving forward
- Explain to patients not only what is happening, but also why it is
- Recognise that what is said to the patient and what is heard by the patient may be different
- Offer support when significant others first see their bodily alterations
- The need for touch and closeness on the part of the nurse is a model for carers and relatives
- Be aware of the point that the patient has reached in the grieving process (as there are fluctuations between stages)
- Be aware of patients/relatives progressing in their acceptance (or otherwise) of the condition at different rates
- Be alert to the patient who may be having a bad day, does not interact with others or has limited or no social support network
- Be aware of the 'passive' patient who appears to accept everything
- Compliment patients on natural traits and accentuate body image parts that have not changed; that is, emphasise the good points
- Be aware of further onslaughts of altered body image on patients undergoing adjuvant treatment
- Be aware of a conspiracy of pretence, false laughter, etc.
- Give time out for patients/relatives to cope (e.g. to have time alone in the sitting room) after being told bad news
- Ask non-invasive questions on follow-up, for example 'Do you mind if I ask whether...you go out shopping/see your friends/have returned to work/planned a meal out, a holiday?
- Facilitate the acceptance of possible role changes
- Encourage self-empowerment as appropriate
- Take note of the use of humour, which is appropriate sometimes but can be devastating if used inappropriately
- Assess and encourage appropriate coping strategies with the patient
- Work with the patient to make living more meaningful and personally fulfilling (Price, 1990)

Table 10.3 Nursing interventions to facilitate adaptation in patients undergoing changes in body image – sexuality issues

- Enable the patient to realise that even if sexual function is altered, this should not destroy sexuality
- Suggest alternative ways of expressing/making love
- Reduce embarrassment for patients who may find it difficult to talk about sex activity
- Demonstrate sensitivity and receptiveness to persons who are same-sex orientated
- Review medication that may interfere with sexual function
- Have no preconceived ideas of the sexual needs of elderly, single and homosexual patients (Booth, 1990)

Conclusion

What is normal? What is an intact body image? Society appears to dictate the normal and the eccentric. Those nurses who truly understand their patients may be able to help them make some sense and adjust to their new self. However, they cannot go through the circumstances instead of the patient. But with the right help, the pain and outrage of a changed body image may bring insight and growth (Salter, 1997). Each individual has particular ways of accepting his or her change in body image, and the age at the time of body image change is important (Stewart, 1981)

Adaptation is not always positive because there are individuals who will permanently avoid the reality of having undergone changes in their body. Such people will continue to deny changes and remain regressed or develop a psychosis (Murray, 1972). Adaptation can be helped by using a model for body image care (Price, 1990) and by measuring and assessing body image (Price, 1990; Frank-Stromberg, 1992; Dolan and Birtchnell, 1997). However, one has to also bear in mind that this group of patients often face a limited future, and if cognitive difficulties are present this may mean that they are unable to be fully helped or to achieve full adaptation. Expectation is very important to the process of coping with a defect and prepared individuals adapt more easily to body image changes than do those in whom alteration occurs without warning (Donovan and Pearce, 1976; Smitherman, 1981; Wassner, 1982)

Sacks (1986) asks if there is any 'place' in the world for a person who is like an island, who cannot be made part of the main? Can 'the main' accommodate, make room for the singular? It is imperative that, when considering body image changes in the person with a CNS tumour, we offer a resounding acceptance of each individual and that our nursing care helps them see themselves as indeed part of 'the main'. Health care professionals can make a difference to patients by supporting them through their illness trajectory and assuring them that 'to me you are still you' (Tschudin, 1981).

References

Amato C (1991) Malignant glioma: coping with a devastating illness. Neuroscience Nursing 23(1): 20–2.

Batchelor D, Grahn G, Oliver G, Pritchard P, Redmond K, Webb P (1991) Cancer Care Priorities for Nurses: Altered Body Image. London: European Oncology Nursing Society.

Blackmore C (1988) Cited in Salter M (Ed) Altered Body Image: The Nurse's Role. Chichester: John Wiley & Sons.

Booth B (1990) Does it really matter at that age? Nursing Times 86(3): 50–2.
Bunuel L (1986) Cited in Sacks O, The Man who Mistook his Wife for a Hat. London: Picador, p 22.
Burnard J, Morrison L (1990) Body image and physical appearance. Surgical Nurse 3: 4–8.
Carlisle A (1993) Cited in Cronan L, Management of the patient with altered body image. British Journal of Nursing 13(5): 257–61.
Charmaz K (1983) Loss of self: a fundamental form of suffering in the chronically ill. Sociology of Health and Illness 5: 168–95.
Cohen A (1991) Body image in the person with a stoma. Journal of Enterostomal Therapy 18(2): 68–71.
Cooper R, Cooper L (1996) Low fat living. Italy: Rodale Books.
Costello B (1976) Cited in Donavon M, Pearce S, Cancer Care Nurs. New York: Appleton-Century-Crofts, p 19.
Daily Mail (1996) Study of 6–11 year olds concerned with dieting. 14 September.
Darbyshire P (1986) When the face doesn't fit. Nursing Times 82: 28–9.
Davis P (1997) Cited in Salter M (Ed.) Altered Body Image: The Nurse's Role, 2nd edn. London: Baillière Tindall., pp 267–85.
Denning D (1982) Head and neck cancer: our reactions. Cancer Nursing (August): 269–73.
Die-Trill M, Straker N (1992) Psychological adaptation to facial disfigurement in female head and neck cancer patients. Psycho-Oncology 1: 247–51.
Dolan B, Birtchnell S (1997) Measuring body image. In Salter M (Ed.) Altered Body Image: The Nurse's Role. London: Baillière Tindall, London, pp 51–74.
Donovan M, Pearce S (1976) Cancer Care Nursing. New York: Appleton-Century-Crofts.
Erwin-Toth P, Spencer M (1991) A survey of patient perception of quality of care. Journal of Enterostomal Therapy Nursing 18(4): 122–5.
Ettinger F (1995) Bags of urine don't have to be on display. Nursing Standard 10(3): 41.
Frank-Stromberg M (1992) Instruments for clinical nursing research. New York: Boston Jones and Bartlett.
Freedman T (1994) Social and cultural dimensions of hair loss in women treated for breast cancer. Cancer Nursing 17(4): 334–41.
Freeedman T (1997) Cited in Salter M (Ed) Altered Body Image: The Nurse's Role, 2nd edn. London: Baillière Tindall, p 79.
Goffman E (1963) Notes on the management of spoiled1 identity. New York: Prentice Hall.
Harter S (1985) Cited in Eisenberg N (Ed.) Contemporary Topics in Developmental Psychology. New York: Wiley-Interscience, p 286.
Hayward J (1975) Information – a Prescription against Pain. London: Royal College of Nursing.
Horowitz M (1966) Body image. Archives of General Psychiatry 14: 213–20.
Janelli L (1986) Body image in older adults: a review of the literature. Rehabilitation Nursing 11(4): 6–8.
Janelli L (1993) Are there body image differences between older men and women? Western Journal of Nursing Research 15(3): 327–39.
Kelly M, May D (1982) Good and bad patients: a review of the literature and a theoretical critique. Journal of Advanced Nursing 7(2): 147–56.
Krumm S (1982) Psychological adaptation of the adult with cancer. Nursing Clinics of North America 17(4): 729–37.

Kuykendall J (1988) Teenage trauma. Nursing Times 85(27): 26–8.

Lindsay M (1989) Communicating with Neurological Patients: The Nurse's Role. London: Scutari Press.

MacElveen-Hoehn P (1985) Sexual assessment and counselling. Seminars in Oncology Nursing 1(1): 69–75.

McKeag G (1995) The role of the neuro-oncology liaison nurse. Paediatric Nursing 7(10): 24–6.

Mock V (1993) Body image in women, treated for breast cancer. Nursing Research 42(3): 153–7.

Morse J, O'Brien B (1995) Preserving self: from victim, to patient, to disabled person. Journal of Advanced Nursing 21: 886–96.

Mulgrew B, Dropkin M (1991) Coping with craniofacial resection. A case study. Journal of the Publ. Soc. Otorhinolaryngeal Head and Neck Cancer 8: 10.

Murray R (1972) Principles of nursing intervention for the adult patient with body image changes. Nursing Clinics of North America 7(4).

Newton C, Mateo M (1994) Uncertainty: strategies for patients with brain tumor and their family. Cancer Nursing 17(2): 137–40.

Peplau H (1969) Professional closeness. Nursing Forum viii(4): 343–60.

Price B (1990) Body Image: Nursing Concepts and Care. London: Prentice Hall.

Ross M, Tait R, Grossberg G, Handal P, Brandeberry L, Nakra R (1989) Age differences in body consciousness. Journal of Gerontology 44: 23–4.

Sacks O (1986) The Man who Mistook his Wife for a Hat. London: Picador.

Salter M (1995) Body image study shows most patients need support. Eurostoma 12: 18–19.

Salter M (1997) Altered Body Image: The Nurse's Role, 2nd edition. London: Baillière Tindall.

Scrambler G, Hopkins A (1986) Being epileptic: coming to terms with stigma. Sociology of Health and Illness (1): 26–43.

Smith J (1997) Cultural issues associated with altered body image. Cited in Salter M, Altered Body Image: the Nurse's Role, 2nd edn. London: Baillière Tindall.

Smitherman C (1981) Nursing Action for Health Promotion. London: FA Davis.

Stewart WHF (1981) Finding feelings behind the words. Nursing Mirror 153: 43–51.

Thompson J (1990) Sexuality: the adolescent and cancer. Nursing Standard 4(37): 26–8.

Tschudin V (1981) Counselling Skills for Nurses, 2nd edn. London: Baillière Tindall.

Wassner A (1982) The impact of mutilating surgery or trauma on body image. International Nursing Review (29 March): 86–90.

Wichowski H, Kubsch S (1997) The relationship of self-perception of illness and compliance with health care regimens. Journal of Advanced Nursing 25: 548–53.

Wilson-Barnett J (1980) Prevention and alleviation against stress in patients. Nursing 2: 432–6.

Chapter 11
Psychological support

Sue Kibler

Introduction

I think, therefore I am.

This famous philosophical statement by René Descartes (1596-1650) (Magee, 1987, p 83) gives an indication of the value of the human brain. It is the seat of personality, the organ of the body that more than any other is linked to our sense of self. We are born helpless and unconscious into a world of material objects and people. Our early development as babies and children is all about learning to experience this world, to see, hear, smell, taste and touch. What we experience through these senses, we learn to call 'reality'. As motor skills develop, we learn that we can have an impact on the world. We can mobilise within it; we can manipulate objects and affect people in order to achieve our goals. Our sense of purpose and meaning in the world is based on who we are and what we can do. We feel we are in control of our lives and our destinies. All perception of reality and purposeful function in the world is dependent on the healthy functioning of the CNS. The diagnosis of a malignancy of the CNS can mean the beginning of the end of the known and valued world.

The impact of diagnosis

Most people live within a network of individuals and groups. This often includes family members, that is, a spouse or partner, parents, siblings and children. However, not everyone shares their life with blood relatives or enters into committed partnerships. For the purposes of this chapter therefore, 'family' will indicate those who are nearest and dearest to the patient, whose proximity results in involvement in the disease process.

The diagnosis of a CNS tumour is a devastating life event, throwing both the patient and the family into a crisis. It comes as a sudden and unexpected intrusion into normal life, turning the whole world upside down. Suddenly, everything seems out of control and overtaken by the tumour. Hospital appointments for investigations become the order of the day, taking the place of normal routines. There may be admission for surgery and/or daily attendance for radiotherapy. What was an ordinary lifestyle becomes fraught with chaos and uncertainty on both practical and emotional levels (Kibler, 1996).

Uncertainty is something every human being has to learn to deal with. None of us can see the future or know what will happen tomorrow. However, most of us can be fairly sure that what we plan, we have a reasonable chance of being able to achieve, at least in the short term. We have a sense of having choice and control over our future. The diagnosis of a CNS tumour produces for both patient and family a state of complete uncertainty, in which nothing can be assumed, no plans can be made and the future is an awesome and frightening unknown, dreadful in its threat of the extinction of meaning, purpose and fulfilment.

The cognitive state of uncertainty, which results when there is not enough information to define or categorise an event adequately (Newton and Matteo, 1994), is experienced by patients with CNS tumours and their families, with extensive and potentially catastrophic effects. It is the underlying condition, a major source of stress, that produces crisis. Uncertainty strikes at many levels. The disease may affect areas of the brain controlling mobility, perception, cognition and emotion (Salander, 1996). The patient may experience hemiplegia, hemiparesis, seizures or other physical deficits that make normal physical functioning impossible. There may be visual or auditory disturbances that not only compromise safety, but also result in a loss of pleasurable pursuits such as reading or listening to music (Guerrero, 1996).

Cognitive impairment can impinge on communication, especially if memory and speech are affected, leaving the patient feeling isolated and alone. Going to work or driving a car may be eliminated from daily life, with resultant economic threat and uncertainty. Emotional lability, frustration, anger and a sense of loss are common features of what the patient and family have to bear. There can be existential questioning, trying to make sense of the catastrophe. The patient, disabled and unable to go to work, may feel socially dead (Guerrero, 1996). The workplace provides, for many people, a sense of identity outside the family. Also, in our culture, to be socially valuable one must be economically productive (Lindsay, 1990). Being unable to work produces feelings of uselessness and the stigma of not being a whole person. Thus physical, cognitive, emotional, social and spiritual functioning are all threatened.

The family as well as the patient experience the CNS tumour. Family members have to find a way of integrating the disorganisation that illness brings into other normal aspects of life and coping with the resultant feelings. Wanting to comfort and relieve the anguish of the patient, family members often feel powerless and helpless. The disruption to routine can cause ambivalence and resentment towards the situation, which then can result in feelings of blame, guilt and shame (Robinson, 1992). The whole network and matrix of the family can be shaken and the psychological health of the family unit strained.

Roles and relationships within the family have to change, sometimes drastically. The duties and responsibilities of the person with the tumour often have to be taken over by someone else. This can leave the patient with a sense of loss and decreased value, whilst the other person may feel burdened and resentful (Robinson, 1992). Children sometimes have to assume responsibilities beyond their years, including helping with the care of the ill parent. Strain in relationships easily arises. If clear communication is not possible, either because of the effects of the illness or because of family dynamics, enormous misunderstandings and problems can arise. The family gets its sense of purpose and direction from being able to have dreams and goals for the future. These are severely disrupted by the diagnosis, causing frustration, anger and grief (Robinson, 1992).

Personality change is one of the most difficult aspects of the illness to cope with and can be particularly hard for the spouse or partner, for whom the patient seems to be no longer the person they made a commitment to. The relationship changes from one of mutuality to one of unequal caring. The patient can have bouts of dysphoria, becoming demanding and dominating. Dependency increases, with the caring spouse left feeling as if a child to be cared for has replaced the previously equal partner (Salander, 1996).

Loss is the predominant theme throughout the course of the illness, from diagnosis to death. Recovery to full health is rarely achieved (Salander et al, 1996a). The losses may initially be minimal, with family and friends sharing hopefulness about the outcome.

Gradually, as deterioration increases, losses accrue, losses of memory, strength, endurance, physical capacity, gait and independence (Amato, 1991). Grieving goes on throughout the illness at each loss, accompanied by anger and sadness. Death often comes as welcome release from a terrible prison for both patient and family. Sometimes there can be a secondary bereavement for the family, when the professional carers that have been so involved for so long are no longer part of everyday life.

Addressing the diversity of problems

CNS tumours are responsible for over 3000 deaths each year in the UK (Oswin, 1992). Some present few symptoms until diagnosis, which comes as a cataclysmic event. Other people can have symptoms for a long period of time before they grow severe enough to motivate the person to seek medical advice. Some are even misdiagnosed, their symptoms, such as cognitive impairment, being put down to stress or even psychiatric disorders (Oswin, 1992). The site, grade and type of tumour will determine the prognosis and symptoms likely to be experienced (see Chapter 3). The nurse has a key role in helping both patient and family cope with and endure the disease process. As prognosis is poor, death is usually the expected long-term outcome. In some cases, however, the course of the disease extends over several years, with vacillations in improvement and deterioration. The needs of the patient and family will vary according to stage of illness and whether the patient is in hospital or at home.

A multidisciplinary team approach is essential and cannot be overemphasised. The skills of many groups of health professionals are required, including nurses, doctors, physiotherapists, speech therapists, occupational therapists, social workers, clinical psychologists and counsellors, all with good links to their colleagues within the primary health care team in the community (see Chapter 9). However, nurses have a key role in the care of patients with CNS tumours. Nursing assessment, intervention and evaluation of care is core to the whole process of treatment for this group of patients.

The most important task of the nurse is to establish and develop a relationship of trust with the patient and family. This is done through honesty and consistency throughout the course of the illness. Having someone who is reliable, sensitive to needs and able to be with the patient and family throughout the ups and downs of the disease process is an important factor in their coping.

Assessment of needs

The needs of patients with cancer fall into five broad categories (Kibler, 1996):

1. information;
2. symptom control;
3. practical help;
4. communication;
5. psychological adjustment.

Patients with CNS tumours and their families have specialised needs relating to all of these categories.

Information

Patient and family education, giving information about the illness, treatment protocols and side-effects, is an important part of comprehensive and individualised patient care. Having information and understanding empowers the patient and family, and enhances their coping (Newton and Matteo, 1994). This is especially important during the crisis stage of the disease at the time of diagnosis, when the patient and family are feeling very frightened, overwhelmed, confused and vulnerable. At this point, denial is often one of the strategies used against the sense of disaster; information given may seem not to be taken in. There can be a fine line between breaking down denial and giving information; this important coping strategy needs to be recognised and respected, especially in the early stages, when the patient and family are in shock. Professionals need to be honest, accurate, open and trustworthy (Amato, 1991) but also sensitive to how much information the patient and family want and need. Throughout the illness, there may be variance between patient and family in the type and amount of information needed, and these differences should be acknowledged and respected. If asked, people can often give an indication of their informational needs. Some need to know everything possible to have a sense of empowerment and control; others prefer to know as little as possible – 'what you don't know, you can't worry about'.

There may be physical and cognitive deficits, such as visual or hearing impairment, receptive or expressive dysphasia, memory loss or personality change, that make information-giving difficult (Gardner, 1992). Families' and patients' abilities to assimilate information may vary from day to day depending on anxiety levels, fatigue and other factors. The nurse should assess the patient's and family's needs for information, addressing their concerns and queries first, using judgement on how much can be taken in at a particular time. Consistency in information given by more than one health care professional is crucial, especially if there are deficits that make assimilating information difficult. Having several professionals involved can be overwhelming and confusing, and a consistent approach is essential. This may be achieved by limiting those who give information to a small group within the larger multidisciplinary team, for example the clinical nurse specialist, neurosurgeon, and neuro-oncologist (Newton and Matteo, 1994). The help and advice of speech and occupational therapists may be required to maximise the potential of effective communication of information.

Symptom control

Patients with CNS tumours may suffer a wide range of physical symptoms, both from the disease itself and from the side-effects of treatment. Pain, including headaches and vomiting (as a result of raised intracranial pressure), sensory loss including smell, taste, vision and hearing, hemiparesis/hemiplegia and weakness, and so on (Guerrero, 1996; see also Chapters 1 and 3) can result from the disease itself. Treatment with radiotherapy can cause an initial worsening of symptoms, which raises anxiety levels in both patient and family. The nurse has an important role of education and reassurance that these do not reflect disease progression and will be transient (Guerrero, 1996). Fatigue and/or somnolence can be a major problem. Treatment usually involves steroids, which can cause gastric irritation, euphoria, insomnia, dysphoria, weight gain and depression (see Chapter 8). Hair loss can be an especially distressing side-effect of radiotherapy or chemotherapy; steroid-induced acne can be equally embarrassing (see Chapter 10). The nurse has a responsibility to inform the patient and family of probable side-effects and to give them appropriate support as these occur. This may involve referral to others such as clinical nurse specialists dealing with altered body image or counselling.

For the patient, an important aspect of support when facing distressing symptoms is the feeling of being heard and understood. Giving false reassurances or advice that tries to 'make it better' is not helpful. For example, if a patient is upset about hair loss, reassuring them that the wig-maker is available is not enough. The patient needs to know that someone understands what hair loss means for them and that grief for this loss is a normal part of the process of adjusting to the illness. If the distress is severe and ongoing, referral for psychological care may be appropriate.

Patients with CNS tumours can also suffer from more mundane side-effects of illness and treatment such as constipation, oral thrush or skin breakdown, especially if mobility is severely decreased. The nurse should be attentive to these seemingly minor symptoms. Patients will often suffer in silence under the assumption that nothing can be done to relieve relatively insignificant discomforts. Paying them heed and relieving them will increase not only the patient's comfort, but also trust in the nurse as well.

Practical help

The amount and type of practical help required by the patient and family will depend on a variety of factors. The extent of physiological and neurological deficit, the functional level of the patient both physically and mentally, and the level of support available within the family will be important variables to consider (Coyle et al, 1985). Socioeconomic factors will play an important part as well. In assessing the patient and family, the nurse and others in the multidisciplinary team must consider how independent the patient is safely able to be and what support is needed. Who are the primary caregivers, and where are the physiological, psychological and social limits of care (Coyle et al, 1985)?

There are several areas that need careful forethought when planning for the care of the patient at home. The need for household help, including assistance with shopping and child care, must be considered. Planning help for the patient's physical care must bear in mind such things as the need for the caregiver to try to continue to work outside the home, and having to prepare special meals, as well as the amount of help needed to manage the patient's physical needs for bathing, toiletting and transferring. The needs of the primary caregivers must also be addressed. They may have health problems that must be taken into account. There may be anxieties about being left alone with the patient, fears concerning lack of knowledge in caring for the patient, fatigue due to loss of sleep, and worry about expenses (Cawley and Gerdts, 1988).

The diagnosis of a CNS tumour causes severe disorganisation within the family unit on a practical as well as an emotional level, and the resulting needs must be addressed. Economic factors can be a major consideration for the patient and family, especially if the patient's financial contribution to the family has been significant. Financial worries can usurp emotional energy, making it more difficult to cope with physiological deficits and difficulties. The patient's sense of self-esteem and the family's lifestyle can be threatened by loss of income. Deep depression because of a sense of social worthlessness can ensue.

The nurse needs to bear in mind the practical impact of the illness on the patient's and family's way of living. Encouraging the expression of anxieties and worries will diminish the sense of isolation and will give the nurse the opportunity to refer the patient and family to the appropriate professional resource for help. Many people are unaware of what financial benefits they may be entitled to and are relieved to learn that assistance is available. In addition to government benefits, organisations and charities such as Macmillan Cancer Relief can sometimes provide additional help.

The multidisciplinary team approach is particularly important in sorting out practical problems. Good communication between nurse, social worker, physiotherapist, speech and occupational therapists, psychologist, counsellor and medical staff/general practitioner, including the patient and family in the discussion whenever possible, is essential for maintaining optimum quality of life over the course of the disease, whatever the outcome (see Chapter 9).

Communication

Good communication is essential to effective coping, improving quality of life by reducing levels of anxiety and depression. However, there are as many styles and ways of communicating as there are patients and families. The nurse's role lies in assessing the communication needs of patients and families, and obtaining the appropriate resources where necessary.

Some people are very open, communicating easily about their problems and difficulties; others rarely express their feelings even to their nearest and dearest (Kibler, 1996). Within families, patterns of communication are usually set long before a life-threatening illness strikes. Some families cope best by freely airing their fears and worries, whereas others prefer to 'bottle things up'. There can be a conspiracy of silence that stems from a need to protect but results in more acute isolation (Curtis and Kibler, 1990). Patterns of communication cannot be expected to change in the face of malignancy, but the nurse can become aware of how the family operates and facilitate the best communication possible. Poor communication is second only to pain in causing more suffering than any other problem (Gardner, 1992).

Tiredness, weakness, nausea, headache and other discomforts may diminish the patient's will to communicate. If personality changes have occurred, the clarity of communication is even more uncertain. The family may feel that the person they wish to communicate with is no longer there. Trying to communicate can be risky, as the patient's response is unknown and may be abusive or angry. As the disease progresses and the emotional and physical energy resources of the carers become less robust, verbal communication with the patient may become less of a viable option. Non-verbal communication, especially touch, may be the best vehicle for conveying love and care as death approaches. The help of speech and occupational therapists can be invaluable in helping the family to learn ways of communicating with the patient if neurological deficits are a major problem (see Chapter 9).

Regardless of the patient's capacities for communication, the family will need the support that talking about their situation can bring. If there are difficulties within the family, referral to a counsellor or clinical psychologist may be appropriate. The nurse can be an empathic listener, bringing the relief that comes from being heard and understood.

Psychological adjustment

Every person is a unique individual with their own way of coping with the diagnosis of a CNS tumour. Likewise, each family member will have to find his or her own way of dealing with the devastation and disorganisation to the family unit that the diagnosis brings. Relationships, sexuality and children must also be considered in the equation.

The family, as an interactive network of relationships, is a living system that has its own way of structuring roles and responsibilities, and of handling demands, conflicts and crises (Robinson, 1992). Throughout the stages of the illness, the patient and family must find ways of adjusting to uncertainties about the future, the strong feelings including fear and anger that the illness and treatment bring, and the sense of grief and loss that can at times be overwhelming.

In the initial stages of shock and disbelief, a common coping strategy is denial. There is a sense of 'this can't be happening to me/us' and an attempt to reinterpret negative information positively or to reject bad news. Later, as reality dawns, there can be a steady state of coping: what was once unthinkable disruption to life becomes 'normal'. The patient and family seem to plod on despite the barrage of overwhelming difficulties.

In some cases, life returns to normal, at least outwardly, and it may seem hard to believe that there is within the patient's CNS a malignant growth that may ultimately prove fatal. In such cases, recurrence brings its own crisis like the bursting of a bubble, when the patient and family have to regroup their coping resources to face the inevitable. During the end-stages of the disease, there can be a letting go, an acceptance on the part of both patient and family that death is the inevitable outcome, and appropriate preparations can be made.

One of the essentials of life for many people is a sense of meaning and purpose, and alongside that a feeling of hope. People with CNS tumours and their families can often go a long way towards healthy psychological adjustment if these two conditions are met, and a large part of the adjustment process will be in trying to maintain a sense of meaning and purpose despite the reigning chaos, and in continuing to have hope.

People with CNS tumours and their families, like all who suffer with cancer, seem to struggle universally with two ubiquitous difficulties: the uncertainty of the outcome of the disease, and the sense of loss of control. These go hand in hand with the search for meaning and purpose, and the desire for hope. Nurses who are sensitive to these universal needs can facilitate patient and family adjustment by taking the time to listen to their perspective on the situation, identifying the patient's and family's personal meaning of the illness (Amato, 1991).

Greer and Watson (1987) and Moorey and Greer (1989), working with patients with cancer, have described five ways in which people react to the threat of uncertainty and feelings of loss of control that the illness brings. These also apply to patients with CNS tumours and their families, especially when cognitive impairment and personality changes are minimal. Most people will employ several of these coping styles at various times and with varying intensity over the course of the disease:

1. Fighting spirit: the patient/family see the illness as a challenge and have a positive attitude towards the outcome.
2. Avoidance/denial: the impact and threat of the disease are denied and minimised.
3. Fatalism: an attitude of passive acceptance, with no fighting strategies.
4. Helplessness/hopelessness: the person(s) feel overwhelmed by the enormous threat and want to give up without a fight.

5. Anxious preoccupation: an obsession with anxious thoughts, constantly seeking reassurance.

Patients and families can employ differing coping styles at the same time, the patient for example having a fighting spirit while the partner is feeling helpless and hopeless. The nurse needs to be aware of the individuality of coping strategies and that patients and families will not always be coping in the same way. It may be helpful for the nurse to explain these differences to patients and families as a means of enhancing understanding and communication between them.

Robinson (1992) describes three stages of coping that families of patients with cancer experience: an initial phase, an adaptation phase and a terminal phase. In the initial phase, the patient and family are informed of the diagnosis and experience shock, anxiety and fear. Struggling with the threat of despair, the family searches for meaning and hope. This often takes the form of having a great need for information and can result in demands on health care professionals. The nurse who understands that what may seem unreasonable or unrealistic demands for information by the family can in fact be a desperate attempt to search for meaning and hope, can respond with appropriate empathy and sensitivity. This will avoid leaving the family feeling that they have to 'fight the system'.

In the adaptation phase, the patient remains 'the patient' while the family has to reorganise itself and its roles to accommodate change. Other family members have to find a way of balancing the time spent on the patient with that for other pursuits. If needs go unmet, there can be anger and resentment, which can then lead to guilt. The uncertainty of the disease process is an added anxiety at this time. The nurse can be of help by listening to the frustrations and anxieties of the family and by normalising their experiences and feelings. The family may be able to resolve some of their dilemmas regarding time by talking through options with the nurse who is willing to listen and help them to consider the best means of managing the situation.

The terminal phase is spent dealing with approaching death and the separation and grief that this will bring. It is often heralded by the onset of recurrence and the realisation that no more treatment aimed at cure can be offered. Patients and families are sometimes less disturbed by the thought that the tumour has recurred than by the fear of no more treatment being offered. The family will often have strong feelings of loss and may begin the process of grieving during this phase.

Some families will want to talk about death with the patient and may need the help of someone outside the family to do this. If the nurse does not feel confident in facilitating this communication, referral to a clinical psychologist or counsellor may be appropriate. When both patient and family are willing to talk but find it too difficult, often all that is needed to open communication is the presence of a third party. This person can sensitively ask the questions of patient or family that need to be answered. For example, if patients want the family to know that they realise they are dying but find it too difficult to say so, the nurse can, in the presence of the family, ask the patient 'How ill do you think you are at the moment?' Patients will find it possible to tell the nurse they know they are dying, and as the family are there to hear the response, it can open the much-needed discussion between them all.

Relationships

One of the most profound effects of the diagnosis of a CNS tumour can be on relationships within the family. Salander (1996) conducted a study on the spouse's perspective of the disease experience in patients with malignant glioma. He interviewed patients and their spouses at intervals during the disease process and found three different trajectories of crisis: crisis delayed until the disease progressed, immediate crisis and crisis delayed until the patient returned home.

In the first group, where crisis was delayed until disease progression, the family returned to more or less normal life after diagnosis and treatment, with some bearable deficits. There was a mutual collusion between patient and spouse in the illusion of a hopeful future. However, when relapse occurred, spouses had to abandon the alliance in favour of their own reality, in order to prepare for the separation of death, but overtly continued to support the patient's illusion.

In the second group, when the crisis was immediate, the patients were neurologically disabled with marked reductions in physical capacity from the outset of the illness. This broke the continuity of family life. The spouse perceived the patient as cognitively impaired, and the mutuality of the marriage relationship altered as the patient became passive towards and dependent on the spouse. These spouses were unable to build an alliance with the patient's illusion; the process of mourning for the loss of the patient began then, with the change in personality and character. For some, it felt that the person they were caring for was not the same person they had married.

In the third group, the crisis was delayed until the patient returned home. In this group the patients were in good physical condition on discharge from hospital. They tended to be euphoric and overly optimistic about their futures, however, and became demanding and dominating towards their partners, which eventually resulted in a loss of mutuality within the relationship. As the patients' disease progressed, they became dysphoric and agitated; it seemed that they could not tolerate their increasing loss of function and became demanding rather than dependent. The spouses responded by increasing the emotional distance; in these cases, death was a welcome release from an unbearable prison.

Salander's study highlights three coping styles for spouses, each related to a trajectory of events. Where patients are relatively well and able to function with an acceptable degree of normality, the gravity of the situation is ignored in favour of an alliance of illusion until the disease progression makes this impossible. Spouses then distance themselves, accepting reality while continuing overtly to collude with the illusions of patients. Where the neurological deficits are significant from the outset, patients become dependent on spouses and the relationship changes; for the spouses, mourning begins immediately. Where patients are physically well but suffer from emotional disturbances and personality changes related to the disease, the situation becomes untenable for the spouses, who resort to emotional distancing.

Sexuality

The sexual aspect of being is of great importance to most people. It seems that the enormity of its importance to patients is inversely proportional to the frequency of its mention to them by nurses and other health care professionals. It is no less important to partners and patients with CNS tumours and needs to be addressed appropriately in this client group.

Sexual expression, like other aspects of personality, is highly individual. Some people particularly value sexual aspects of their body image, and the threat that illness and treatment brings can be overwhelming. Because physical attractiveness is so highly valued in Western society (Newell, 1991), it can seem to be an attack on the most essential part of the self. If patients feel that an important part of their identity is being lost, the not inappropriate response can be anger, grief or depression (see Chapter 10).

Similarly, sexuality plays a unique part in any close relationship. Where sexual intercourse is part of the expression of intimacy and love between two people, its disruption by illness can have a devastating effect on the relationship. In some relationships, the act of sex is of major importance and forms the core of the connection. For others, it is a less important aspect and is one of many ways of connecting and sharing intimacy. The emphasis and importance placed on sex will have an effect on the adjustments the relationship has to make as result of the CNS tumour and its treatment.

The effects of CNS tumours can cause sexual difficulties. If seizures have been one of the symptoms, there may be fear of provoking an attack through orgasm. Fatigue caused by the illness and/or treatment can limit desire; the patient may feel it best to preserve limited energy for other more essential activities. Salander et al (1996b) found that physical deficiencies and overall fatigue limited sexual activity. Where the patients evidenced a personality change, they found that partners often expressed a decline in sexual attachment. The change in relationship from mutual loving to one-sided caring took sexual togetherness off the agenda.

It is important for the nurse to be aware of the effects on sexuality that partners and patients with CNS tumours may experience. The opportunity to discuss these concerns and difficulties with an understanding listener and the chance to express painful feelings can help to relieve the tensions that arise. Although it can be difficult to broach and takes courage for the nurse to bring up, the patient and family will often be relieved to find this sensitive yet very important aspect of the illness process addressed.

Children

The disruption to family life that CNS tumours cause can have its most powerful effect on children. Children who are too young to understand cognitively what is going on will nonetheless pick up the distress and anxiety in adults around them and will respond in their own ways. Adults often feel overly protective of children and try to exclude them from knowledge of the illness as a means of reducing the child's experience of trauma.

There is no easy way to deal with children in the families of patients with CNS tumours. Families have their own dynamics, which will be affected by the upheaval that illness brings. The most important need of children is to feel secure. They need to know that, no matter what happens, they will be loved and cared for, and that they are accepted regardless of other circumstances. If this attitude can be maintained despite the vacillations to daily routine that the illness brings, the trauma will be minimised.

Children, just like adults, need a certain amount of knowledge to manage their anxieties. If they can be given information appropriate to their level of understanding, they will usually find ways to cope. Adults often try to protect children by withholding information from them. This may make it easier for the adult, but the fantasies of a child are often much worse than reality. Visiting parents in hospital or seeing parents partly bald can be a new and strange experience for children. Explanations before they occur can prepare children and give them the resources to deal with potentially frightening situations. Children are often very resilient and can quickly accept changes as being normal. They should be included in the disease process as much as possible. If they are old enough, they should be given a choice of how much to be involved so that their sense of being out of control is minimised.

Behaviour problems including sleep disturbances can occur when normal family life is disrupted. This may be a reaction to feeling excluded or insecure, or a way of expressing anger because of their sense of loss or because their own needs are going unmet. Children are not always able to verbalise their concerns and needs, and may act them out instead. When the parents of badly behaved children are themselves stressed by illness, it can all become too much. The nurse should be aware of the need for children to be included in the family's process of coping with a CNS tumour and be ready to offer help and support to parents. This may include referral to a social worker or child psychologist if available and appropriate. Giving parents the space to air their concerns and frustrations about their children and helping them to formulate a plan for meeting the practical demands that children make will help them to cope.

Children need most to be included as death approaches. They too need to grieve and to prepare for separation. Explanations of death should be made in ways that they can understand. Adults should be careful that their explanations do not prejudice children adversely. For example, if a child is told that 'Mummy is going to heaven' or 'God is taking Mummy away to be with Him' without also explaining that Mummy does not want to leave but has an illness that is causing this, the child may grow up feeling rejected by Mummy or hating God for taking her away. Adults should explain changes in appearance and activities so that the child does not feel abandoned or rejected as attention from the ill parent diminishes. Children also need to experience the reality of death. If they can see the body and attend the funeral, their imaginations will have less fuel for later nightmare fantasies about what the dead parent was really like and what happened to the body.

Children will often ask questions, and these can be a good indicator of how much they want and need to know. However, in the presence of anxious adults, children will sometimes not dare to voice their queries. If adults can offer opportunities for children to ask questions and provide them with answers appropriate to their level of understanding, their anxiety levels will usually be reduced.

Maintaining the normality of family life and activities as far as possible will also help to reduce stress. Like adults going to work, children will find that going to school and other usual events gives them something else to think about and relieves some of the burden of anxiety.

Supporting patients and families – the use of counselling skills

Throughout the course of the illness, patients with CNS tumours and their families require support both from health care professionals and from other friends and family members around them. It is difficult to define exactly what support is, but it unquestionably involves the feeling of being heard and understood. The nurse's role in offering psychological support to patients with CNS tumours and their families involves having the confidence to approach this client group with the necessary skills of listening. The pressure of time and demands of work often make it virtually impossible for nurses to spend the time they would like talking to patients and families, but a few moments well spent can have a therapeutic effect. There are many books and courses on counselling skills available (see Useful Addresses). Space here does not permit an exhaustive review of counselling skills, but a few of the important ones are outlined (Kibler, 1996).

Attending and listening

A large part of communication takes place non-verbally. Patients and families are quick to notice nurses' body language and by it to discern how willing they may be to listen. How nurses sit and hold themselves says a great deal about what they are feeling and to what extent they are engaging with the person being listened to. If nurses stand at the end of the bed, fiddling with a chart or with something else in their hands, the message to the patient and family may be 'There is something else I would rather be doing; I do not really have time for you.' If, however, nurses sit down (preferably at the same level as the patient), make eye contact and sit in an open relaxed way, the message will be 'I am here for you; I am ready to really listen to what you have to say.'

Listening means more than just hearing the words that are said; it includes noticing the patient and family's body language, eye contact and tone of voice. It also means hearing what is not being said. Patients and families may ask indirectly for what they need, or give non-verbal cues rather than asking outright. The nurse who is able to really listen will be aware of all of the communication going on, both verbal and non-verbal.

Questioning

How a question is phrased makes a significant difference to the response returned. There are essentially two types of question: open and closed. A closed question can be answer yes or no, whereas an open question invites the respondent to reveal something of themselves. For example, 'Do you have a headache today?' may be the shortest route to the information the nurse is seeking, but to ask 'How are you feeling today?' invites the patient to say a bit more. It may be not only the headache, but also the frustration of being ill that the patient will feel better for having communicated.

In patients with CNS tumours, questioning can be very difficult if there are cognitive, memory or personality changes. Especially in the face of receptive or expressive dysphasia, communication can be very limited. The nurse needs to listen extremely attentively, watching for gestures or other non-verbal cues that might shed light on what the patient is trying to say. The help and advice of occupational and speech therapists is valuable. A few guidelines are to ensure maximum attention from the patient, which may mean reducing external stimuli (turning off the TV, drawing the curtains around the bed and so on). Simple language should be used, supplemented with writing if appropriate. Closed questions that require only a nod or a shake of the head may be the best means of communicating when there are speech problems.

Empathy

Empathy means seeing things from the other person's perspective and involves true understanding. It differs from sympathy, which is having compassionate feelings for someone else. Although it is impossible to understand completely how it is to be in someone else's situation, and never possible truly to say 'I know just how you feel', empathy is the ability to perceive the other's way of looking and feeling. It is understanding, and communicating that understanding.

Reflecting and paraphrasing are two skills of empathy. Reflecting means saying back what the person has said in order to indicate he or she has been heard. Paraphrasing goes a step further and means putting into other words what has been said. For example, if a patient says, 'I hope the radiotherapy doesn't make me feel sick today', to reflect would be to say, 'You hope the radiotherapy doesn't make you feel sick.' To paraphrase would be to say 'You're worried the radiotherapy may make you feel sick.' Either response will tell patients that they have been heard, and the response to empathy will not uncommonly be more disclosure on the part of the patient.

Summarising

At the end of a conversation with patient or family, it is often useful to summarise what has been said. This reassures them that they have been heard and also clarifies what, if any, action has been agreed upon as the outcome. Especially if there is cognitive impairment in the patient, or significant anxiety in the patient or family, summarising can reinforce what has been said.

Perhaps the most important skill of communication with patients with CNS tumours and their families is that of approachability. No matter how great the demands and pressures on the nurse, if the patient and family have a sense that they will be heard and, within reason, their needs met, much anxiety and demanding behaviour can be avoided. A nurse who gives the impression of being too busy and stressed to be approached will engender a sense of anxiety in the patient and family. One who gives the impression of availability, even if that availability is limited, gives the patient and family a sense of being cared for. The health care system can be a huge, amorphous, impersonal organism that the patient and family are left feeling they have to fight in some way. To have an alliance with someone within it who is available to hear, understand and be an advocate can significantly reduce the stress of being ill.

Nurses sometimes feel that they have to employ the coping strategy of avoidance in dealing with patients and families whom they know to be demanding or time-consuming. When nurses feel pressured and time is limited, it can seem the best strategy. However, this can leave patients and families feeling neglected, which only increases their anxiety. One way of managing this dilemma is to assert clear and realistic time boundaries. If, at the outset of a potentially involved and lengthy conversation, nurses state clearly that they can only give a certain amount of time at that point, patients and families are under no illusions as to what is on offer. When the available time has passed, nurses can then extricate themselves without guilt. Because no unreasonable expectations have been fostered, patients and families will have had some of their needs met and will have experienced nurses as reliable. Nurses will have given what is realistic without unduly adding to their own stress.

The role of therapists

Not infrequently, the scope of psychological support required by patients and families with CNS tumours is beyond the remit of the nurse. The nurse's role then becomes one of referral to the appropriate resource. Depending on the structure of the service providing health care, the patient and/or family may be referred to a social worker, counsellor, clinical psychologist or psychiatrist.

It is sometimes difficult to ascertain whether a symptom is of physiological or psychological origin. For example, if a patient shows lack of concentration, it could be stress related or it might be cognitive impairment resulting from the tumour. To discern the difference, simple tests can be applied (Folstein et al, 1975). The Mini Mental State checks patients' orientation by asking them the name of the ward they are on, which hospital they are in or who the current Prime Minister is. They might also be asked to count backward from 100 in sevens, or to spell a word backwards. If they are unable correctly to perform these simple tests, cognitive impairment rather than stress is the probable cause. This is one means by which nurses can know when it is appropriate to refer to a clinical psychologist.

It can also be difficult to discern when the symptoms of anxiety or depression indicate that referral is appropriate. Symptoms of clinical depression include anorexia, insomnia or change in sleep pattern, and low mood. These may be difficult to separate from the effects of illness or treatment. Patients with anxiety states may exhibit unrealistic fears, irrational thoughts or feelings of panic. When any of these symptoms are pronounced or persistent, the patient should be referred for psychological assessment.

Patients with CNS tumours may very rarely be so depressed they become suicidal. Threats of suicide can provoke extreme anxiety in carers, both family and professional. However only a tiny percentage of patients actually take their own lives; a threat of suicide is usually a cry to have the awfulness of the situation understood. Nurses can perform a suicide risk assessment, which will ascertain whether further psychological intervention is required. The first principle is not to be afraid to mention suicide. Talking about it will reduce rather than increase the likelihood of its occurrence. The patient can be asked 'Do you ever get so low that you think of taking your own life?' If the response is affirmative, the next step is to ask whether this is just a fantasy or an actual plan. If it is a plan, then ask how it would be done (drugs, hanging, car exhaust fumes and so on). Are the means available? If the patient has decided how to do it and has access to the means, ask what is keeping him or her from doing it. It will often be some good reason such as not wanting to hurt their family that makes the actual act an impossibility. However, it may be a serious threat, and further help should be obtained through referral to a clinical psychologist or psychiatrist. In most cases, patients do not actually want to kill themselves, but they want someone to take notice of how terrible they feel. Talking with them about suicide will let them know that they have been heard. However, it may still be appropriate to refer on for the assessment and treatment of depression.

Clinical psychologists or psychiatrists will be able to administer psychological tests to determine the level of anxiety or depression and whether the cause is physiological or psychological. Appropriate medication, such as anxiolytics or antidepressants, can then be recommended. Beyond assessment, the overall aim of these therapists is to enhance the coping skills of the patient and family, encouraging independence (Newell, 1991). A number of different approaches, frequently cognitive-behavioural in orientation, may be used. These will challenge negative thought patterns, promote a greater sense of control and help the patient and family to identify strategies for coping and attaining agreed goals (Coyle et al, 1985; Watson et al, 1988; Moorey and Greer, 1989).

Support groups for patients and/or families of patients with CNS tumours have been found to be helpful (Amato, 1991; Leavitt et al, 1996), although a group setting is not everyone's cup of tea and individual preferences must be respected. Through the group, the sharing of experiences, information and feelings reduces the sense of isolation and adds normality to the illness experience. Coping skills can also be identified and improved, and emotions validated (Amato, 1991).

Leavitt et al (1996) conducted a descriptive, exploratory study of support groups and found five thematic categories that emerged: telling the story, managing medical advice, information-seeking and exchange, the long haul and family life changes. They also found two major categories of supportive mechanism: finding a safe haven and maintaining morale. Support groups help by minimising the sense of isolation, serving as a buffer against stress, fostering self-awareness and providing socialisation and affirmation (Johnson and Lane, 1993).

Staff support

An important and easily overlooked aspect of caring for patients with CNS tumours and families is the support needs of health care professionals themselves. Nurses in particular can become very close to patients and families, and the death of the patient is a bereavement for them as well as for the family. The sense of loss and grief in the nurse is often ignored, but perpetual bereavements over time can mount up and result in 'burnout' (Amato, 1991).

Awareness of the need for staff support is gradually awakening within the NHS, along with a recognition of stress as an organisational issue (Tschudin, 1996). However, nurses have a responsibility to look after themselves and to take appropriate steps to manage stress. The first step is awareness of the problem, and becoming cognisant of the grief that caring for patients with CNS tumours and their families can bring. Time should be taken to acknowledge the loss, both as an individual and within the nursing and multidisciplinary teams. There should ideally be a forum for reviewing the illness process, looking not only at what could have been done better for the patient and family, but also at what was done well. Valuing others and feeling valued is an important part of support (Tschudin, 1996).

The ideal is often far from the norm, but even where nurses work in unsupportive environments, there may be opportunities for individual support. NHS Trusts are increasingly using counsellors as a measure to address stress, both within and outside the occupational health services. The Royal College of Nursing provides free, confidential, short-term counselling for its members. The National Association for Staff Support (NASS) produces literature and holds conferences and other events to help nurses raise awareness of the need for and take steps to implement support initiatives in their areas of work.

Conclusion

The diagnosis of a CNS tumour is a life-shattering event, throwing both patient and family into a state of potentially overwhelming uncertainty. The prognosis is often uncertain, and for those patients with high-grade glioma, the incidence of recurrence is quite high. There are often many problems to be dealt with along the way, including neurological deficits and personality changes, and many losses – of the sense of self, of body image, of career, of a role in the family and society. The whole family is affected by the illness and must adapt and change with the disease process. The need for psychological support is paramount.

A multidisciplinary approach is essential, and the nurse has an important role within the team as carer, advocate and assessor of need, providing support and referring to other professionals as necessary. The nurse can also suffer bereavement and has needs for support that should not be overlooked.

References

Amato CA (1991) Malignant glioma: coping with a devastating illness. Journal of Neuroscience Nursing 23(1): 20–3.

Cawley MM, Gerdts EK (1988) Establishing a cancer caregivers program. Cancer Nursing 11(5): 267–73.

Coyle N, Monzillo E, Loscalzo M, Farkas C, Massie MJ, Foley KM (1985) A model of continuity of care for cancer patients with pain and neuro-oncologic complications. Cancer Nursing (April): 111–19.

Curtis T, Kibler S (1990) Counselling in cancer care. Nursing Times 86(51): 25–7.

Folstein MF, Folstein SE, McHugh PR (1975) Mini mental state: a practical method for grading the cognitive state of patients for the clinician. Journal of Psychological Research 12: 189–98.

Gardner R (1992) Psychological care of neuro-oncology patients and their families. British Journal of Nursing 1(1): 553–6.

Greer S, Watson M (1987) Mental adjustment to cancer: its measurement and prognostic importance. Cancer Surveys 6: 439–53.

Guerrero D (1996) Brain tumours. In Tschudin V (Ed.) Nursing the Patient with Cancer, 2nd edn. London: Prentice Hall, pp 146–61.

Johnson J, Lane C (1993) Role of support groups in cancer care. Supportive Care in Cancer 1: 52–6.

Kibler S (1996) Counselling. In Tschudin V (Ed.) Nursing the Patient with Cancer, 2nd edn. London: Prentice Hall, pp 452–67.

Leavitt MB, Lamb SA, Voss BS (1996) Brain tumor support group: content themes and mechanisms of support. Oncology Nursing Forum 23(8): 1247–56.

Lindsay M (1990) Communicating with Neurological Patients: The Nurse's Role. London: Scutari Press.

Magee B (1987) The Great Philosophers. Oxford: Oxford University Press.

Moorey S, Greer S (1989) Psychological Therapy for Patients with Cancer: A New Approach. Oxford: Heinemann Medical Books.

Newell R (1991) Body-image disturbance: cognitive behavioural formulation and intervention. Journal of Advanced Nursing 16: 1400–5.

Newton C, Mateo MA (1994) Uncertainty: strategies for patients with brain tumor and their family. Cancer Nursing 17(2): 137–40.

Oswin M (1992) The quiet menace. Nursing Times 88(34): 40–1.

Robinson S (1992) The family with cancer. European Journal of Cancer Care 1(2): 29–33.

Salander P (1996) Brain tumors as a threat to life and personality: the spouse's perspective. Qualities in the Short Life: Psychological Studies Relevant to Patient and Spouse in Malignant Glioma. Umea University Medical Dissertations. Department of Oncology, Umea University, Sweden.

Salander P, Bergenheim T, Henriksson R (1996a) The creation of protection and hope in patients with malignant brain tumours. Social Science Medicine 42(7): 985–96.

Salander P, Karlsson AT, Bergenheim T, Henriksson R (1996b) Sexuality, psychosocial well-being and cognitive function in patients with malignant glioma treated with estramustine in addition to radiotherapy. Qualities in the Short Life: Psychological Studies Relevant to Patient and Spouse in Malignant Glioma. Umea University Medical Dissertations. Department of Oncology, Umea University, Sweden.

Tschudin V (1996) Staff support. In Tschudin V (Ed.) Nursing the Patient with Cancer, 2nd edn. London: Prentice Hall, pp 468–75.

Watson M, Greer S, Young J et al (1988) Development of a questionnaire measure of adjustment to cancer: the MAC scale. Psychological Medicine 18: 203–9.

Further reading

Giovagnoli AR, Tamburini M, Bioardi A (1996) Quality of life in brain tumour patients. Journal of Neuro-oncology 30: 71–80.

Salander P, Karlsson T, Bergenheim T, Henriksson R (1995) Long term memory deficits in patients with malignant glioma. Journal of Neuro-oncology 25: 227–38.

Weitzner MA, Meyers CA, Byrne K (1996) Psychosocial functioning and quality of life in patients with primary brain tumors. Journal of Neurosurgery 84: 29–34.

Useful Addresses

British Association for Counselling
1 Regent Place,
Rugby,
Warwickshire CV21 2PJ
Tel: (01788) 550899

National Association for Staff Support (NASS)
9 Caradon Close,
Woking,
Surrey GU21 3DU
Tel: (01483) 771599

Royal College of Nursing Counselling Service
8–10 Crown Hill,
Croydon,
Surrey CR0 1RZ
Tel: (0345) 697064

Chapter 12
Future planning of care

Mave Salter

Introduction

The aim of this chapter is to encourage awareness of the importance of future care planning for the patient with CNS malignancies. Care does not cease when all hope has gone; instead, it continues to involve agencies to support the patient and family. As such, arrangements must be undertaken with the involvement of both patients and their families/carers, while also involving both the multidisciplinary team and the primary health care team so that health care professionals can plan care using a team approach. Some CNS tumours, in particular high-grade gliomas, generally have a poor prognosis. Therefore the aim of future care planning for this group of patients is to enable them to remain at home for as long as possible.

The patient within the family

Following a diagnosis of a CNS tumour, life for the patient and family will never be the same again. Diagnosis generates real anxiety within a family and alters communication patterns, roles and relationships between its members (Robinson, 1992). Yet the burden of care often falls solely on the family's shoulders (McKeag, 1995). Many patients with cancer, not least patients with CNS tumours, must continue to struggle daily with disease, the residual effects of treatment or the sense of incompleteness or loss when treatment is completed (Morra, 1988).

Patients and their families often attempt to protect each other. This means that they have to deal with their fears and anxieties on their own when they are in most need of mutual support (Altschuler, 1997).

This results in stressful outcomes both for the person who has cancer and for the other family members (Robinson, 1992). Rather than being passive observers, family members are active, vital participants in the patient's treatment and care (Lewandowski and Jones, 1988; Woods et al, 1989). Thus professionals must identify the patient's and family's personal meaning of the disease in order to enable them to adjust (Amato, 1991).

The role of the nurse is to facilitate self-care and care by the family, and this is where education and continuing care in symptom managemement are a planned component of care. Cancer, particularly CNS tumours, is a potent agent of change, consistently disrupting a family's established patterns of daily living. As patients find themselves facing a life defined by uncertainties, remissions, exacerbations and changes in treatment, the family is similarly confronted with continual change (Robinson, 1992). Therefore support by provision of community services as well as follow-up care by hospital personnel is necessary.

Role changes

If a family member changes, some compensatory change must occur in the rest of the family, and if the role of that individual is seriously altered, this may require a complete reorganisation of family life (Lindsay, 1989). Role change is a common occurrence for patients and families affected with CNS tumours. In role change, one person feels a sense of loss while another feels burdened by the added responsibility. Uncertainties about the future, survival and treatment outcomes, anticipatory grief, feelings of injustice, and fear and anger regarding the management of treatment are often experienced (Cassileth and Hamilton, 1979; Johnson, 1988; Lewandowski and Jones, 1988; Woods et al, 1989; citation in Robinson, 1992).

In one study on brain tumour support groups, family roles changed following diagnosis (Leavitt et al, 1996). Changes included parents having to care for their adult children and grandchildren or spouses of patients becoming totally responsible for the family and taking on new responsibilities. Adult children discussed their hesitation to assume the role of decision-maker for a newly disabled parent, and many family members described the stresses of trying not to take over or speak for the patient. Also of concern was the need to adjust to differences in family life on a daily basis, with a disabled or demoralised spouse now perhaps home all day instead of being out. Coupled with this is the stress of needing to be strong on the one hand but feeling selfish on the other. Along with this role reversal is the fear of job loss (for both the patient and partner) with concerns about the effects of disability on close relatives and friends (Lindsay, 1989). Thus the inevitable 'role reversal' that the disease imposes may lead to tension. It is in this context that clinicians have the job of enabling patients to get as much enjoyment out of life as possible and to prevent future regret on the part of the person surviving that the last months together were not better spent (Davies and Clarke, 1993). As such, supporting the patient and family in the community is of paramount concern.

The carers' perspective

Patients with CNS tumours will experience various disabilities. Studies addressing the impact of disability on family members reveal that, when one member of a family becomes disabled, the entire family experiences the disability (Hart, 1981; Miller et al, 1983; Watson, 1987).

Caring produces guilty feelings about not doing the job to perfection. Carers may, at times, wish that they might die so they would not have to cope any longer, and later experience awful guilt at the thought of wishing themselves dead (Lindsay, 1989). Similarly, Northouse (1988) found that, following a cancer diagnosis, more effective communication between the family was associated with a better negotiation of altered family roles. Northouse suggests that some family members question whether they are doing enough and feel guilty when mishaps, such as a patient falling, occur. Dangerous and irresponsible behaviour can threaten disaster to the patient and others, but practical measures such as turning off gas supplies and locking outside doors can be taken (Lindsay, 1989). However, such measures do little, in reality, to allay anxiety. Thus careful, individual assessment needs to be made of whether the patient can be left alone or whether their 'at-risk' category means that there is a need for constant supervision. Family members often report that the emotional energy associated with providing care outweighs the physical energy required. Therefore referral for psychological help to facilitate improved coping mechanisms for the carer and the emotional help offered by a hospice home care or Macmillan nurse, are important in monitoring those patients at home (see Chapter 11).

Incapacity of the breadwinner may lead to a reduction in the family's standard of living. Practical advice and access to financial support in the way of state benefits should be discussed. Most people do not like to call attention to themselves by having to ask for help. The person with a CNS tumour often has to resolve the conflict between two antagonistic situations: the desire to achieve maximum independence and to be treated like anyone else while requiring help that others may not need. This proves to be a fine balance and a dilemma.

A single carer should not try to carry the whole load of the illness either. There is a tendency for caregivers to become quite isolated, receiving fewer and fewer visits from friends and going out less (Lindsay, 1989). It is understandable for carers to get the impression that they are isolated, with no-one to turn to, and that little can be done for the patient with a CNS malignancy. Support from the community services is therefore important.

A major source of uncertainty for the primary caregiver is never knowing what is coming next in the (often) downward slide of the patient with a CNS tumour. The amount of care a patient requires depends on the severity of the deficits. Newton and Mateo (1994) found that even simple caretaking tasks required significant changes in lifestyle and that, although caregivers need respite time, this is often difficult to achieve because getting someone to assume care for only a few hours is not easy. Support outside the immediate family may be limited, and the caregiver may have others in the family, such as small children, who also require care and attention. However, when a temporary replacement is found, the primary caregiver may experience guilt at leaving the patient. With families that include young children/teenagers, supporting the family thus requires the participation of a health visitor/school nurse. The assistance of a social worker as well as community nursing support involving the primary health care team, palliative care services and voluntary organisations is imperative.

Partners may be at different levels of coping, family members blaming themselves if they feel they cannot manage. This is a major issue for families of patients with CNS tumours as the aetiology of these malignancies is unknown. One husband declined counselling because he felt he should be able to cope with balancing his full-time job, which meant that he was away from home for 14 hours each day, with that of caring for his young children and also his wife. He denied the difficulties, feeling that if he went for counselling, an admission of not coping, his children would be taken away from him. Somnolence after his wife's cranial radiotherapy treatment meant they both thought the tumour was recurring. To patients and families this phenomenon, if unexplained, leads to the fear of treatment failure and disease recurrence (see Chapter 6). Somnolence added to the tension within this family. A case conference/family meeting assisted in addressing some of the problems. The patient's husband was helped to recognise that it was acceptable to feel overwhelmed and ask for help.

Chronic caring may lead to the patient being abused, be it physically or emotionally. For example, a dominant wife refused to permit her husband to have a commode in the house. Their teenage children also treated their father badly, because his incapacity meant he could no longer stand up for himself. This led to his morale and self-esteem being destroyed by the attitudes of his family members. Personality changes on the part of the patient are often the breaking point for some families (McKinlay et al 1981; Brooks, 1985; Liss and Willer, 1990). Therefore an opportunity to address such problems within a counselling session may help the family to cope better (see Chapter 11).

Spousal concerns

Personality change, more than somatic deficiency, is the crucial issue with which spouses must cope (McKinlay et al, 1981; Brooks, 1985; Liss and Willer, 1990). Marital disharmony, breakdown and divorce are not uncommon results (Bomford et al, 1993). However, it is also not uncommon for a couple whose relationship has dissolved to come back together again for the duration of the illness. Salander (1996, p 6) quotes a patient's wife whose husband had a CNS tumour:

> I knew that time was limited, but we couldn't make use of it. With another cancer disease, that would have been possible. He was so changed, he wasn't his normal self, so it was impossible...It wasn't B who died, but the one I took care of – the other one. Sometimes it strikes me that my real husband is gone, and not just the one that was so changed.'

At times, patients do not wish to face their diagnosis and therefore deny it, to the detriment of their partners, who desperately want to support them but feel unable to because of the patient's denial. This can lead to isolation for both patient and partner. As Salander (1996) states, these spouses know that the disease is a threat to their loved one but they also know that it affects their children, friends, daily routines, finances, social life, work and, last but not least, prospects for the future. This practical and social turmoil was the spouses' burden, and the future was unpredictable.

For most people, interpersonal relationships are essential to their happiness. The support of family, friends and health care professionals can be of inestimable value to patients in enabling them to cope (Bomford et al, 1993). However, their previous ability to socialise, whether as a spouse or parent or in peer groups, may be altered by illness.

Assisting the family

Intensive treatment programmes for people with CNS tumours and their families need to be matched by a concern for their psychological and social well-being. This may best be achieved by a key worker liaising between tertiary and community settings, drawing on the resources of, for example, counselling, supportive care and, if necessary, psychiatric services (Davies and Clarke, 1993). The concept of a key worker is also highlighted by Amato (1991), who states that communication during the process of illness is important.

The advocacy role of the nurse

The amount of support needed by each family will vary according to the situation at the time and also their wishes. Specific issues of care may vary because of physical and cognitive disabilities, age, gender orientation, relationships and so on (McKeag, 1995). Professionals need to be honest, open, accurate and trustworthy. Patients are most likely to align with someone on the treatment team, and the team needs to be flexible about who that identified person is.

Care in the community

At the root of all community care policies, there seems to be the firm, unequivocal assumption that family members, usually female, provide most informal care in the care of the young, the elderly and the sick. This has been repeatedly borne out by research. This situation has arisen since the distinction between 'care in the community' and 'care by the community' has become meaningless in the light of insufficient statutory resources, such as hostels, home helps, respite care, day care and personal care, even when voluntary organisations contribute (Wade, 1992). When at home, many patients and families prefer to press on without nursing intervention. Families may therefore decline the services offered because they prefer to deny the illness themselves or to pretend to their neighbours that all is well (Salter, 1997). It is therefore of paramount importance to plan for continuity of care in the community.

Discharge planning

The frequently used phase 'quicker and sicker' increasingly describes the hospital discharge planning for the 1990s (Jackson, 1994). However, despite more than 20 years of research, literature and government guidelines, there are still crucial gaps in knowledge of the use and effectiveness of particular strategies to produce 'ideal discharge planning' (Tierney and Closs, 1993).

Hence planning for discharge has been highlighted as a problem in patient care for some decades now, communication breakdown between hospital and community staff being the main area of concern (O'Leary, 1988). In the past few years, there has thus been more emphasis on discharge planning, key documents including the Department of Health circular (1989) stating that discharge planning should have a multidisciplinary approach, and the NHS and Community Care Act (1990, which came into being in 1993). This latter document highlights the need for 'seamless care', meaning that there should be complete continuity of care from hospital to community and vice versa.

The Patient's Charter (Department of Health, 1991) states that 'Before you are discharged from hospital, you can expect a decision to be made about how to meet any needs you may continue to have. Your hospital will agree arrangements with agencies such as Community Nursing Services and Local Authority Social Services departments. You and, if you agree, your carers will be involved in making these decisions.'

Much of the emphasis of the NHS and Community Care Act 1990 (see below) is placed on discharge policies as hospital discharge has long been recognised as paramount to the success or failure of the Act. Therefore, if a comprehensive assessment of a client's needs can take place in hospital and adequate preparation be made for the appropriate care after discharge, the central elements of care in the community start to fall into place (Cole, 1992).

Discharge planning is a process and service in which patients' needs are identified and evaluated, and assistance is given in preparing to move from one level of care to another, that is, hospital to home, or hospital to another care facility. The process involves arranging that phase of care, be it self-care, care by family members, care by a professional health provider or combinations of these options (Bristow et al, 1986). Discharge planning can be defined as a systematic multidisciplinary process by which the needs and resources of patients and their carers are assessed. This assessment enables a comprehensive discharge and the arrangements of appropriate community support and services on discharge from hospital (Tierney and Closs, 1993).

Discharge planning should thus start either before (for example, in the outpatient department), or on admission to hospital. A multidisciplinary meeting or case conference/family meeting in which a patient's discharge needs can be discussed is helpful, and community staff can also identify additional educational needs arising in the care of patients with neuro-oncological problems (Coyle et al, 1985). Glavassevich et al (1991) found that community health nurses identified a need to have more information with respect to care after discharge and closer affiliations with hospital nurses. Hence the hospital visit is an ideal opportunity to fulfil this.

When a package of care is arranged for a patient on discharge, a written list of those involved, with contact names and telephone numbers should also be made available. It also helps for the patient and family to know when to expect the first visit from a health care professional. Research indicates that the development of standardised, written discharge guidelines is important in the provision of concrete information to patients and their families (Glavassevich et al, 1991). Equally important is clear, accurate patient documentation in the process of discharge. When planning discharge, options such as day care, hospice or respite care to provide relatives with a planned break should be considered. If necessary and available, an evening service should be provided to ensure that the patient is settled at home on the day of discharge. Additionally, some areas will have an on-call contact number for patients to telephone during the night.

Discharge arrangements and a proposed care package should be confirmed with the community on the day of discharge. When 'complex' discharges occur, a telephone call to the family the day after the discharge is usually welcomed to ensure that all the services arranged are going to plan. Different types of patient and family require varying levels of support. If possible, care more locally, whether inpatient or outpatient care, means that patients do not have to travel long distances to an oncology centre (Bomford et al, 1993).

The NHS and Community Care Act (1990)

In 1993, the local authorities assumed a major new responsibility for the community care of vulnerable adults, in particular the responsibility for assessing needs and for funding provision of residential and nursing home care. The Act also includes eligibility criteria for residential, nursing home and hospital care, the respective responsibility of each authority (health and local authorities) and the arrangements for assessment and discharge from hospital.

The present Act represents an attempt to tackle the issue within a model of 'mixed economy of welfare', that is, plurality of service providers. This should be provided by a number of sources in the voluntary and private sectors and, as a last resort, the public sector. However, the people providing the main bulk of care will, as always, be the informal carers in the family (Cole, 1992).

The Act also includes guidelines on ensuring that the package of care will be appropriate for the patient's/carer's needs. Inherent in the Act is the aim of social services and health authorities working together to promote greater use of domiciliary, day and respite care. Thus the emphasis is on care at home, thereby reducing institutional care.

Local authorities are able to charge clients for non-health services that they provide (George, 1993). This has further implications for clients in that there is a fine line between health and personal social service needs, some patients being expected to pay for some of the services that will keep them at home (Salter, 1996).

Continuing health care needs

Some patients can now be cared for under the category of continuing health care needs (with health care free at the point of delivery), providing they meet certain criteria. This followed a 'test' case brought to the Health Ombudsman in which a patient who had had a stroke was discharged from hospital and the family had to pay for his care in a nursing home (Giles, 1994). In patients with CNS tumours requiring palliative care, a decision must often be reached between the local authority and health authority as to who will provide and pay for their care.

Community care

It is often the GP, in conjunction with the district nurse and hospice home care team or Macmillan nurse, who is the predominant carer at home. Marie Curie nurses, arranged through the district nurse, offer a sitting service during either the day or night to give carers a break. However, this is dependent on the health status of the patient and may be limited in terms of its availability. Some areas offer 'Hospital at Home' schemes, working in close liaison with district nurses and offering additional help for those patients recently discharged from hospital. In neuro-oncology, community physiotherapists, occupational therapists and speech therapists are vital members of the community team, especially as many patients with CNS tumours have cognitive and/or physical deficits (see Chapter 9). Another important member of the primary health care team is the community psychiatric nurse, especially where there may be personality changes or aggressive tendencies in the patient with a CNS tumour.

One family carer suggested that professionals do not always make it possible for relatives to manage the nursing of a patient with a brain tumour at home. Carers may be told that they will not manage and that the care and lifting of a heavy, helpless patient will be too difficult. However, families should be given all support in providing care for a patient at home if this is the option they choose:

> The hospital provided a special bed, a hoist and a hammock for lifting Nita, a large adjustable armchair for her and a special mattress to prevent pressure sores. The district nurse...taught me home nursing techniques. (Oswin, 1992, p 41).

Discharge planning and palliative care are within the realm of expert nursing practice. Future planning is often left until the occurrence of a major crisis, as nurses may be uncertain when best to plan future care (Guerrero, 1996). For many patients with CNS malignancies, there is a quick trajectory from diagnosis to palliative care, and many patients may have severe physical and psychological deficits. Therefore the involvement of the primary health care team and hospice/Macmillan teams at an early stage is a consideration when planning care.

Professionals should be concerned with how to improve the remaining time rather than with how many months an individual has left to live (Dudas and Carlson, 1984). Possibly, the most frightening situation for patients with CNS tumours is to have to live with the fear of recurrence or progression.

Thus the role of the nurse in identifying specific patient and family needs is crucial. Providing the appropriate support and education on how best to care for the patient therefore means that patients can remain at home and need not be admitted to hospital purely for social reasons.

The psychological well-being of children is paramount, and it is vital to ensure they have access to support. The school nurse provides liaison between the school and primary health care team members, and the family. For example, one patient's daughter did not want to go to school in case 'mummy had another fit'. The school nurse worked alongside the class teachers to enable this child to feel secure at school in the knowledge that someone was caring for her mother at home.

Finances

Whilst health care is free at the point of delivery, social care is means-tested and requires payment. However, certain benefits, such as Disability Living Allowance (DLA, for patients under 60 years of age) and Attendance Allowance (AA, for people over retirement age), could be used to offset some of the cost. In the case of patients with high-grade gliomas, DLA and AA are obtainable under special rules. This means that patients do not require a lengthy medical examination and allows for financial assistance at an earlier stage. It is also backdated to the date of application.

Social services packages of care

Packages of care are arranged through care managers in local authority social services departments and include arrangements for personal care, help with meals, housework, shopping and laundry. Some health authorities may also have crisis care or immediate response teams for patients being discharged home. It is therefore worth exploring what is available within each health authority in relation to patient and family support.

Voluntary organisations

National Support Groups such as the British Association of Cancer United Patients (CancerBACUP) provide people with a telephone link for information and counselling, whilst the National Cancerlink organisation provides information and advice, and may offer local support groups for the patient and family.

Although many people find support within their family structure, participation in a support group can assist patients and families to cope with the uncertainties of the disease process along with others who have successfully coped with a similar situation (Hilton, 1992; Newton and Mateo, 1994). Organisations such as Crossroads provide sitters to give the carer a break during the day or night.

Hospices

Palliative care is about the relief of physical and psychological distress. The period of palliative and continuing care incorporates the time from the diagnosis of incurable malignancy to death. The skills of palliative care teams are paramount when dealing with patients with malignant brain tumours. Patients and families need support and guidance about their disease, with constant advice on symptom and medication management, aiming to maintain quality of life.

Hospices provide a more informal, less institutional and quieter environment than an acute ward. A high staff-to-patient ratio gives more time for patient care, bearing in mind the complex needs of the patient with a CNS tumour. Palliative care medicine is now recognised as a separate specialty with specific training requirements. This has improved the provision of high standards nationally and encouraged research into palliative care. If necessary, hospices can arrange for respite care, which may provide relatives with an opportunity for a much-needed rest. Support for caregivers is crucial and can make a difference if a patient is to stay at home. Alternatively, day care within the hospice environment may provide company and psychological as well as nursing support. Day care allows some patients who would otherwise require hospitalisation to remain at home (Topliss, 1979).

Final stages of care

The final stage of neurological cancer is heralded by increasing neurological deficits and disabilities. At this stage, drug therapy may need reviewing, especially as there is a tendency to prescribe increased doses of dexamethasone during decline, with decreasing effect (Amato, 1991).

Optimistic attitudes are now difficult to maintain. Questions of reoperation and further treatment with, for example, chemotherapy may need to be addressed (see Chapter 7). The maintenance of independence and dignity must be the clinical goal. If, from the outset, contact has been maintained with local services, care can probably be organised at the community level and the patient remain at home.

The carer will need help both emotionally and physically. Insomnia, for example, is common with steroids; this will at times tend to disturb the carer as well and Marie Curie night-sitters may be required. Personality and severe cognitive change in a loved one is particularly distressing whatever the cause (Davies and Clarke, 1993).

For those patients unable to speak, caregivers who have spent many hours with patients in better times interpret moods, movements, sounds and looks in order to facilitate survival. The goal in promoting quality of life becomes death with dignity. Patient survival becomes family survival. Life's unfinished business may be completed while coping with the present and preparing for the future. Hospice/home care teams can help both the emotional and physical problems of the family (Amato 1991).

During the final stages, support for the patient changes from that of active treatment to that of more active symptom control (Bass and Windle, 1972). A high staff-to-patient ratio gives more time for patient care, often requiring a constant anticipation of patients' needs. The primary health care team has by now built a strong relationship with the patient and carer. Therefore, at the time of greatest distress and vulnerability, new primary health care relationships do not have to be established. If this is not the case, the nuance of such a transfer may well be interpreted by the patient and family as abandonment, loss of interest, lack of concern and loss of hope on the part of the hospital team. As well as symptom control, a support network for the patient and family is the essence of successful home management. Telephone calls initiated by the hospital nurse specialist to the patient, family or community health care team member are extremely effective in monitoring symptoms, anticipating problems and decreasing anxiety (Coyle et al. 1985).

If the patient is a child or adolescent, the grief, guilt and anger not only of the parents but also of any siblings must be acknowledged and dealt with. Similarly, if the patient is an adult, it is not just the partner, but the wider family, especially children, whose feelings need to be addressed. This is also of paramount importance when the patient dies (Coyle et al, 1985).

Bereavement

Bereavement counselling should be offered to all families. Studies of adult bereavement are increasingly suggesting that survivors' grief is more likely to run a disabling and chronic course if they have received little or no warning of imminent or probable death, have not discussed death with their spouse and have felt helpless to deal with distressing symptoms (Ransford and Smith, 1991) (see also Chapter 11).

Conclusion

All patients should have access to a uniformly high quality of care in the community or hospital wherever they may live, in order to ensure the maximum possible cure rates and best quality of life. Care should be provided as close to the patient's home as is compatible with high-quality, safe and effective treatment (Calman and Hine, 1995). But let the carers also have their say: 'Although Nita's long illness is now in the past, I can still recall my exhaustion, my hopes...and I think about other brain cancer patients and their relatives – those who have just been told the news...those beginning sessions of treatment with hope, those struggling to adjust to changes in appearance and loss of their abilities, those trying to accept that all hope has gone...' (Oswin, 1992, p 41). As such, future planning of care must always remain a major concern.

References

Altschuler J (1997) Family relationships during serious illness. Nursing Times 93(7): 48–9.

Amato C (1991) Malignant glioma: coping with a devastating illness. Neuroscience Nursing 23(1): 20–2.

Bass R, Windle C (1972) Continuity of care: an approach to measurement. American Journal of Psychology 129: 196–201.

Bomford C, Kunkler I, Sherriff S (1993) Quality of life. In Walter and Miller's Textbook of Radiotherapy, Radiation Physics, Therapy and Oncology. Edinburgh: Churchill Livingstone, pp 559–64.

Bristow O, Stickney C, Thompson S (1986) Discharge Planning for Continuity of Care. Publication No. 21. 1604. New York: National League of Nursing. In Salter M, Nursing the patient in the community. In Tschudin V (Ed.) Nursing the Patient with Cancer. London: Prentice Hall.

Brooks N (1985) Head injury and the family. In Brooks N (Ed.) Closed Head Injury: Psychological, Social and Family Consequences. Oxford: Oxford University Press, pp 123–45.

Calman K, Hine D (1995) A Policy for Commissioning Cancer Services. London: Department of Health.

Cassileth B, Hamilton J (1979) The family with cancer. In Cassileth BR (Ed.) The Cancer Patient: Social and Medical Aspects of Care. Philadelphia: Lea & Febiger.

Cole A (1992) Confidence trick. Social Work Today 25(5): 3.

Coyle N, Monzillo L, Loscalzo M, Farkas C, Massie M, Foley K (1985) A model of continuity of care for cancer patients with pain and neuro-oncologic complications. Cancer Nursing 8(2): 111–19.

Davies E, Clarke C (1993) Malignant cerebral gliomas: rehabilitation and care. In Greenwood et al, Neurological Rehabilitation. Edinburgh: Churchill Livingstone, pp 535–43.

Department of Health Circular (1989) Caring for People: Community Care in the Next Decade and Beyond. London: HMSO.

Department of Health (1991) The Patient's Charter. London: HMSO.

Dudas S, Carlson C (1984) Cancer rehabilitation. Oncology Nursing Forum 15(2): 183–8.

George M (1993) Funding the Act. Nursing Times 89(3): 24–5.

Giles S (1994) News focus: Why no one wants to bite the bullet. Health Service Journal (10 March): 11.

Glavassevich M, Thomas S, Galloway S (1991) An educational program to improve quality of life for individuals with acoustic neuroma. Journal of Neuroscience Nursing 23(4): 231–4.

Guerrero D (1996) Brain tumours. In Tschudin V (Ed.) Nursing the Patient with Cancer. London: Prentice Hall, pp 146–61.

Hart G (1981) Spinal cord injury: impact on clients' significant others. Rehabilitation Nursing 6(1): 11–15.

Hilton B (1992) Perceptions of uncertainty: its relevance to life threatening and chronic illness. Critical Care Nursing 12: 70–3.

Jackson M (1994) Discharge planning: issues and challenges for gerontological nursing. A critique of the literature. Journal of Advanced Nursing 19: 492–502.

Johnson J (1988) Cancer: a family disruption. Recent Results in Cancer Research 108: 306–10.

Leavitt M, Lamb S, Voss B (1996) Brain tumor support group: content themes and mechanisms of support. Oncology Nursing Forum 23(8): 1247–56.

Lewandowski W, Jones S (1988) The family with cancer: nursing interventions throughout the course of living with cancer. Cancer Nursing 11(6): 313–21.

Lindsay M (1989) Communicating with Neurological Patients: The Nurse's Role. London: Scutari Press.

Liss M, Willer B (1990) Traumatic brain injury and marital relationships: a literature review. International Journal of Rehabilitation Research 13: 309–20.

McKeag G (1995) The role of the neuro-oncology liaison nurse. Paediatric Nursing 7(10): 24–6.

McKinlay W, Brooks D, Bond MD, Martinage D, Marshall M (1981) The short-term outcome of severe blunt head injury as reported by relatives of the injured persons. Journal of Neurology, Neurosurgery and Psychiatry 44: 527–33.

Miller P, McMahon M, Garret M, Johnson N, Ringel K (1983) Family health and psychosocial responses to cardio-vascular disease. Health Values: Achieving High Level Wellness. 7(6): 11–18.

Morra M (1988) Choices: who's going to tell the patients what they need to know? Oncology Nursing Forum 15(4): 421–25.

Newton C, Mateo M (1994) Uncertainty: strategies for patients with brain tumor and their family. Cancer Nursing 17(2): 137–40.

Northouse L (1988) Family issues in cancer care. Advanced Psychosomatic Medicine 18: 82–101.

O'Leary J (1988) A period of transition. Nursing Standard (3 July): 51.

Oswin M (1992) The quiet menace. Nursing Times 88(34): 40–1.

Ransford HE, Smith ML (1991) Grief resolution among the bereaved in hospice and hospital wards. Social Science and Medicine 32: 295–304.

Robinson S (1992) The family with cancer. European Journal of Cancer Care 1(2): 29–32.
Salander P (1996) Brain tumours as a threat to life and personality: the spouse's perspective. Journal of Psychosocial Oncology 14(3): 1–16.
Salter M (1996) Nursing the patient in the community. In Tschudin V (Ed.) Nursing the Patient with Cancer. London: Prentice Hall.
Salter M (1997) Altered Body Image: The Nurse's Role. London: Baillière Tindall.
Tierney A, Closs J (1993) Discharge planning for elderly patients. Nursing Standard 7(52): 30–3.
Topliss E (1979) Provision for the Disabled, 2nd edn. Oxford: Blackwell/ Robertson.
Wade D (1992) Measurements in Neurological Rehabilitation. Oxford: Oxford University Press.
Watson P (1987) Family participation in the rehabilitation process: the rehabilitators' perspective. Rehabilitation Nursing 12(2): 70–3.
Woods N, Lewis F, Ellison E (1989) Living with cancer: family experiences. Cancer Nursing 12(1): 28–33.

Index

abducens nerve (CN VI) 12, 19, 23, 41–8
abduction 56, 62
abscesses 103, 202
accelerated radiotherapy 156–7, 160
accessory nerve (CN XI) 12, 23, 41–3, 51
accommodation 45, 62
acetylcholine 22
acidosis 144
acne 205, 212, 276
acoustic nerve (CN VIII) 12, 19, 23, 41–3, 49–50, 108, 135
acoustic neuromas 67, 134, 135
  neuro-imaging 92, 106, 108–9
acoustic schwannomas 106, 108–9
action potentials 4
acute lymphoblastic leukaemia 80
acute reactions to radiotherapy 165–6
Addisonian crisis 166, 202–3, 204
adenocarcinomas 102, 103
adenomatous polyposis 67
adolescents 257–8, 306
adrenal insufficiency 202–3, 204
adrenaline 22
adrenocorticotrophic hormone (ACTH) 77
afferent fibres 1, 10, 43
ageusia (loss of taste) 173
AIDS 100
alcohol 206, 207, 212, 215
alkylating agents 180, 181, 194
allergies 83, 91, 126
alopecia *see* hair loss and alopecia
alphafetoprotein (AFP) 78, 185
amygdaloid complex 25
anaemia 186, 212, 213
anaesthesia 8–4, 71, 85, 86, 90, 236
  neurosurgery 126, 127, 141
  see also general anaesthesia
analgesia 140, 142, 145, 172–3, 193, 206–8, 217–18
  pupil constriction 46
anaphylaxis 86, 187
anaplastic astrocytoma 67, 74, 93, 96–7
anaplastic ependymoma 67
anaplastic ganglioglioma 68
anaplastic meningioma 69, 79
anaplastic oligoastrocytoma 67
anaplastic oligodendroglioma 67, 75, 190
aneurysms 46, 107
angiography 81, 82–4, 92, 104, 105
angular gyrus 26
anhydrosis 46, 63
anopia 24
anorexia 169, 173, 187, 193, 259, 289
anosmia 25, 42, 62, 79, 174
anoxia 236
anterior cerebral arteries 12, 13
anterior commissure 5, 6, 25
anterior communicating arteries 12, 13
anterior cranial vault meningiomas 79
anterior fossa 127
anterior inferior cerebellar artery 13
anterior insular 25

anterior spinal artery 13
anthracenediones (mitozantrone) 181
anthracycline antibiotics (bleomycin) 181, 192, 195
antibiotics 142, 181, 195
  prophylactic 126
anticonvulsants 144
antidepressants 290
antimetabolites 180–1
antisense and gene therapy 183
anxiety and fear 8, 48, 216, 235, 245
  altered body image 254, 261, 264–5
  care planning 294–5, 196, 306
  family 247
  neurosurgery 125, 127, 140–1, 145, 147–8
  psychological support 275–6, 278–9, 281, 284–6, 288–90
  radiotherapy 161, 163, 164, 165–8, 170–1, 174, 176
  teamwork 221–2, 247
anxiolytics 170, 290
aphasia 38, 62
aplastic anaemia 213
apnoea 53
apoptosis 152, 180
apraxia 39, 62
aqueduct stenosis 133
arachnoid cysts 116
arachnoid granulations 103
arachnoid mater 15
arachnoid villi 15
arachnoiditis 196
archicerebellum 10
aromatherapy 173, 207, 216
arrhythmias 139–40, 205, 217
arteriovenous malformations (AVMs) 156
aseptic meningitis 137
association areas 7–8
astroblastoma 68
astrocytes 3, 93, 98
astrocytomas 67, 73–5, 93–6, 99–100
  anaplastic 67, 74, 93, 96–7
  children 109, 110, 111, 113–16
  radiotherapy 158
  spinal cord 122
  surgery 133
asynergia 11
ataxia 20, 54, 62, 70, 238, 242
  medication in symptom management 212, 213, 215
atrophy 55, 196
atropine 46
Attendance Allowance (AA) 304
attention *see* concentration and attention
auditory nerve *see* acoustic nerve (CN VIII)
aura before seizures 25, 72, 143, 144
autonomic functions 9, 41, 43
autonomic nervous system 10, 16, 21–2, 23, 26
axons 2–4, 16, 18, 20–1, 26, 63
  sight 23, 25
  smell 25
azoospermia 187, 197

Babinski response 60, 61, 62
balance and equilibrium 10, 11, 53–4, 237, 261
  cranial nerves 23, 43, 49
  vestibular system 19–20
basal cisterns 119
basal ganglia 9, 10, 100, 241
baseline assessments 30, 34, 35, 59, 126
  height and weight 185, 193
basilar arteries 12, 13
basophilic tumour cells 77
behaviour 32–3, 40, 70, 238, 263, 285
Belbin's teams 227, 228, 229, 230
Bell's palsy 48
benzodiazepines 144
bilateral acoustic neuroma 67
biopsy 75, 78, 158, 236
  neuro-imaging 81, 92, 106, 114, 118
  neurosurgery 124–5, 128, 131–2
bitemporal hemianopia 24, 45, 70, 79
bladder function 21, 30, 31, 54, 138, 195–6
  myelography 91
  seizures 143, 144, 261
  urinary retention 60, 141
  see also incontinence
bleomycin 181, 192, 195
blinking 18, 45, 47
blood-brain barrier 3, 13, 85, 89, 98
  chemotherapy 180, 181, 182–3, 184
  medication in symptom management 205–6, 216
blood chemistry 126, 185, 192
blood clotting screen 83
blood count 83, 174, 185, 192, 194
blood gases 139

blood pressure 21, 61, 140
blood-tumour barrier 182, 183
body image 70, 126, 145, 168, 204, 253–70
  psychological support 276, 292
body language 27, 286–7
bone flaps 128, 129
bone marrow 76, 78, 174
  spinal metastases 120, 121
  suppression 186–7, 194, 259
bowel function 30, 31, 54, 71, 138, 194, 217–18
  myelography 91
  seizures 143, 144
  see also incontinence
brachytherapy 155, 159
bradycardia 61, 140, 211
brain metastases 66, 78–80, 158–9, 192
brain stem 19–21, 32, 34, 52–3, 59, 61, 70
  circulation 13
  cranial nerves 41, 46, 49
  death 52–3
  gliomas 74, 75, 134
  neuro-imaging 108, 109, 110, 114–15
  neurosurgery 129, 130, 132, 134
  pupillary light reflex 25
  reflexes 25, 49
  speech and language therapy 240, 244
brain structure 1, 5–13, 14–15, 19–20, 23–5
  cranial nerves 40–52
  neuro-imaging 85, 88, 89, 92–109
  neurosurgery 124, 127–48
  radiotherapy 152, 153–4, 158–9
  reticular system 26
breast cancer 54, 80, 100, 102, 120, 134, 158
breastfeeding 209, 217, 218
British Association of Cancer United Patients (CancerBACUP) 304
Broca's area 8, 37–8
Brown-Sequard-type syndrome 72
bulbar palsy 51
Burkitt's lymphomas 80
burr holes 129, 131–2
busulphan 180, 195
calcification 75, 82, 84, 99–100, 103, 104, 107
  paediatric neuro-imaging 113–14, 116–18
caloric testing 49, 52
candidiasis 173, 201, 203, 219, 277
  radiotherapy 166, 173, 174
carbamazepine (Tegretol) 212–14, 215
carboplatin 181–2, 191, 192
carcinomatous meningitis 80, 102, 103
cardiac arrest 33, 52, 144
cardiac function *see* heart and cardiac function
cardiovascular instability 139–40
care in the community 299–300, 301, 302–4
carmustine (BCNU) 180, 186
carotid artery 105
cataracts 46
cauda equina syndrome 71
cavernous sinus 47, 77, 106
cavitron ultrasonic surgical aspirator (CUSA) 135
cefuroxine 126
central nervous system structure 1–2, 3–4, 25
  neurological assessment 30–1, 33, 55
central neurocytomas 68
central neurofibromatosis 67
central sulcus 7–8
cerebellar infiltration 76
cerebellopontine angle cistern 108
cerebellopontine region 108, 129
cerebellum 5, 7, 10–11, 19–20, 49, 68, 70, 80
  neurological assessment 1, 53–4
  neurosurgery 129, 132, 134
  speech and language 11, 244
cerebral angiography 81, 82–4, 92, 104, 105
cerebral convolutions 6
cerebral cortex 6, 7–8, 9–10, 12, 21, 32, 63
  neuro-imaging 92
  neurosurgery 135
  reticular system 26
  speech and language therapy 241
cerebral function 31, 32–40
cerebral hemispheres 40, 66, 70, 73, 74, 80, 133

neuro-imaging 93, 94, 102, 109–11, 114–15
see also dominant hemispheres
cerebral motor cortex 9, 11, 19, 20–1, 72
neuro-imaging 96
neurosurgery 135, 143
cerebropontine angle 48
cerebrospinal fluid (CSF) 15, 61, 75–6, 78, 80
chemotherapy 185
leakage 91, 142
neuro-imaging 85, 88, 91, 99, 111–13, 116–17, 119–21
neurosurgery 137–8, 139, 142
radiotherapy 158
raised intracranial pressure 73, 202
seeding 76, 111–13, 117, 119
shunting 69
cerebrum 5–9, 13, 25
cervicomedullary junction 130
chemoradiotherapy 78
chemotherapy 78, 179–200, 276, 305
administration routes 183–4, 186–7, 189
altered body image 259–60
neuro-imaging 81, 92, 100
oral hygiene 219
radiotherapy 158, 159, 174, 190–2, 195–6
chiasmatic cistern 107
children 66, 70, 71, 106, 109–19, 159, 189, 284–6
altered body image 257–8
angiography 83
care planning 295, 297–9, 304, 306
chemotherapy 189
craniopharyngiomas 77, 109, 115, 116–17
CT scans 85, 110–11, 113–14, 116–19
gliomas 73–5, 93, 109, 110, 114–16
medication in symptom management 209, 214, 218
medulloblastomas 76, 109–14, 118, 134
meningiomas 103
MRI scans 89, 110–12, 114, 116–19
myelography 90
neuro-imaging 92, 93, 109–19
neurosurgery 110, 112, 114, 115, 133, 134
psychological support 271, 273, 277, 279, 284–6
radiotherapy 114, 158, 159, 174, 175
spinal tumours 120
chlorambucil 180, 197
chondroma 69
chondrosarcoma 69
chordoma 69, 120, 130
choriocarcinoma 68
choroid plexus 15, 68
papilloma 68, 109, 115, 119
chromophobe adenomas 77
cimetidine 208, 209, 214
cingulate 9
circle of Willis 12, 13
cisplatin 181–2, 195–6
claustrophobia 86, 162
clinical nurse specialist 233, 276
clinical psychologists 146, 233
psychological support 274, 278, 279, 282, 285, 289, 290
clival chordomas 130
clivus 130
clumsiness 31
cochlear division (CN VIII) 43, 49–50
co-danthramer 194, 217, 218
codeine 145, 207
codeine phosphate 194
co-dydramol 206
cognition 234–5
altered body image 253–4, 255, 257, 260, 262, 268
care planning 299, 303, 306
informed consent 188
neurological assessment 32, 34, 37, 40
neurosurgery 125, 145–6, 147, 148
psychological support 272–5, 280, 282, 284, 287–9
teamwork 221, 233–6, 238–9, 242, 249
colloid cysts 133
colour 44
coma 33–7, 49, 51, 52, 186
Glasgow Coma Scale (GCS) 33–7, 41
communication 241–4, 278–9
aids 146, 244
altered body image 259, 260
care planning 294, 296, 299, 300
psychological support 272–3, 275–6, 278–9, 281–2, 286–8

speech and language therapy 240–4
teamwork 223, 226, 232, 240–6, 249
see also speech and language
computed tomography (CT) 84–6, 91
acoustic tumours 108
chemotherapy 185, 198
children 85, 110–11, 113–14, 116–19
intracranial malignancies 94–5, 97–8, 100–33, 107
medulloblastoma 76
meningiomas 104
neuro-imaging 81–2, 84–6, 89–90, 110–11, 113–14, 116–19, 122
neurosurgery 128, 131, 132, 137, 143
pituitary adenomas 107
radiotherapy 154, 157, 164, 175
spinal tumours 122
concentration and attention 38–9, 145, 289
neurological assessment 32, 34, 38–9, 45
teamwork 234–6, 242, 244
conflict within team 223, 225–6, 229
consciousness level 32–3, 70, 208, 238
neurological assessment 29, 31, 32–7, 61, 62
neurosurgery 136, 137, 140, 141, 143, 144
radiotherapy reaction 173
reticular system 26
seizures 143, 144
consensual reaction of pupils 25, 45
consent 125, 126, 188–9
constipation 145, 217–18, 277
chemotherapy 186–7, 194
medication in symptom management 201, 207, 208, 217–28
contraceptive pills 212, 215
contralateral hemiparesis 70
contrast medium 92, 94, 97–8, 101–4, 107–8
angiography 83
children 110–14, 117
CT scan 85–6
MRI scan 89
myelography 90–1
spinal cord 122
control and autonomy 248
altered body image 255–6, 259, 260–1
psychological support 272, 280, 290
conus medullaris 71, 122
conventional brain scan 82, 89, 90
co-proxamol 206, 214
cornea 23, 43
reflexes 18, 47, 52, 60, 138
corpus callosum 5, 6, 70, 98
cortical mapping 135
cortical motor integration 39
corticobulbar tract 21
corticopontocerebellar tract 11
corticospinal tract 16, 20–1
corticosteroids 77, 185, 191, 195, 255
medication for symptom management 202, 204, 208, 219
radiotherapy 165, 166, 170, 171, 173
corticovestibulospinal 64
cotton buds 32
cotton-wool 32, 47
cough reflex 50–1, 53
counselling 145, 146, 196, 286–9
altered body image 265, 266
care planning 297–8, 299, 306
psychological support 274, 276, 278–9, 282, 286–9, 291
cranial germinoma 157
cranial nerves 1, 16, 23, 40–52, 59, 63, 69, 244
I (olfactory) 23, 25, 41–3, 174
II (optic) 23, 24, 41–5, 67, 75, 77, 115, 158, 176
III (oculomotor) 10, 19, 23, 41–3, 45–7
IV (trochlear) 10, 19, 23, 41–3, 45–7
V (trigeminal) 12, 18–19, 23, 41–3, 47–8, 51, 135
VI (abducens) 12, 19, 23, 41–8
VII (facial) 12, 23, 41–3, 48, 51, 135
VIII (acoustic) 12, 19, 23, 41–3, 49–50, 108, 135
IX (glossopharyngeal) 12, 23, 41–3, 50–1, 135
X (vagus) 12, 23, 41–3, 50–1
XI (accessory) 12, 23, 41–3, 51
XII (hypoglossal) 12, 23, 41–3, 51–2
meningiomas 79
neurological assessment 29, 31
neurosurgery 135, 138, 141

palsies 70, 77, 80, 110, 186
voluntary muscle activity 20–1
craniectomy 129, 134
craniopharyngioma 29, 68, 77, 107, 116–17
children 77, 109, 115, 116–17
radiotherapy 157, 158
craniospinal axis radiotherapy 153–4, 158, 162, 174, 175
medulloblastoma 76
PNETs 191
craniotomy 124, 128–9, 130, 131, 133, 140, 145
body image 259, 263
image guided 131, 132
creatine kinase 144
Crossroads 305
cushingnoid effects 256, 257
Cushing's response 61, 140, 206
cyanosis 143
cyclizine 216, 217
cyclophosphamide 180, 191, 195–6, 197
cystic cerebellar astrocytomas 74
cystic neoplasms 77
cystitis 180, 196
cysts 69, 99, 107, 133
children 110–11, 114, 115–16, 117, 118
spinal cord 122
cytidine analogues (cytarabine) 180
cytons 2–3
cytotoxic drugs 186–7
chemotherapy 180–200
resistance 182–3
trials 198

dacarbazine 180
danthron 218
daunorubicin 195
death 52–3, 124, 305, 306–7
psychological support 273–4, 279–83, 285–6, 291–2
debulking tumours 74, 75, 81, 124–5, 134, 158, 236
decussation 12, 20
dehydration 141, 145, 193, 194
dementia 175
dendrites 2–3, 4
depression 27, 145, 196
altered body image 254, 255, 257
medication in symptom management 204, 205, 217
psychological support 276, 278, 283, 289, 290
dermatomes 17, 59
desmoplastic infantile ganglioglioma 68
dexamethasone 126, 202–5, 305
radiotherapy 166, 170, 173
symptom management 202–5, 208, 216, 217
dextropropoxyphene 206, 214
diabetes 52, 141, 166, 257
steroid-induced 166, 173, 204, 257
diagnosis 30, 147, 271–4
body image 254
care planning 294–6, 298, 303, 305
neuro-imaging 81–123
neurosurgery 124, 125, 128, 131, 147
psychological support 271–4, 275, 277, 279, 281–2
teamwork 221, 233, 235, 242, 245–8
diarrhoea 186–7, 194, 217
diazemuls 144
diazepam 86, 144, 209
diencephalon 5, 9–10, 25
dihydrocodeine 207
diltiazem 214
diplopia 45, 46, 62, 79, 186, 213
disability *see* loss of function and disability
Disability Living Allowance (DLA) 304
discharge 300–2
gradual 265, 266
planning 234, 235, 300–2, 303
diversional therapy 193
DNA 151–2, 179–81
doctors 227, 248, 274, 276, 278, 302
documentation for neurosurgery 126
doll's eyes (oculocephalic reflex) 49, 52, 62
dominant hemispheres 8–9, 26–7, 37, 70, 135
speech and language therapy 240–1
domperidone 216, 217
dorsal root ganglia 14, 16, 17, 18
dorsiflexion 62
downward gaze 23, 43
doxorubicin 181, 191, 195
dressing 39, 40, 61, 235
dry desquamation 168, 169
dura 13, 23
neuro-imaging 92, 101, 102, 103

neurosurgery 129, 133, 134, 140, 142
spinal tumours 120, 134
dura mater 15
dural sinuses 13, 15
dysarthria 52, 62, 242, 244
dyscalculia 242
dysdiadochokinesia 11
dysembryoplastic neuroepithelial tumour 68
dysgerminoma 78
dysgraphia 241
dyslexia 241
dysmetria 11
dyspepsia 166, 201, 203, 208–9, 215
dysphagia 51, 62, 175, 187, 193, 244–5
dysphasia 38, 62, 70, 146, 260, 275, 287
radiotherapy 165
speech and language therapy 241, 242, 243–4
dysphonic speech 11
dysphoria 273, 276, 283
dysplastic gangliglioma of cerebellum 68
dyspnoea 204
dyspraxia 70, 241–2
dysuria 186

early delayed reactions to radiotherapy 165, 166–75
ears 19, 23, 43, 171
eating 39, 60, 61, 138, 141
see also nutrition and diet
economic factors 277–8, 297, 302, 304
efferent fibres 2–3, 26, 43
electrocardiogram 126, 185, 195
electrolyte imbalance 52, 141, 205
electrophysiological monitoring 135
embolisation 83–4, 105, 135
embryonal tumours 68, 152
emotions 8, 9, 10, 40
empathy 287–8
employment 145, 243, 273, 292, 296
body image 254, 260, 263–4
encephalitis 80, 94
encephalopathy 196
endocrine 10, 52, 71, 75, 77, 106, 204
radiotherapy 159, 176
endocrinologists 159, 176
endoscopic techniques 131, 133
eosinophilic tumour cells 77
ependymal cells 67, 93
ependymoblastoma 68, 76, 158
ependymoma 67, 76, 112–14, 133–4, 153, 158
children 109–15
spinal cord 76, 122
epidural space 119
epilepsy and seizures 72–3, 142–5, 160, 209–15, 260–1
aura 25, 72, 143, 144
blood-brain barrier 182
body image 256, 260–1, 264
chemotherapy 186
gliomas 74
hydrocephalus 73
manifestation of tumours 69, 70, 72–3
medication in symptom management 201, 209–15
meningioma 79
neurological assessment 31
neurosurgery 138, 142–5, 209
oligodendroglioma 75
physiotherapy 236
psychological support 272, 284
radiotherapy 166
removal of hippocampus 27
epirubicin 181, 195
equilibrium *see* balance and equilibrium
erythema 168–9, 171
erythema multiforme 213
erythromycin 214
etoposide (VP16) 181, 187, 191, 195
European Organisation for Research and Treatment of Cancer (EORTC) 190
Ewing's sarcoma 120
expressive dysphasia 38, 70, 146, 165, 244, 260
psychological support 275, 287
extension 35, 37, 56–8, 60, 62–3
external beam radiotherapy 153–5, 156–8
extradural spinal tumours 71, 119, 120, 134
extramedullary tumours 71, 91, 120, 134
extrapyramidal system 9, 26
extravasation 184–5, 186–7
eye opening 34, 35
eyelids 43, 46, 48, 63, 138
eyes 11, 23–5, 42–7, 49, 62, 62, 90

medication in symptom management 205, 211–12, 215, 217
reflexes 18, 25, 47, 49, 52, 60, 62, 138
vestibular system 19–20
see also pupils; vision and sight

face 18–19, 23, 43
expressions 32, 40, 43, 48
face masks 161–3, 164
facial nerve (CN VII) 12, 23, 41–3, 48, 51, 135
facial palsy 138
falls 31
falx 104, 133, 140
family and carers 245–50, 282–3, 286–9, 294–307
altered body image 253–8, 260, 263–7
care planning 294–307
chemotherapy 185–8, 189, 192, 197
history 31–2, 37, 83, 126, 128, 266
medication for symptom management 205
neurological assessment 31–2, 36, 38
neurosurgery 125, 127, 145–8
predisposition to tumours 66, 67, 115
psychological support 271–92
radiotherapy 151, 157, 160–1, 164–6, 168, 170, 174–6
teamwork 221–2, 231, 233–6, 239–40, 243–50
famotidine 208
fasciculation 55, 63
fear *see* anxiety and fear
fibrillary astrocytomas 67, 93–7
Grade II 94–6
paediatric 109, 114, 116
fibrosis 186, 195
filum terminale 122
first cervical vertebra (atlas) 130
fissures of the brain 6, 7, 10, 47
flaccid paralysis 51
flexion 35, 37, 56–8, 60, 63
fluid imbalance 141, 205
fluoropyrimidines 180
folinic acid rescue 181, 186
foramen of Luschka 119
foramen magnum 10, 12, 14, 15
forebrain 5
Foster-Kennedy syndrome 79
fourth ventricle 5, 11, 15, 129, 134, 137
children 110, 111, 112–14, 119
fractionation 152–3, 156, 176
stereotactic radiotherapy 155–6, 163
frank anaplastic change 75
freehand technique 131, 132
frontal lobes 7, 20, 70, 75, 241, 264
neurological assessment 36, 37, 40
neurosurgery 128, 130, 133, 143, 146
frontotemporal region 79, 141
functional imaging 92

gabapentin (Neurontin) 215
gadolinium 103
DTPA (Gd-DTPA) 89, 95, 97, 104, 112, 120
gagging 43, 50–1, 53, 60, 138
galactorrhoea 217
Galveston Orientation and Amnesia Test 40
gamma rays 151, 153
ganglia 2, 14, 16, 17, 18
gangliocytomas 68, 118
gangliogliomas 68, 109
ganglioneuromas 118
gastrointestinal tumours 21–2, 43, 100, 101
gemistocytic tumours 67
gender 78, 103, 116, 299
body image 258, 260
general anaesthesia 133, 135, 136, 138–9, 141, 259
angiography 83–4
children 112, 159
myelography 90
genetic predisposition to tumours 66, 67, 115
genitourinary tract tumours 100, 101
germ cells 68, 69, 78, 116
chemotherapy 185, 191–2
radiotherapy 78, 152, 153–4, 158
germinomas 68, 78, 109, 179, 191
giant cell astrocytomas 67, 93
giant cell glioblastoma 67
glands 2, 22, 23
Glasgow Coma Scale (GCS) 33–7, 41
glial cells 4, 28, 115, 118, 154
glioblastomas 106, 133

multiforme 67, 73, 93, 96–9, 103
gliomas 66, 73–5, 92, 93, 94–100, 114, 157–8, 190–1
brain stem 74, 75, 134
care planning 294, 304
chemotherapy 179, 184, 190–1
children 73–5, 93, 109, 110, 114–16
ependymoma 76
mixed 67
psychological support 282, 292
radiotherapy 152, 154, 155, 157–8, 160, 176
spinal 71, 122
gliomatosis cerebri 68
gliosarcoma 67, 74
glomus jugulare 51
glossopharyngeal nerve (CN IX) 12, 23, 41–3, 50–1, 135
glucocorticoid therapy 172
steroids 202, 208
glucose 12, 13, 22, 52, 139, 142
glycogen 22
gonadotrophins 77
Gorlin's syndrome 67
Gradenigro's syndrome 48
granisetron 216, 217
granulocytic sarcoma 68
granulocytopenia 187
grasp reflex 36, 70
gravity 10, 55
grey matter 2, 6, 9, 20
neuro-imaging 102, 103, 107
spinal cord 14, 16, 18
gross tumour volume (GTV) 152
growth 71, 77, 159
gustatory cortex 25
gynaecomastia 217
gyri 6, 9, 16, 18, 20, 26

haemangioblastoma 67
haematomas 137, 139, 140, 202
haemopoietic neoplasms 68, 69
haemorrhage 44, 52, 70
neuro-imaging 93, 97, 103, 107, 114
neurosurgery 124, 130, 138, 142, 143
hair loss and alopecia 166–7, 195, 260, 276, 285
body image 256–60, 266
chemotherapy 187, 195
radiotherapy 166–9
shaving for surgery 126
hamartomas 75
head turning 23, 43
headaches 19, 31, 36, 172–3, 201–8
chemotherapy 186
epilepsy 73
gliomas 74
manifestation of tumour 70, 73
pituitary tumours 77
post-myelography 91
psychological support 276, 279, 287
radiotherapy 166, 172-3
raised intracranial pressure 19, 73, 201-2, 205-6, 209
symptom management 201-8, 209, 212, 213, 215, 217
Health Ombudsman 302
health visitors 297
hearing 7-8
acoustic schwannomas 108
chemotherapy 185, 186
cranial nerves 16, 23, 43, 49-50
neurosurgery 146
psychological support 272, 275, 276
radiotherapy reaction 171
heart and cardiac function 2, 12, 21, 22, 43, 195
arrhythmias 139–40, 205, 217
chemotherapy 185, 187, 195
electrocardiogram before treatment 126, 185, 195
medication in symptom management 205, 206, 217
hemianopia 24, 45, 70, 79
hemiparesis 70, 73, 79, 272, 276
hemiplegia 33, 55, 234, 236, 239
psychological support 272, 276
hepatotoxicity 206
high-dependency unit (HDU) 136
higher functions 5, 8, 26–7, 31, 70, 112, 145
judgement and reasoning 39–40
hindbrain 5
hippocampus 9, 27
hirsutism 204, 212
history 31–2, 37, 83, 126, 128, 266
HIV 66, 77–8
homonymous hemianopia 24, 70
hope 280, 281
hormones 77, 107
Horner's syndrome 46, 63
hospices 305
care planning 297, 301–3, 305, 306

hospitalisation 124, 125
human chorionic gonadotrophin (HCG) 78, 185
hydrocephalus 70, 71, 73, 77, 133, 137, 202
children 109, 110, 113, 115, 119
hydrocortisone 168–9, 192
hyoid 43
hyperfractionation 156–7
hypernatraemia 52
hyperostosis 79
hyperpyrexia 187
hyperreflexia 71
hypersensitivity 187
hypertension 143, 186, 205
hypertonia 55, 63
hypertonus 238, 239
hypnotics 170
hypofractionated radiotherapy 157
hypoglossal nerve (CN XII) 12, 23, 41–3, 51–2
hypoglycaemia 33, 144, 204
hypokalaemia 196, 218
hypomagnesaemia 196
hyponatraemia 213
hypotension 186–7, 204, 211
hypothalamus 5, 9, 10, 21–2, 71, 77, 115–16
children 110, 115–16
gliomas 74
radiotherapy reaction 172, 176
reticular system 26
hypothermia 52
hypotonicity 55
hypoxia 33, 139, 144, 145

idarubicin 181, 195
ifosfamide 180, 195–6
immune deficiency 66, 77, 100
immunotherapy 183
incontinence 70, 186, 218, 262
infarction 48, 70, 93, 94–5, 137
infection 91, 142, 168, 169, 171, 203
chemotherapy 193, 194–5
inferior frontal lobe 118
infertility 154, 159, 187, 197
infratentorial approach 128, 129, 131, 133
insomnia 205, 212, 306
psychological support 276, 285, 289
intention tremor 11
intensive care unit (ICU) 136
internal carotid artery 12, 13
interstitial radiotherapy 154–5, 159
intradural extramedullary tumours 91, 120
intradural spinal tumours 71, 134
intramedullary tumours 71, 120, 122, 134
intraventricular neuro-imaging 109
involuntary movements 9, 26, 55
iodine-125 radiotherapy 155
ionizing radiation 151–2
iridium-192 radiotherapy 155

Jacksonian march 72, 143
jaundice 214
joints 1, 11, 15, 18, 63, 234, 261
neurological assessment 55–7, 59–60
physiotherapy 237, 238, 239
judgement and reasoning 39–40

key worker 299
kidney cancer 102, 134

lacrimation 43, 47
laminectomy 134
lamotrigine (Lamictal) 215
language *see* speech and language
lansoprazole 209
larynx 23, 43, 50–1
late delayed reactions to radiotherapy 159, 165, 175–6
lateral gaze 23, 43
lateral geniculate body 24–5
lateral medullary syndrome 19
lateral ventricles 118, 119, 128
Le Forte maxillotomy 130–1
leaders of teams 223, 226–7, 230, 232, 249
left vertebral artery 13
leptomeninges 80, 90, 102
leucomalacia 175
leucopenia 186, 212, 213
leukaemia 80, 101, 109, 197
Lhermitte's phenomenon 175
limbic association areas 7–8
limbic system 9, 21, 25, 40
linear accelerators (Linac) 153, 154
liver function 22, 137
medication in symptom management 206, 209, 213–15, 217

lobotomy 27
localising signs 29, 35, 37, 58
logical problems 27
lomustine (CCNU) 180, 186, 190
long tract signs 70, 110
loss of function and disability 235
  altered body image 253–7, 259–64
  care planning 295–7, 299, 303, 305
  neurosurgery 125, 145, 147–8
  psychological support 272–6, 279, 282–4
  teamwork 222, 232–40, 248
lower quadrantinopia 70
lower motor neurones 21, 55, 63
lung cancer 80, 100, 102, 120, 134, 158
  small cell 80, 192
lymphoblastic lymphomas 80
lymphoedema 184, 222
lymphomas 77, 80, 240
  neuro-imaging 92, 93, 101
  radiotherapy 152, 153, 158
  spinal tumours 120
  see also primary lymphomas

Macmillan Cancer Relief 278
  nurses 297, 302, 303
macroadenomas 77, 106–7
macrophages 4
magnetic resonance imaging (MRI) 86–9
  chemotherapy 185, 198
  children 89, 110–12, 114, 116–19
  gliomas 93, 95–8
  medulloblastoma 76
  meningiomas 104–5
  neuro-imaging 81–2, 84, 86–93, 95–8, 100–8
  neurosurgery 128, 131, 132
  radiotherapy 154, 157, 175
  spinal tumours 120
  venography 104–6
magnetic resonance spectroscopy (MRS) 89
mandibular branch (V3) 41, 47
mannitol 202, 205–6, 216
  chemotherapy 183, 187, 196
Margerison and McCann's teams 227, 229–30
margins of radiotherapy 154–5
Marie Curie nurses 303, 306
massage 173, 193, 207, 216, 222
mastoid bone 131
mathematical and numeracy problems 27, 242
maxillary branch (V2) 41, 47
medial gaze 23, 43
medial temporal lobes 39, 99
Medical Research Council (MRC) 55, 59, 190
medication 83, 137, 201–20, 241, 290, 305
  altered body image 263, 265, 267
  neurological assessment 32, 52
  pupil dilation and constriction 46
medulla 41, 114, 216
  oblongata 5, 7, 10, 11, 12, 18–20
  rhythmicity area 12
medulloblastoma 67, 68, 69, 76, 110–12
  chemotherapy 191
  children 76, 109–14, 118, 134
  neurosurgery 134
  radiotherapy 76, 154, 157–9, 163, 176
medulloepithelioma 68
megaloblastic anaemia 212
melanin 103
melanoma 80, 100, 102, 103
melphalan 180
memory 9, 26–7, 39, 145, 215
  altered body image 256, 257
  neurological assessment 31, 37–40
  psychological support 272, 274, 275, 287
  teamwork 234, 235, 238, 242
meninges 14–15, 19, 68–9, 101, 103
  cranial nerve 23, 43
  spinal tumours 119
meningiomas 42, 67, 68–9, 78–9, 103–6
  neuro-imaging 92, 93, 103–9
  neurosurgery 104, 105, 106, 133, 135
  radiotherapy 106, 158
  spinal cord 71, 120
meningitis 137, 142
  carcinomatous 80, 102, 103
menstrual cycle 171–2, 197, 204, 215
mesencephalon 5, 10
mesenchymal 69
Mesna (mercaptoethane sulphonic acid) rescue 180, 196
metastases 66, 69, 76, 78–80, 100–3, 158–9

chemotherapy 192
children 111–12, 113, 117
neuro-imaging 89, 92–3, 98–103, 106, 111–13, 117, 120–1
neurological assessment 54
nuclear medicine 89
radiotherapy 100, 155, 158–9
speech and language therapy 240
spinal cord 54, 66, 71, 80, 103, 120, 121, 134
methotrexate 180, 181, 186, 191, 193, 195–6
metoclopramide 216, 217
microadenomas 76–7, 106
microglial cells 4
midbrain 5, 10, 11, 19, 20, 99, 114
cranial nerves 41, 47
middle cerebral artery 13
midline 70–1, 109, 110, 115
shift 82
mineralocorticoid steroids 202
Mini Mental State Examination 40, 289
minimally invasive techniques 128, 131–3
mitomycin C 180
mitosis 2, 4, 74, 152, 179, 182
mixed germ cell tumours 68
mixed gliomas 67
mixed neuronal-glial tumour 68
mixed oligoastrocytomas 67
moist desquamation 168, 169
monoamine oxidase inhibitor (MAOI) 181, 187
monoclonal antibodies 183
moods 26, 32, 40, 48, 255, 289, 306
morphine 207
motor cortex 9, 11, 19, 20–1, 72
neuro-imaging 96
neurosurgery 135, 143
motor function 1–3, 7–12, 55–9, 237–8, 239
body image 261–2, 263
cranial nerves 23, 41, 43, 47, 51
neurological assessment 29–31, 53, 54, 55–9
psychological support 272, 277
radiotherapy 175
reticular system 26
spinal cord 14, 16–17
surgery 138, 145
vestibular system 19
see also walking and gait
motor response 34, 35, 36–7
mouth 23, 43, 48, 50
mucaine suspension 175
mucositis 186–7, 193–4
Muga (multigated acquisition) scan 195
multifocal glioblastoma 73
multiple sclerosis 48, 103, 175
muscles 1, 2, 7, 10–12, 14–21, 145, 234
body image 261
cranial nerves 23, 48, 50–1
medication in symptom management 203–4
metastases 80
myelography 91
neurological assessment 48, 50–1, 53–60, 62, 63
physiotherapy 237–40
reticular system 26
speech and language therapy 242
tone 10–11, 55, 71, 234, 237–40
music 27
myalgia 204
myelin 3–5, 6, 169, 175
myelitis 80
myelodysplastic syndrome 197
myelography 82, 90–1, 120
myelopathy 176
myelosuppression 186–7
myocardial contraction 12
myxopapillary ependymoma 67

nadir count 185, 186–7, 192, 194
nail bed pressure 36, 58, 60
National Association for Staff Support (NASS) 291
National Cancerlink 304
nausea and vomiting 16, 73, 193, 216–17
body image 259, 260
chemotherapy 186–7, 188, 193
medication in symptom management 201–2, 204, 207–8, 212–17, 219
neurological assessment 31
neurosurgery 137, 141
radiotherapy 174
raised intracranial pressure 73, 202, 216
psychological support 276, 279
necrosing encephalopathy 196
necrosis 74, 133, 137, 184
neuro-imaging 90, 97, 98, 103, 111

neocerebellum 11
neocortex 25
neoplasms 4, 68–9, 77, 202
  neuro-imaging 81, 92, 120
nerve palsy 46
nerve sheath tumours 120
neuroblastoma 68, 120
neurocytoma 68, 118
neuroepithelial tumours 67–8, 73–5
neurofibroma 69, 71
neurofibromatosis 67, 75, 115
neuroforamen 120, 122
neuroglia 2–5, 13, 92, 182
neurological deterioration 69–72, 136–8, 196, 305
  medication in symptom management 202, 205, 208
  psychological support 282–3, 292
  radiotherapy reactions 172, 173
  surgery 124, 136–8, 148
neurones and neuronal tumours 2–5, 6, 19–20, 25–8, 182
  children 115, 118–19
  epilepsy 72
  lower motor 21, 55, 63
  neurological assessment 41, 55, 63
  sight 23, 25
  spinal cord 14, 16–17, 18
  upper motor 20–1, 55, 61, 63–4, 71
neurosurgery and surgery 40, 76, 78, 79, 124–50, 259
  acoustic schwannomas 108
  body image 256, 258, 259, 263
  chemotherapy 184, 190, 191, 192
  children 110, 112, 114, 115, 133, 134
  debulking tumours 74, 75, 81, 124–5, 134, 158, 236
  epilepsy 138, 142–5, 209
  intracranial metastases 103
  meningiomas 104, 105, 106, 133, 135
  postoperative management 136–47
  psychological support 272
  radiotherapy 151, 154, 158, 165, 175
  rehabilitation 147–8
  teamwork 236, 241
  see also resection of tumours
Neuro-tip 32
neurotransmitters 2, 4
neutropenia 186–7, 194, 259
NHS and Community Care Act (1990) 300, 302
nitrogen mustards 180
nitrosoureas 180, 190, 194
nizatidine 208
nodes of Ranvier 3, 4
non-germinomas 78, 191
non-glial tumours 92
non-haematological tumours 66
non-Hodgkin's lymphoma 77
non-meningothelial tumours 69
non-small cell lung cancer 80
noradrenaline 22
nose 25, 42, 130
nuclear medicine 82, 89–90
nutrition and diet 141
  body image 257, 263
  chemotherapy 181, 187, 188, 193, 194
  medication in symptom management 204, 207, 218, 219
  neurosurgery 141, 142, 145
  radiotherapy reactions 174
  teamwork 222, 245
nystagmus 11, 20, 49, 63, 70, 211
nystatin 193, 219

occipital cortex 42
occipital lobe 7, 10, 13, 25, 70, 127–8, 133
occupational therapists 233–6, 237, 303
  neurosurgery 146, 147
  psychological support 274, 276, 278, 279, 287
oculocephalic reflex (doll's eye) 49, 52, 62
oculomotor nerve (CN III) 10, 19, 23, 41–3, 45–7
oculovestibular reflex 49, 52
odontoid peg 130
oedema 33, 73, 75, 241
  medication in symptom management 202, 205–6, 213, 214
  neuro-imaging 95, 97, 100, 102–4, 111
  neurosurgery 126, 128, 131, 137–41, 144, 145
  radiotherapy 165, 166, 171
  raised intracranial pressure 202, 205–6

oesophagitis 175
olfactory groove 25, 42, 79
olfactory gyrus 25
olfactory nerve (CN I) 23, 25, 41–3, 174
olfactory neuroblastoma 68
oligoastrocytomas
  (oligodendroastrocytomas) 67, 75, 99
oligodendrocytes 3–4, 93, 98
oligodendroglial cells 67, 169
oligodendrogliomas 67, 75, 98–100, 133, 190
  anaplastic 67, 75, 190
omeprazole 209
ondansetron 216, 217
oopheropexy 154
open surgical techniques 128–31
ophthalmic assessment 78
ophthalmic branch (V1) 41, 47
ophthalmic complications 205
ophthalmoplegia 79
ophthalmoscope 32, 44
opiates 46, 194, 207, 215
opioids 140, 145, 217
optic chiasm 5, 23–5, 41, 45, 71, 115–16
  craniopharyngiomas 77
  gliomas 74, 75
  meningiomas 79
  neuro-imaging 107, 110, 115–16
optic nerve (CN II) 23, 24, 41, 42–5
  children 115
  craniopharyngiomas 77
  gliomas 67, 75, 158
  radiotherapy 176
optic pathway gliomas 109, 115
optic tracts 115
organ donation 53
  transplants 66, 77, 100
orientation 34, 35, 37
osseous spine 119
osteoblastic change 79
osteogenic sarcomatous metastases 103, 120
osteonecrosis 204
osteoplastic flaps 129
osteoporosis 203, 204
otitis externa and media 171
otoscope 32
ovaries 78, 102, 154
oxygen 2, 12, 13, 21, 53
  neurosurgery 138, 139, 141, 144
  radiotherapy 152
pain 16–18, 71, 72, 80, 140–1
  anxiety 264, 265
  body image 264–5, 268
  chemotherapy 184, 186–7, 193–4
  cranial nerves 45, 48
  medication in symptom management 202, 203, 208
  neurosurgery 125, 140–1
  psychological support 276, 278
  radiotherapy 164
  sensation 15–19
  stimulus for neurological assessment 35–8, 53, 58, 59
  teamwork 221–2, 234
paleocerebellum 10
palliative care 297, 302, 303, 305
  chemotherapy 190, 191, 192, 197
  radiotherapy 157, 159, 161
  teamwork 221, 236
pantoprazole 209
papilloedema 44, 63, 73, 79
paracetamol 206
paraesthesia 196, 256
parafalcine 103, 104
paraganglioma 69
parahippocampus 9
paralysis 11, 51, 54, 58, 63, 71–3, 91
  body image 259, 264
  chemotherapy 186
  physiotherapy 238
  radiotherapy 176
  Todd's 73, 144
  vocal cords 50
parasagittal region 142
parasagittal meningiomas 79
paraspinal soft tissues 119
parasympathetic nervous system 21, 22
parenchyma 68, 76, 79
parietal lobes 7, 40, 70, 241
  neurosurgery 128, 133, 142, 146
parieto-occipitotemporal association areas 7–8
Parinaud's syndrome 71
parosmia 42, 63
parotid gland 23
patent airway 139, 143, 144
patient abuse 298
Patient's Charter 300
patterns and intellectual function 27
payment for community care 302, 304
pen-torch 32
perianal reflex 60

perianal "saddle" anaesthesia 71
periaventricular areas 77
peripheral nervous system (PNS) structure 1, 4, 80
cranial nerves 41
spinal cord 14, 18
peripheral neurofibromatosis 67
peristalsis 22
personality changes 40, 70, 79, 145, 188
body image 257, 264
care planning 298, 303, 306
psychological support 273, 275, 279–80, 282–4, 287, 292
petroclival meningiomas 133
petrous bone 109, 131
petrous temporal bone 47, 48
pharynx 23, 43, 51
phenobarbitone 215
phenytoin (Epanutin) 144, 205, 209, 211–12, 214, 215
phlebitis 184
physiotherapists 233, 236–40, 274, 278, 303
neurosurgery 139, 147, 148
pia mater 13, 15
pilocarpine 46
pilocytic astrocytomas 67, 74, 93, 110, 111
children 109, 110–11, 114, 115
pineal tumours 10, 71, 78, 116–18
calcification 82
children 109, 111, 115, 116–18
parenchymal 68
radiotherapy 158, 176
pineoblastoma 68, 109, 111, 118, 158
pineocytoma 68
pituitary 5, 24, 41, 68, 70–1, 76–7
adenomas 29, 45, 68, 71, 76–7, 92–3, 106–8, 157–8
apoplexy 70
diabetes 141
meningiomas 106
neurosurgery 130, 141
radiotherapy reactions 172
stalk 99
plain films 81, 82, 122
planning target volume (PTV) 152
plantar reflexes 60–1, 63, 71
plasmacytoma 68
platinum 185
play therapy 159, 189
pleomorphic xanthoastrocytoma 67, 93
podophyllotoxins 181
polar spongioblastoma 68
polyuria 186
pons 5, 7, 10, 11–12, 19, 41
gliomas 75, 114–15
positioning 9, 10, 127, 143–5, 238–9, 261
coma patients 51
neuro-imaging 82–4, 86
post-myelography 91
postoperative 138, 139, 140, 145
physiotherapy 237, 238–9
radiotherapy 159, 162–3, 164
positron emission tomography (PET) 82, 90, 175
postcentral gyrus 16, 18
posterior cerebral arteries 12, 13
posterior communicating arteries 12, 13
posterior fossa 10, 13, 70, 76, 244–5
children 66, 109–15, 118
neuro-imaging 89, 93, 101, 105, 109–15, 118
neurosurgery 127, 129, 133–4, 137, 139, 141–2
radiotherapy 163
posterior inferior cerebellar artery 13
precentral gyrus 20
prednisolone 191
prefrontal association areas 7–8
prefrontal cortex 26–7
pregnancy 171–2, 197, 209, 211, 217, 218
premedication 126
preoperative care 125–7
prepiriform area 25
pressure sensation 16, 18, 19
primary areas 7–8
primary lymphomas 66, 68–9, 77–8, 93, 100, 101
chemotherapy 179, 185, 191
radiotherapy 77–8, 153
primary tumours 66, 67, 69, 79–80, 115, 133
ependymomas 76
gliomas 66, 73, 93
melanocytic lesions 69
neoplasms 92, 120
occipital 70
spinal 66, 71, 76, 120, 134
see also primary lymphomas

primitive neuroectodermal tumours (PNETs) 68, 76, 191
  chemotherapy 179, 191
  children 109, 110, 111, 115, 118
  radiotherapy 154, 157, 158
procarbazine 181, 190, 197
prognosis 92, 100, 110, 111, 243, 294
  chemotherapy 184, 189, 191
  coma 33
  germ cell tumour 78
  glioma 74
  medulloblastoma 76
  meningioma 79, 106
  primary lymphoma 78
  psychological support 274, 292
  radiotherapy 157, 159, 161, 176
prolactin 77, 217
pronator drift 55
prophylactic H_2 antagonist 166, 173, 203, 208
proprioception 18, 59–60, 63, 72, 237, 261
proptosis 45, 79
prosencephalon 5
prostate cancer 54, 101, 120, 134
protoplasmic tumour 67
proximal myopathy 203
pruritus 187
psychiatrists 289, 290, 299
psychosis 27, 187, 268
  steroid-induced 166, 205
ptosis 45–6, 63, 71
puberty 71
pupils 22, 23, 25, 29, 46, 52, 71
  brain stem death 52
  cranial nerves 43, 45
  opiates 207
  seizures 143, 144
pyogenic abscesses 103
pyramidal system 9, 12, 20, 61

quality of life 144, 189, 232, 243–4, 278
  body image 253, 258, 259, 260
  care planning 305, 306, 307
  chemotherapy 179, 189, 190–2, 197–8
  medication in symptom management 217, 220
  radiotherapy 155, 157
  rehabilitation after surgery 147–8

radical radiotherapy 156–7
radionecrosis 89, 153, 175, 176
radiosensitivity 152
radiotherapy 151–78, 259
  care 159–65, 298
  chemotherapy 158, 159, 174, 190–2, 195–6
  children 114, 158, 159, 174, 175
  efficacy 157
  germ cell tumours 78, 152, 153–4, 158
  medulloblastoma 76, 154, 157–9, 163, 176
  meningiomas 106, 158
  metastases 100, 155, 158–9
  neuro-imaging 81, 92, 100, 106, 114
  oral hygiene 219
  primary lymphoma 77–8, 153
  psychological support 272, 276
  raised intracranial pressure 40, 165, 170, 172, 174
  speech and language therapy 165, 241, 242, 244
  techniques 153–7
  treatment related problems 165–76
raised intracranial pressure 69, 73, 201–2, 255, 276
  cardiac problems 139–40
  children 109
  glioma 75
  headaches 19, 73, 201–2, 205–6, 209
  medulloblastoma 76
  meningioma 79
  metastases 80
  nausea and vomiting 73, 202, 216
  neurological assessment 35, 40, 44, 46, 61
  neurosurgery 124, 136–41
  oligodendroglioma 75
  radiotherapy 40, 165, 170, 172, 174
  steroids 202
ranitidine 208–9
rashes 208, 213, 215, 217
Rathke's pouch 77
Raynaud's syndrome 187
reaching 54
reading 27, 241
receptive dysphasia 38, 70, 146, 244, 260
  psychological support 275, 287
recurrence of tumours 90, 201, 247
  acoustic schwannoma 108
  care planning 298, 303

chemotherapy 190, 191
children 112, 114, 119
meningioma 104, 106
psychological support 280, 281, 292
radiotherapy 161, 165, 175
reflex hammer 32, 60
reflexes 17, 18, 60–1, 63, 70, 237
brain stem 25, 49
chemotherapy 196
cornea 18, 47, 52, 60, 138
cranial nerves 47, 49, 50–1
gagging 43, 50–1, 53, 60, 138
neurological assessment 31, 36, 47, 49, 50–1, 52–3
oculocephalic 49, 52, 62
oculovestibular 49, 52
spinal cord 14, 53
vestibular system 19
rehabilitation 147–8, 256, 266
teamwork 221–2, 232–7, 239–40, 249
relaxation 140, 193, 234, 235–6
renal function 144, 195–6, 209, 217
chemotherapy 182, 185, 186–7, 195–6
test (EDTA) 196
resection of tumours 124–5, 127, 130, 132–5, 137
acoustic schwannoma 108
children 112, 119
meningiomas 104, 106
neuro-imaging 81, 93, 96, 99
radiotherapy 151
respiratory function 2, 12, 21, 22, 138–9, 144, 236
chemotherapy 186, 195
medication in symptom management 204, 206
neurological assessment 52, 53, 61
respite care 299, 301, 302, 305
reticular formation 10, 12, 26
reticular system 26, 32
reticulospinal tract 16, 20
retinoblastoma 68
retromastoid craniectomy 134
rhabdomyosarcoma 120
rhombencephalon 5
Rinne's test 50
Romberg test 54
Rosenthal fibres 74
Royal College of Nursing 291
sagittal sinus 79, 104, 105
salicylates 214, 215
salivation 43, 48, 143
saltatory conduction 4
scalp shielding 166–7
Schwann cells and schwannomas 3, 4, 69, 106, 108–9
school nurses 297, 304
secondary areas 7–8
seeding 76, 111–13, 117, 119, 158
seizures *see* epilepsy and seizures
self-care 222, 234, 265, 295
self-esteem 278, 298
body image 254, 255, 256, 261, 267
sella turcica 106–7, 130
sellar region 68
seminiferous epithelium 197
sensory function 1–2, 7, 10, 11, 15–21, 23–5, 59
cranial nerves 23, 41, 43, 47, 49, 50
neurological assessment 30–1, 41, 43, 47, 49, 54, 59
psychological support 276
radiotherapy 175
spinal cord 14, 16
surgery 138
teamwork 234, 237, 239
septum pellucidum 118
sexuality 8, 31, 168, 264, 279, 283–4
body image 254, 264, 267
shoulder shrug and abduction 23, 43, 56
side-effects 165–76, 186–7, 192–7, 202–20
body image 253, 260
chemotherapy 179, 186–7, 188, 192–7
CT scans 86
medication 145, 202–20
MRI scans 89
psychological support 275, 276–7
radiotherapy 156–7, 161, 165–76
speech and language therapy 242, 244
sight *see* vision and sight
simple photon emission computed tomography (SPECT) 82, 90
simulation of radiotherapy 163–4
single-fraction radiosurgery 155–6
sinuses 13, 15, 23, 36, 79, 104–6, 129, 130
skin problems 1, 22, 167, 168–9, 259, 277

skull base approach 128, 130–1
sleep 26
  insomnia 205, 212, 276, 285, 289, 306
small cell lung cancer 80, 192
smell 25, 62, 63, 174, 276
  cranial nerves 16, 23, 42, 43
Snellen chart 32, 44
social services packages of care 304
social workers 147, 233, 297
  psychological support 274, 278, 285, 289
sodium valporate (Epilim) 144, 214–15
somatic cortex 10
somatic nerve 7–8, 18
somnolence 169–70, 242, 276, 298
spasticity 238, 239, 242
spatial perception 40
speech and language 8–9, 26–7, 37–8, 62, 70, 240–5, 260
  altered body image 255, 256, 260
  cerebellum 11, 244
  chemotherapy 193
  cranial nerves 43, 50, 52
  neurological assessment 31, 32, 37–8, 39, 43, 50, 52
  neurosurgery 135, 146, 148
  radiotherapy 165, 241, 242, 244
  psychological support 272, 276, 287
  teamwork 233, 240–5, 246
speech and language therapists 233, 240–5
  care planning 303
  neurological assessment 37–8, 51
  post-neurosurgery 138, 146, 147, 148
  psychological support 274, 276, 278, 279, 287
sphenoid sinus 130
sphenoid wing 79, 106, 133
spina theca 71
spinal cord 1–3, 14–21, 66, 78, 119–22, 134
  body image 259
  brain 7, 11, 12
  compression 54, 62, 71, 119, 120–1, 134, 204
  ependymoma 76, 122
  extradural tumours 71, 119, 120, 134
  intradural tumours 71, 134
  manifestations of tumours 71–2
  meninges 14, 119
  metastases 54, 66, 71, 80, 103, 120, 121, 134
  neuro-imaging 90, 103, 112, 113, 117, 119–22
  neurological assessment 29–30, 36, 54–60, 62, 63
  neurosurgery 124, 127, 134, 138, 142
  primary tumours 66, 71, 76, 120, 134
  radiotherapy 152, 153, 154, 158, 176
  reflexes 14, 53
  reticular system 26
spinal nerves 1, 14, 21, 58, 69
spinal shock 60
spinocerebellar pathways 11
spinothalamic tracts 14, 16, 18
spousal concerns 298–9
staff support 291, 292
stapes 43
status epilepticus 144, 210
stereotactic techniques 92, 125, 131–2, 236
  chemotherapy 183
  frameless 131, 132
  radiosurgery 133
  radiotherapy 155, 159, 162, 163
sternal rub 36
sternomastoid muscle 23, 51
steroid myopathy 203, 204
steroids 48, 59, 100, 195, 276, 306
  altered body image 254, 256, 257
  medication in symptom management 202–6, 208, 209, 216
  neurosurgery 126
  radiotherapy 165, 166, 169, 172–3, 175
  see also corticosteroids
Stevens-Johnson syndrome 213
stigma 222, 254, 261, 262–3, 273
  epilepsy 145, 261
stimuli for assessment 33, 34, 35–8, 53, 58–60
  noxious 37, 58, 60
stomach cancer 102, 103
stomatitis 187
stress 21, 201, 203
  body image 255, 265
  care planning 295, 296

epilepsy 210, 212
headaches 201, 207
psychological support 272, 274, 285–6, 288–9, 291
teamwork 223, 231, 235, 245–7
stroke 83, 124
subarachnoid space 15, 71, 98, 102, 137
children 112, 117
haemorrhage 52
subcallosal gyri 9
subependymal giant cell astrocytoma 67, 93
subependymoma 67
subthalamic nucleus 10
suicide 289–90
sulci 6, 7
summarising 288–9
superior cerebellar artery 13
superior orbital fissure 47
superior sagittal sinus 104, 105
support groups 290–1, 295, 304
supraorbital pressure 36
suprasellar region 71, 79, 109, 116
supratentorial approach 127, 128–9, 131, 133, 138
neuro-imaging 101, 109, 111, 115–18
supratentorial tumours 209
PNETs 76, 191
surgery *see* neurosurgery and surgery
swallowing 62, 138, 141, 175, 193, 205
neurological assessment 31, 43, 50–1
speech and language therapy 240, 244–5
sweating 21–2, 46, 63, 143
sylvian fissure 7
sympathetic nervous system 21–2
synapses 2, 4, 16–17, 18, 20, 27, 63
reticular system 26
sight 25
vestibular system 19
syrynx 71, 122

tachycardia 143
tarsorrhaphy 48, 63
taste 173–4, 193, 276
cranial nerves 16, 23, 43, 48
teeth 23, 43
telencephalon 5
teletherapy 153
temperature 10, 16–18, 21, 47, 72
sensation 15–19, 59
temporal lobes 7, 25, 26, 70, 72, 241
medial 39, 99
neurosurgery 128, 133, 146
temporomandibular joint 141
temporoparietal lobe 38
tendons 18
teniposide (VM26) 181
tension pneumocephalus 137–8
tentorium 128, 129
teratoma 68, 78, 109, 118
testicular seminoma 78
thalamus 5, 9–10, 16, 18, 26, 132, 241
thiopurines 180
third ventricle 5, 9, 15, 71, 77, 115, 128
thrombocytopenia 186–7, 194, 212, 259
thrombosis 105, 145
thyroid cancer 102
thyroid stimulating hormone (TSH) 77
titanium 129
Todd's paralysis 73, 144
tongue 23, 43, 51–2
depressor blade 32, 50
topical nystatin 193
touch 15, 16, 18, 19
transoral approach 130
transplants 53, 66, 77, 100
trans-sphenoidal approach 128, 130
trapezium squeeze 36
trapezius muscle 23, 36, 57
trigeminal ganglion 48
trigeminal nerve (CN V) 12, 18–19, 23, 41–3, 47–8, 51, 135
trigeminal neuralgia 48
trigone 119
trochlear nerve (CN IV) 10, 19, 23, 41–3, 45–7
tuberous sclerosis 67, 93
tumour necrosis factor (TNF) 183
tumour radiosensitivity 152
tuning fork 32, 50
Turcot's syndrome 67
two-point discrimination 15

ulceration 203
uncal (tentorial) herniation 46
United Kingdom Central Council for Nursing, Midwifery and Health Visiting 231

upper motor neurones 20–1, 55, 61, 63–4, 71
upper quadrantinopia 70
upward gaze 23, 43, 71
urea 52
urticaria 86, 187, 213

vagus nerve (CN X) 12, 23, 41–3, 50–1
vascular endothelial hyperplasia 74
vasomotor centre 12, 139
vecuronium 46
venography 104–6
venous sinuses 129
ventricles 110–15, 118, 119, 128, 137
  see also fourth ventricle; third ventricle
verapamil 214
verbal response in neurological assessment 34–6
vertebral canal 14, 15
vertigo 64
vestibular division (CN VIII) 43, 49
vestibular system 19–20
vestibulocerebellar connections 19
vestibulocerebellar tract 11
vestibulocortical connections 20
vestibulo-ocular reflex 49, 53
vestibulo-ocular tracts 19
vestibulospinal tracts 16, 19
vibration 16, 18, 59
videofluoroscopy 51
vigabatrin (Sabril) 215
vinblastine 181
vinca alkaloids 181, 194, 196
vincristine 181, 186, 190–2, 195, 196
vindesine 181
vision and sight 7–8, 62, 78, 137, 205, 234, 256
  cranial nerves 16, 23–5, 42–5
  craniopharyngiomas 77
  fields 23–5
  gliomas 75
  macroadenomas 107
  manifestations of tumours 70, 71, 73
  meningiomas 79
  metastases 80
  neurological assessment 29, 31, 32, 41, 42–5
  psychological support for problems 272, 275, 276
  radiotherapy 175–6
visual cortex 25
vital signs 29–30, 61
vocal cord paralysis 50
voluntary movement 9, 10–11, 17, 20–1, 23, 26
  neurological assessment 53–4, 55–9
von Hippel-Lindau syndrome 67
von Recklinghausen's disease 67

walking and gait 11, 14, 20, 54, 70
  body image 256, 257, 261, 263
  physiotherapy 236, 237, 239
warfarin 137, 209, 212
washing 40, 60, 61, 235, 247, 277
Weber's test 50
weight 126, 185, 193, 254–6, 276
Wernicke's area 8, 26–7, 37, 38
white matter 4, 6, 14, 73, 175
  neuro-imaging 98, 102, 103, 104
wigs 167, 258, 276
World Health Organisation grades 67, 93, 96–9, 110, 111
wound healing 129, 141, 142, 203

X-rays 75, 126, 185, 195
  neuro-imaging 82, 84–5, 91
  radiotherapy 151, 153, 163–4

yolk sac tumours 68